AIDS

Modern Concepts and Therapeutic Challenges

edited by

Samuel Broder
Clinical Oncology Program
National Cancer Institute
National Institutes of Health
Bethesda, Maryland

Marcel Dekker, Inc.　　　　New York and Basel

ISBN 0-8247-7649-6

MARCEL DEKKER, INC.
270 Madison Avenue, New York, New York 10016

Current printing (last digit):
10 9 8 7 6 5 4 3 2 1

PRINTED IN THE UNITED STATES OF AMERICA

To Gail

Preface

The onset of the Acquired Immunodeficiency Syndrome (AIDS) has altered the clinical, scientific, and social perspectives of the American public, probably immutably. First we were required to accept the principle that, even as the twentieth century draws to a close, a surprising pathogen (in this instance, a retrovirus) could still enter the population with deadly force. Then we had to reconcile ourselves to the simultaneous success and limitations of contemporary technology—a technology that has made astonishing progress in understanding the etiology and spread of a new disease but has still not provided a proven means for curing those already afflicted or vaccinating those at risk for infection. Finally we were reminded that the scientific community contains many men and women who are prepared to take intellectual and physical risks, if necessary, in response to a public health emergency.

Those of us currently active in AIDS research are painfully aware that we are only at the beginning of the story. No one doubts that the years to come will expand our knowledge and change our perspectives, perhaps many times before the final chapter is written. This book is an effort to draw together the perspectives and findings of several scientists and clinicians. In some cases, the book deliberately offers the viewpoints of different groups surveying the same field.

On a practical level, the book gives the reader an opportunity to review the molecular, biological, epidemiological, psychosocial, and clinical features of AIDS and its related diseases. We hope that the book will provide the reader with the tools to follow the AIDS saga as it unfolds and that it will serve as a reference from which to weigh and consider new reports in this field.

On a philosophical level, we believe that the book will offer the reader the basis for an informed, albeit cautious, optimism. The data, however preliminary, when taken together, do demonstrate that we are gaining on the virus on several fronts, and in some cases (e.g., the development of practical mass-screening systems to reduce the incidence of transfusion-associated AIDS) significant breakthroughs have been achieved. In addition, our pursuit of the new pathogen that causes AIDS has already yielded a number of novel insights into the regulation and expression of viral and cellular genes, and these insights may have implications in virtually every phase of clinical investigation.

Samuel Broder

Contributors

Marc Alizon   Oncologie Virale, Institut Pasteur, Paris, France

Joseph R. Berger, M.D.   Associate Professor, Departments of Neurology and Internal Medicine, University of Miami School of Medicine, Miami, Florida

Robert J. Biggar, M.D.   Senior Investigator, International AIDS Epidemiology, Environmental Epidemiology Branch, National Cancer Institute, National Institutes of Health, Bethesda, Maryland

Samuel Broder, M.D.   Associate Director, Clinical Oncology Program, National Cancer Institute, National Institutes of Health, Bethesda, Maryland

James W. Curran, M.D., M.P.H.   Director, AIDS Program, Center for Infectious Diseases, Centers for Disease Control, Atlanta, Georgia

Max Essex, D.V.M., Ph.D.   Chairman, Department of Cancer Biology, Harvard School of Public Health, Boston, Massachusetts

Anthony S. Fauci, M.D.   Director, National Institute of Allergy and Infectious Diseases, National Institutes of Health, Bethesda, Maryland

Robert C. Gallo, M.D.   Chief, Laboratory of Tumor Cell Biology, National Cancer Institute, National Institutes of Health, Bethesda, Maryland

Edward P. Gelmann, M.D.   Senior Investigator, Medicine Branch, Clinical Oncology Program, National Cancer Institute, National Institutes of Health, Bethesda, Maryland

Parkash S. Gill, M.D.   Assistant Professor, Department of Internal Medicine, University of Southern California School of Medicine, Los Angeles, California

Jerome E. Groopman, M.D.   Chief, Division of Hematology/Oncology, Department of Medicine, New England Deaconess Hospital, and Associate Professor of Medicine, Harvard Medical School, Boston, Massachusetts

Ann M. Hardy, Dr.P.H.   Epidemiologist, Surveillance and Evaluation Branch, AIDS Program, Center for Infectious Diseases, Centers for Disease Control, Atlanta, Georgia

William A. Haseltine, Ph.D.   Chief, Laboratory of Biochemical Pharmacology, Dana-Farber Cancer Institute, Department of Pathology, Harvard Medical School, and Department of Cancer Biology, Harvard School of Public Health, Boston, Massachusetts

Jay S. Herbst, M.D.   Chief Medical Resident, Department of Internal Medicine, Mount Sinai Medical Center, Miami Beach, Florida

Elaine S. Jaffe, M.D.   Chief, Hematopathology Section, and Deputy Chief, Laboratory of Pathology, National Cancer Institute, National Institutes of Health, Bethesda, Maryland

Russell T. Joffe, M.D.   Staff Psychiatrist, Department of Psychiatry, St. Michael's Hospital, and University of Toronto, Toronto, Ontario, Canada

Phyllis J. Kanki, D.V.M., D.Sc.   Research Fellow, Department of Cancer Biology, Harvard School of Public Health, Boston, Massachusetts

David A. Katz, M.D.   Neuropathologist, Office of the Clinical Director, National Institute of Neurological and Communicative Diseases and Stroke, and Laboratory of Pathology, National Cancer Institute, National Institutes of Health, Bethesda, Maryland

H. Clifford Lane, M.D.   Senior Investigator, Laboratory of Immunoregulation, and Deputy Clinical Director, National Institute of Allergy and Infectious Diseases, National Institutes of Health, Bethesda, Maryland

Alexandra M. Levine, M.D. Professor, Department of Internal Medicine University of Southern California School of Medicine, Los Angeles, California

Abe M. Macher, M.D. Director, Collaborative Center for the Investigation of AIDS, Registry of AIDS Pathology, Armed Forces Institute of Pathology, Washington, D.C.

Makoto Matsukura, M.D. Guest Scientist, Clinical Oncology Program, National Cancer Institute, National Institutes of Health, Bethesda, Maryland

Hiroaki Mitsuya, M.D. Cancer Expert, Clinical Oncology Program, National Cancer Institute, National Institutes of Health, Bethesda, Maryland

Luc Montagnier Oncologie Virale, Institut Pasteur, Paris, France

Wade P. Parks, Ph.D., M.D. Professor, Department of Pediatrics, University of Miami School of Medicine, Miami, Florida

Suraiya Rasheed, Ph.D. Professor, Department of Pathology, University of Southern California School of Medicine, Los Angeles, California

Lionel Resnick, M.D. Chief, Retrovirology Laboratories, Departments of Dermatology and Pathology, Mount Sinai Medical Center, Miami Beach, Florida, and Adjunct Assistant Professor, Departments of Microbiology and Immunology, University of Miami School of Medicine, Miami, Florida

Craig A. Rosen, Ph.D. Instructor, Laboratory of Biochemical Pharmacology, Dana-Farber Cancer Institute, and Harvard Medical School, Boston, Massachusetts

David R. Rubinow, M.D. Chief, Psychiatry Consultation-Liaison Service, Biological Psychiatry Branch, National Institute of Mental Health, National Institutes of Health, Bethesda, Maryland

Bijan Safai, M.D., D.Sc. Chief Attending Physician, Dermatology Service, Department of Medicine, Memorial Sloan-Kettering Cancer Center, and Professor of Medicine, Cornell University Medical College, New York, New York

Gwendolyn B. Scott, M.D. Associate Professor, Department of Pediatrics, University of Miami School of Medicine, Miami, Florida

Joseph G. Sodroski, M.D. Research Associate, Department of Pathology, Dana-Farber Cancer Institute, and Harvard Medical School, Boston, Massachusetts

Pierre Sonigo Unité de Recombinaison et Expression Génétique, Institut Pasteur, Paris, France

Howard Z. Streicher, M.D.   Senior Staff Fellow, Laboratory of Tumor Cell Biology, National Cancer Institute, National Institutes of Health, Bethesda, Maryland

Simon Wain-Hobson, Ph.D.   Research Scientist, Unité de Recombinaison et Expression Génétique, Institut Pasteur, Paris, France

Flossie Wong-Staal, Ph.D.   Section Chief, Laboratory of Tumor Cell Biology, National Cancer Institute, National Institutes of Health, Bethesda, Maryland

Robert Yarchoan, M.D.   Investigator, Clinical Oncology Program, National Cancer Institute, National Institutes of Health, Bethesda, Maryland

Contents

Preface   v
Contributors   vii

1. Human T-Lymphotropic Retroviruses (HTLV-I, II, and III):
    The Biological Basis of Adult T-Cell Leukemia/Lymphoma and
    AIDS   1
    Robert C. Gallo and Howard Z. Streicher

2. Lymphadenopathy/AIDS Virus: The Prototype Human
    Lentivirus   23
    *Simon Wain-Hobson, Pierre Sonigo, Marc Alizon, and
    Luc Montagnier*

3. Molecular Biology of the HTLV Family   39
    Flossie Wong-Staal

4. Progress and Puzzles: Molecular Biology of HTLV-III   53
    William A. Haseltine, Joseph G. Sodroski, and Craig A. Rosen

5. Animal Models of HTLV-III/LAV Infection and AIDS   63
    Phyllis J. Kanki and Max Essex

6. AIDS: A New Kind of Epidemic Immunodeficiency   75
    Ann M. Hardy and James W. Curran

7. Epidemiology of Human Retroviruses and Related Clinical
    Conditions   91
    Robert J. Biggar

8. Psychiatric and Psychosocial Aspects of AIDS   123
    David R. Rubinow and Russell T. Joffe

9. Spectrum of HTLV-III Infection   135
    Jerome E. Groopman

10. Pathology of AIDS   143
    Elaine S. Jaffe, David A. Katz, and Abe M. Macher

11. Infectious Complications of AIDS   185
    H. Clifford Lane and Anthony S. Fauci

12. Kaposi's Sarcoma: An Overview of Classical and Epidemic
    Forms   205
    Bijan Safai

13. Kaposi's Sarcoma in the Setting of the AIDS Pandemic   219
    Edward P. Gelmann and Samuel Broder

14. AIDS-Related Malignant B-Cell Lymphomas   233
    Alexandra M. Levine, Parkash S. Gill, and Suraiya Rasheed

15. An Overview of Pediatric AIDS: Approaches to Diagnosis and
    Outcome Assessment   245
    Wade P. Parks and Gwendolyn B. Scott

16. HTLV-III/LAV-Related Neurological Disease   263
    Joseph R. Berger and Lionel Resnick

17. Dermatological (Non-Kaposi's Sarcoma) Manifestations
    Associated with HTLV-III/LAV Infection   285
    Lionel Resnick and Jay S. Herbst

18. Rapid in Vitro Systems for Assessing Activity of Agents Against
    HTLV-III/LAV   303
    Hiroaki Mitsuya, Makoto Matsukura, and Samuel Broder

19. Strategies for the Pharmacological Intervention Against HTLV-
     III/LAV   335
     Robert Yarchoan and Samuel Broder

Index   361

Human T-Lymphotropic Retroviruses (HTLV-I, II, and III): The Biological Basis of Adult T-Cell Leukemia/Lymphoma and AIDS

Robert C. Gallo
Howard Z. Streicher
Laboratory of Tumor Cell Biology
National Cancer Institute
National Institutes of Health
Bethesda, Maryland

Introduction

The history of retrovirus research is remarkable not only for its insights into basic molecular biology and disease causation, but also for exciting and often unexpected results. Perhaps most interesting is the story of the search for human retroviruses, a saga of frustrations, disbelief, and unexpected findings. A rapid series of discoveries has opened the way to the identification, isolation, and clear link (within the short period of 6 years) of human T-lymphotropic retroviruses as primary causes of at least two fatal human diseases and as more indirect causes of many others.[1] Ironically, all these retroviruses chiefly infect the same cell (the T4-lymphocyte) often with fatal consequences, but with rather opposite effects on the cell. It is also essential not to overly compartmentalize clinical syndromes associated with these retroviruses. The physician will recognize that a spectrum of diseases can occur. Indeed, as with syphilis or tuberculosis, the protean diseases of a previous medical era, retrovirus-associated diseases may take on a multitude of clinical manifestations (see section on HTLV-associated diseases).

Background

Retroviruses (as we now use the term) were first isolated by Peyton Rous from a sarcoma of a chicken in 1911; they were subsequently identified and isolated from many different animals in the ensuing half century. A milestone in this work was the isolation by Ludwik Gross, in the 1950s, of the first mammalian retroviruses from mice with leukemia, and his linking of these murine leukemia viruses to the cause of various types of mouse leukemias.[2] The concept of a leukemia virus in mice met with considerable resistance and also much enthusiasm. Subsequently, they have been associated with malignancies (most frequently leukemias and lymphomas) in many species and with certain nonmalignant disorders.

Retroviruses were first isolated from tumor tissue and recognized by their ability to cause transmissible malignancies. Although all retroviruses share common features, one way of characterizing them is by the type of disease they cause—malignant or nonmalignant (or both) and nonpathogenic. A unique feature of retroviruses is the potential of an infectious agent to be transmitted in the germ line along with normal genetic Mendelian elements. This type is called an endogenous retrovirus and is usually nonpathogenic. A good example of a retrovirus causing only malignant disease in its natural host is the Gibbon ape leukemia virus (GaLV),[3] and an excellent example of one causing both malignant and nonmalignant disease is feline leukemia virus (FeLV). FeLV often causes T-cell leukemia, but more frequently causes a T-cell immunodeficiency disorder mimicking AIDS of man.[4] In fact, many leukemias caused by animal retroviruses also induce some degree of immunosuppression.

Another class of retroviruses was first associated with chronic and progressive disease; they were called lentiviruses to distinguish them from acute viral infections. So far, they are known to cause only nonmalignant disease (e.g., encephalitis, other neurological abnormalities, arthritis, lung disease, hemolytic anemias). The best known example is the visna virus of sheep, which produces a chronic neurological disease ("visna" means "wasting" in Icelandic). Until recently, lentiretroviruses were known only in ungulates. Related retroviruses have been discovered in humans (e.g., HTLV-III, the AIDS virus) and in nonhuman primates (e.g., STLV-III, the simian T-lymphotropic virus III, which also causes an AIDS-like disease).[5,6] STLV-III and related viruses are discussed in other chapters of this book.

General Biology

Retroviruses are enveloped single-stranded RNA viruses. The most common form is the C-type virus, which reproduces by budding from the membrane of an infected cell. The electron-dense viral core contains the single-stranded RNA. A double-stranded DNA form of the virus is used to transcribe new viral RNA genomes and to encode messenger RNA. To enable the virus to do this requires the presence of a special DNA polymerase known as reverse transcriptase (RT), which is complexed to the RNA genome in the viral core. When a retrovirus infects a cell, the reverse transcriptase catalyzes the transcription of the RNA genome into the DNA form (known as the provirus). This DNA form as a double-stranded circular element migrates from the cytoplasm to the nucleus where it can integrate into the host cell DNA. The viral genes may remain integrated for the lifetime of the cell and are duplicated with the host cell genes in all daughter cells. Infection of an organism is generally life-long.

The existence of an integrated DNA provirus derived from the viral RNA genome was predicted by Howard Temin during the 1960s in a moment of brilliant scientific insight. Temin and Baltimore later demonstrated the reality of this prediction during the 1970s, providing both the name and the unifying feature of this group of viruses.[7,8]

Once the retrovirus is integrated into the host cells, expression of viral RNA is under the control of two viral elements called long terminal repeats (LTRs) which define the integration sites of the virus, flanking the viral genome at the 3' and 5' ends. The integrated provirus may be unexpressed, partially expressed, or fully expressed. In the latter case, the viral RNA and proteins will be found in the cell cytoplasm and, under the right circumstances, will assemble at the cell membrane, where budding and release eventually occur, thus completing the virus life cycle (Fig. 1). Because of recombinational events occurring during integration, the provirus may lose portions of its complete genome, but permanently acquire host cell sequences. The subsequent formation of virus with these newly acquired nucleotide sequences, of course, will have some properties that differ from the original virus. (Teich and co-workers[9] have dealt with these features in detail.)

Major progress has come from studies of retrovirus genomes in recent years, and their properties can also be used in classifying these viruses. Structural features of their genome govern the basic type of molecular mechanism by which these viruses alter a cell. The most common type of retroviral genome contains only three essential genes for virus replication, referred to as *gag*, *pol*, and *env* (Fig. 2). Retroviruses like this are important causes of animal disease. The *gag* gene codes for the viral internal structural proteins, the *pol* gene for reverse transcriptase, and the *env* gene for the outer glycoprotein envelope of the virus. The envelope may bind to a cell membrane receptor and

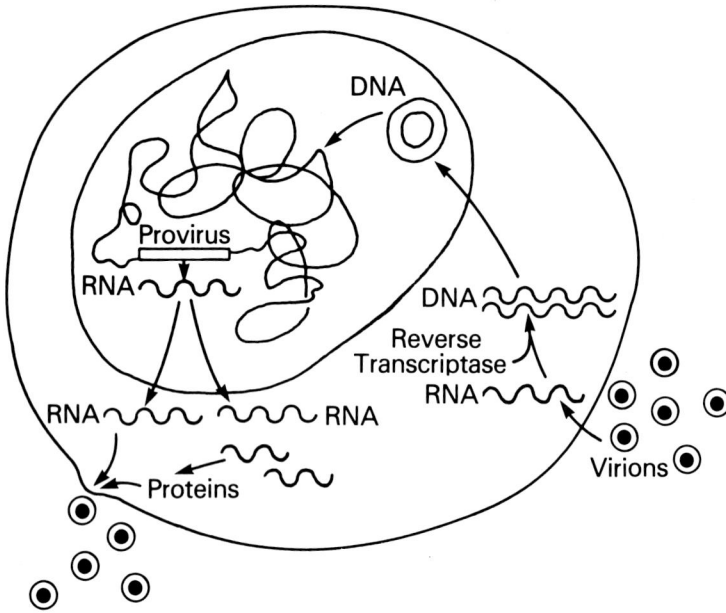

FIGURE 1 Life cycle of a retrovirus. Intact virions are endocytosed via a specific cellular receptor. The uncoated viral single-stranded RNA is then transcribed into double-stranded DNA, enters the cell nucleus, and integrates into the host genome. The DNA provirus in some conditions is unexpressed. In other cases, it is transcribed, giving rise to viral RNA encoding viral proteins and to genome length viral RNA molecules, which then reassemble with viral proteins to make complete virions. These progeny are released by budding from the cell membrane.

mediate penetration of the cell. Therefore, the properties of the envelope can be one major factor determining the kind of cell the virus can infect. Antibodies directed against the envelope of a virus are one of the essential features sought for in a vaccine.

The three viral genes are flanked at their ends by sequences called long terminal repeats or LTRs. These sequences do not code for viral proteins, but instead consist of regulatory elements (conceptually similar to promotor and enhancer elements of cellular genes), including sequences that influence the expression of the viral genes and sometimes of nearly cellular genes. In addition, the LTRs form the sites of integration into the host cell DNA (i.e., the cellular sequences are covalently linked to the LTRs). Viruses with this type of genome are usually called chronic leukemia viruses. Examples are FeLV, mouse leukemia virus (MuLV), avian leukosis virus (ALV), and GaLV. These

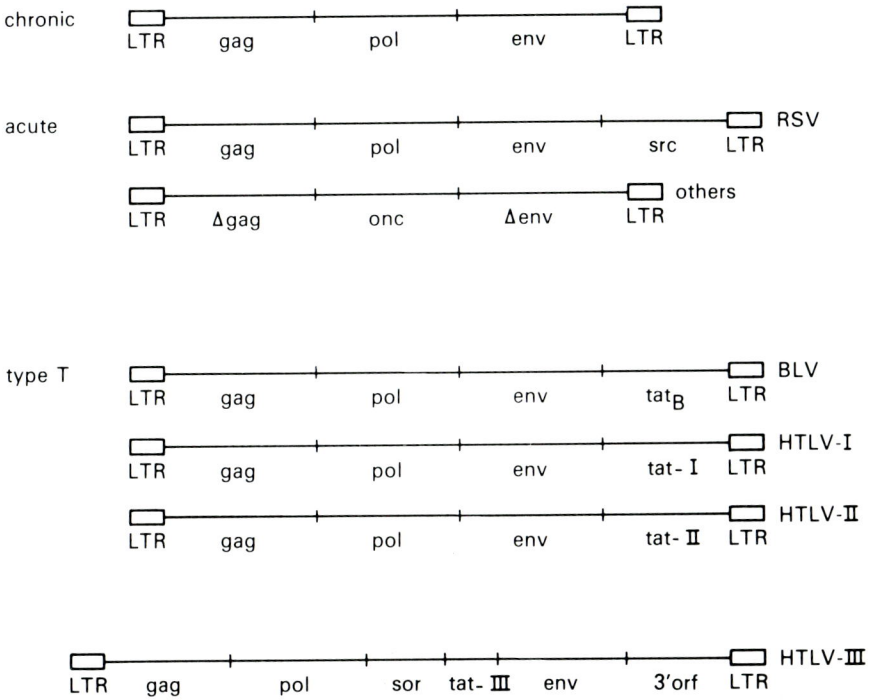

FIGURE 2 Genetic structure and proposed classification of different groups of retro-viruses. *gag* = core proteins; *pol* = reverse transcriptase; *env* = envelope; LTR = long terminal repeat; Δ*gag* and Δ*env* = incomplete genes; src = one of the *onc* genes; BLV = bovine leukemia virus; *tat* = transacting transcriptional activator gene; *sor* = short open reading frame; 3'*orf* = 3' open reading frame. The latter two are genes in HTLV-III of unknown function.

viruses replicate extensively in the host prior to their induction of leukemia, and there is evidence that they cause leukemia by integration within a certain region of a chromosome; thus, an LTR may promote extensive and continual expression of a juxtaposed cellular gene involved in growth. The best example of this so-called *cis* mechanism (the term *cis* is used to contrast with *trans*) is in chickens where the LTRs of the ALV promote cellular oncogene expression, which is believed to be the first step in the leukemic process induced by this virus. Because integration by retroviruses is random, the need to integrate in a specific region for induction of disease may explain the apparent need for viremia and extensive virus replication to promote malignancy. A high rate of replication should favor the chance of integration into regions sufficiently near the cellular oncogene to enable the LTR to activate this gene.

As noted, sometimes retroviruses acquire a host cell gene. When this gene gives the virus the property of rapidly transforming cells and inducing acute malignancies, the virus is often called an acute leukemia or sarcoma virus, and the gene a viral *onc* gene (Fig. 2). Viruses with *onc* genes are fortunately rare and have never been identified in humans. When found in animals, they are of interest chiefly for studying mechanisms of neoplastic transformation, but not as causes of naturally occurring cancer. Every cell infected by these viruses can be transformed (polyclonal) because the product of the viral *onc* gene is directly transforming. Therefore, a common site of integration is not needed. The other categories of known retroviral genomes are described in the following sections.

General Features of Human Retroviruses

A third category of retrovirus genomes was only recently discovered. It consists of all known human leukemia viruses—human T-lymphotropic (or leukemia) virus types I and II (HTLV-I and HTLV-II). It also encompasses bovine leukemia virus (BLV). The third known human retrovirus, human T-lymphotropic virus III (HTLV-III), forms a special subcategory, and although not yet known, it is likely that the lentiretroviruses will be closer to this group and HTLV-III than to other retroviruses. The genomes of all these viruses have the following: (1) in addition to the viral replication genes (*gag, pol, env*), they contain one or more extra genes; (2) the extra gene(s) is (are) not homologous to a mammalian gene cell (i.e., not an *onc* gene)—like the DNA tumor virus-transforming genes, the origin of the extra gene(s) is (are) unknown; and (3) at least one of these extra genes codes for a protein that is involved in activating the expression of other viral genes (likely by binding to the viral LTRs) and probably of certain cell genes (presumably by binding to regulatory enhancer elements in the cell that are similar to the viral LTRs). Recent results have indicated that major aspects of the biological effects of these viruses are mediated by this gene, called a *trans* (see earlier use of the term *cis*) activator or *tat,* which acts by either enhancing transcriptional or post-transcriptional (translational) events. Since *tat* codes for a nuclear protein that can activate other genes, these viruses do not have to integrate in a special region to induce disease. This may be why extensive virus replication is not needed for them to cause neoplastic or nonneoplastic disease in humans. A similar phenomenon is seen in lymphoma of cows induced by BLV. In addition to the genes discussed above, HTLV-III, also known as lymphadenopathy-associated virus or LAV, contains genes of as yet undefined function (3'*orf* and *sor*).

The electron micrographic features of HTLV-I and HTLV-II are similar. HTLV-III differs in its mature form, showing a highly condensed cylindrical core structure (Fig. 3). HTLV-I, the first known human retrovirus, was first isolated in Gallo's laboratory in 1978 and reported in 1980 after its characterization.[10] It was isolated from a young black man with an aggressive T-cell malignancy (now called adult T-cell leukemia) from the United States. The methods developed by Gallo and co-workers for isolation of human retroviruses depended on their idea that a retrovirus might cause disease without an earlier viremia or without evident extensive replication of the tumor. Therefore, sensitive means of virus detection and careful growth of the putative target cells were developed in this laboratory during the 1970s.[11] The sensitive assays were based on the use of the enzyme, reverse transcriptase (RT), as a "footprint" of a retrovirus because this assay can be made several orders of magnitude more sensitive than electron microscopy. A breakthrough in the growth of the target cells was achieved with the discovery of T-cell growth factor (interleukin-2 or IL-2).[12] The combination of growing mature T cells with IL-2 and the use of RT assays eventually led to the routine isolation of HTLV-I. This is the same basic technique used for the isolation of the virus that causes AIDS (HTLV-III or LAV) in various laboratories (see below).

One of the most remarkable features about the currently recognized human retroviruses is their tropism for the T4-helper lymphocyte. Although other cells can be infected, this post-thymic mature T cell is by far preferentially infected in vitro in a mixed cell population by all three types of known human retroviruses. The primary disease caused by each of them almost always involve this cell. Since the T4 cell regulates many of our immune functions and may even regulate some functions of nonlymphoid cells, it is not difficult to understand why these viruses induce such profound clinical disease.

Another extraordinary feature of the human retroviruses is their ability to cause T4 cell alterations in vitro. Infection of T4-lymphocytes by HTLV-I or HTLV-II leads to the immortalized growth of a small number of these cells, and the properties of the transformed cells are very similar to the primary HTLV-I-positive leukemic cells from an ATL patient. Other T4 cells and other T cells infected by HTLV-I may not be transformed, but exhibit impairment of one or more T-cell functions. In vitro infection of T4 cells by HTLV-III can lead to the premature death of these cells when they are activated and the viral genes are expressed, resembling what we assume to be the case in vivo in patients with AIDS.[14,15] This affords us a unique opportunity in medicine—the laboratory study of the molecular and cellular mechanisms of induction of two forms of fatal human disease utilizing the precise target cell and the known causative agents.

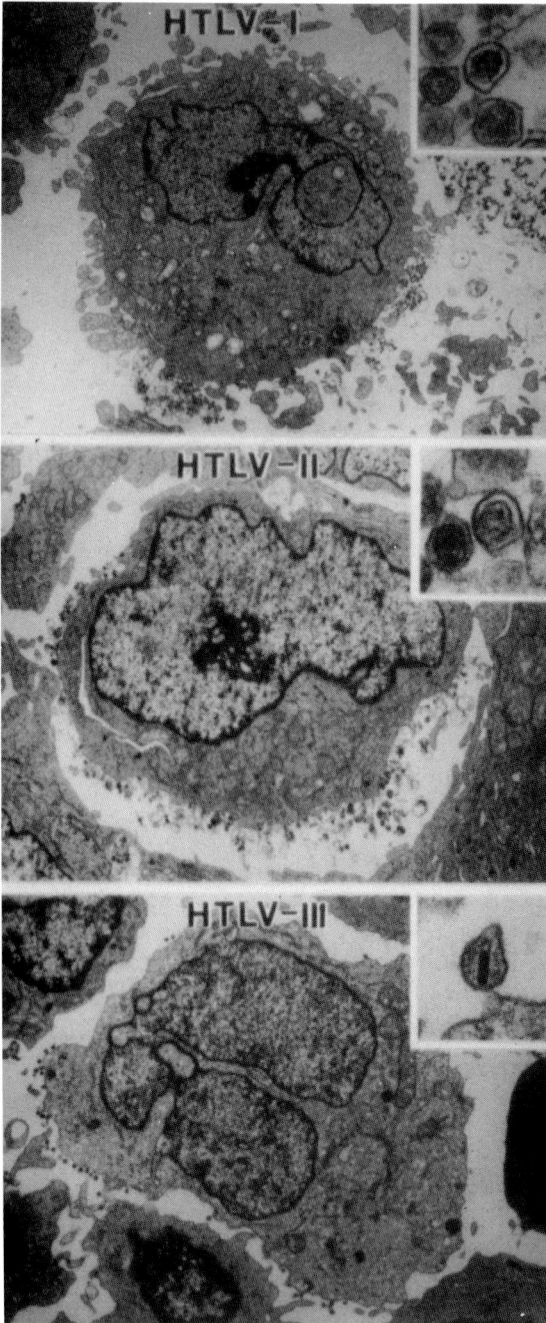

Characteristics of Leukemic Cells and of the Disease Associated with HTLV-I

As noted, the vast majority of known HTLV-I-induced leukemias or lymphomas involve the T4 cell. These cells often exhibit characteristic morphological changes consisting of extensive lobulation of the nuclei and giant multinucleated forms. The latter are probably formed by HTLV-I-induced syncytial formation. In some cases, however, no distinctive morphological changes are evident. A major and apparently consistent difference between the HTLV-I-positive leukemic T cells and normal T cells is the constitutive expression and increased number of receptors for IL-2 in the former.[16] Receptors for the growth factor are present in normal T cells only after they are activated, and then are normally down-regulated. Their continued expression and abundance in the leukemic cells may be central to the abnormal growth of these cells. Despite their T4 characteristics, the virus-positive leukemic cells generally do not have detectable helper function, and some function as suppressor T cells. Also, in vitro infection of cloned functional T cells of different types leads to changes or loss of function. These findings may be reflected in the immune defects and opportunistic infections that occur in these viral leukemias.

Leukemias/lymphomas caused by HTLV-I are usually clinically identified as a particular form of lymphoid malignancy known as adult T-cell leukemia/lymphoma (ATLL), characterized by its aggressive course (median survival about 4 months), hypercalcemia (mechanism unknown), and several forms of skin abnormalities that occur in over half the cases.[17] The disease has many similarities to cutaneous T-cell lymphomas (mycosis fungoides and Sézary leukemias) except for the more aggressive course, and without the presence of the characteristic morphological changes in the T cell or the positive virological studies for HTLV-I, the clinician may not always confidently make the distinction. HTLV-I can also be involved in T4-cell leukemias and lymphomas that exhibit a more chronic "smoldering" course (15 to 20% of cases) with other features differing from ATLL. These may not be pathologically or clinically distinguishable from T-cell CLL, diffuse histiocytic lymphoma, large and mixed cell lymphomas, and typical mycosis fungoides or Sézary leukemias in individual cases. In the United States, only a small

---

FIGURE 3 Composite of cells showing the expression of the HTLV-I, HTLV-II, and HTLV-III viruses demonstrated in the inset in each case. HTLV-I and HTLV-II are similar in appearance, but HTLV-III has a characteristic rod-shaped core. (Figure supplied by S. Z. Salahuddin, Laboratory of Tumor Cell Biology, National Cancer Institute.)

percentage of these diseases are HTLV-I-positive. In contrast, in typical ATLL, close to 100% are virus-positive. Rarely, cases of T8 leukemia have been found, similar to the rare induction of T8-transformed cell lines in vitro by HTLV-I or HTLV-II.

In areas of the world where HTLV-I is endemic, some B-cell lymphoid malignancies, like B-CLL and certain other cancers, have been associated with HTLV-I infection much more frequently than expected from the prevalence of the virus in the general population. Studies of healthly Jamaicans suggest an incidence of HTLV-I infection of 2 to 3% of people, HTLV-I was found in close to 30% of the B-CLL cases.[18] In virus-positive T-cell leukemias, the viral genes are integrated onto the DNA of the leukemic cell. HTLV-I was not found in the B-cell tumor, but was present in the normal T cells of these B-CLL patients. Using cell fusion to "rescue" immunoglobulin products, the malignant B cells of some of these patients make a single type of antibody directed against a protein of HTLV-I.[19] These malignancies, therefore, arise by different mechanisms. In the T-cell malignancies, virus integrates into the DNA of the initial transformed cell, and viral sequences are, therefore, found in all T cells of the tumor. The B-cell tumors may arise in part by an indirect effect of HTLV-I. Chronic antigenic stimulation by viral proteins combined with diminished T-cell immune surveillance may increase the chance for a neoplastic transformation in the expanding B-cell compartment. Therefore, we emphasize that although neither HTLV-I nor HTLV-II can cause AIDS per se, there is much in vitro evidence suggesting that both of these can impair T-cell function, and substantial in vivo evidence suggesting that HTLV-I infection increases the risk of opportunistic infections and certain malignancies.

Origin and Spread of HTLV-I and Epidemiology of ATLL

The first isolates of HTLV-I were from two sporadic cases of T-cell malignancies in U.S. blacks, and the first clusters of ATL were described in Japanese and subsequently in Carribean-born blacks.[20,21] The speculation by Gallo and co-workers[22] that the virus originated in Africa was based on several observations. Studies of the geographic distribution of HTLV-I serology demonstrated that it is widely distributed throughout Africa, especially in central Africa among certain tribes. Moreover, ATLL in the Americas and Europe is present chiefly in immigrant blacks and their descendants, although there are many exceptions. Finally, a highly related virus, termed simian T-cell leukemia (lymphotropic) virus-I or STLV-I, has been found in old world monkeys.[23] In Japan, HTLV-I is prevalent in the two small southwestern islands, Kyushu and Shikoku. We suspect that it was brought there by the 16th century arrival of European adventurers who came with African blacks and monkeys. Unlike ubiquitous viruses such as EBV and the papilloma viruses, the geographic distribution of HTLV-I has been very restricted. For example, far less than 1% of the white U.S. and European populations are infected. It is also very unusual in most of Asia. The establishment of an epidemiological link between this virus and the disease it causes was relatively uncomplicated. The incidence of HTLV-I infection can vary dramatically over small distances. For instance, in some areas of Kyushu, 15 to 20% of the population may be positive, and in nearby towns, the incidence may be less than a few percent. Transmission of this virus is not casual but by intimate contact (by blood or blood products) and, as some studies show, by infection of the developing fetus in utero and perhaps perinatally by breast feeding. Some epidemiology has led to speculation that the virus may also be transmitted by insect vectors, but there are no data bearing on this important question. Finally, it seems that HTLV-I is usually not transmitted as an extracellular virus, but with the infected T4 cell.

Because of the increase in travel, changes in sexual habits, drug abuse (blood in contaminated needles), wide use of blood and blood products in transfusions, and increased recognition, it is likely that problems with HTLV-I will increase in the future. At the moment, it may cause more than 50% of all adult lymphoid malignancies in some endemic areas of the world.

Mechanism of HTLV-I T-Cell Transformation

Much has been learned about the mechanism by which HTLV-I initiates T-cell transformation, but nothing is known about the mechanisms involved in maintenance of the transformed state. After infection of T cells in vitro with HTLV-I (or HTLV-II), a small number (oligo- or monoclonal population) of T cells rapidly become immortalized. In this process, they constitutively express IL-2 receptors, but lose their need for exogenous IL-2 to maintain growth. The *tat* gene product is believed to bind to cellular as well as viral regulatory elements in T cells, which in turn will activate the expression of gene(s) involved in T-cell proliferation. One such gene may be the IL-2 receptor which, as noted earlier, is constitutively expressed in high numbers on the surface in these transformed cells. Although other cells can be infected, infection of a mixed cell population in vitro usually results in the transformation of T4 cells. The striking consistency of the leukemias involving the T4 cells is, thus, understandable but challenging. Perhaps the *tat* binding site in T4 cells differs from that in other cells and facilitates binding of *tat* with greater efficiency, or its position in T4 cells is closer to genes involved in proliferation so that it can more efficiently induce their expression.

We assume that the maintenance of malignancy requires additional genetic changes in the cell because generally after ATLL develops, the HTLV-I genes are not expressed in fresh tumor tissue in (more than 80% of cases). Therefore, it appears that the expression of a viral gene product is not necessary to maintain the malignancy. Several investigations of chromosomal changes in ATLL have pointed to frequent trisomy 7 and a 14q abnormality. However, the situation is currently confused, and there is no agreed upon consistent chromosomal change.

Seeking additional viral isolates from T-cell malignancies, HTLV-II was described by Gelmann and co-workers in 1981.[24] A cell line, developed by Saxon and Golde from a young man with a T-cell variant of hairy cell leukemia, yielded the first isolate of HTLV-II. The disease was not aggressive. The virus has been isolated from several other patients, again from adult T-cell malignancies. All isolates have been from Caucasians. Considerable details exist on the nature of HTLV-II genome and on its in vitro effects. It is overall about 50% homologous to HTLV-I. Few major biological differences have been found, and clinical data are limited to the few case reports available. However, recent seroepidemiology indicates that HTLV-I and HTLV-II may be transmitted among drug addicts. Although it is very likely that this virus was involved in these few leukemias, there is as yet insufficient data to conclude that it is a cause of human leukemia. It is clear that HTLV-II is rare in the general U.S. and European populations.

Concluding Remarks on HTLV-I and HTLV-II

The first known human retroviruses (HTLV-I and HTLV-II) probably came to central African man from monkeys directly or via intermediaries in the distant past. A precise time for this is unknown, but must be many centuries ago. HTLV-I has been linked to the cause of some T-cell malignancies in a way that provides the clearest evidence we have on the direct cause of a human cancer. This evidence includes: (1) epidemiological results clearly linking the two; (2) in vitro transformation of primary human T-cells; (3) lymphoma induction in monkeys with the very closely related STLV-I; (4) molecular biological results showing a monoclonal distribution of the viral genes (provirus) in the tumor cell DNA and no viral sequences in other tissues, providing evidence that the virus entered the patient before or at the time of the first T-cell neoplastic transformation and not later as a passenger virus; and (5) numerous animal models (chicken, mouse, rat, cat, cow, and Gibbon ape) showing that leukemias and lymphomas may be induced by retroviruses. HTLV-I also appears to play an indirect role in the cause of some other malignancies such as some B-cell tumors in HTLV-I endemic regions. HTLV-II has only been isolated a few times. It too probably causes some malignancies, but more evidence is needed.

For review on HTLV-I, and HTLV-II, refer to the reports by Gallo[25] and Broder and Gallo.[26]

HTLV-III and the Origin of AIDS

In 1981, a new immunodeficiency was described in homosexual men with opportunistic infections and malignancies. Subsequently, certain other risk groups have been identified in the United States, notably those exposed to blood products by transfusion, factor VIII, and contaminated needles, recent immigrants to the United States from Haiti, and children of infected parents. A similar disease was emerging at the same time or earlier in parts of central Africa, especially among promiscuous heterosexuals, including prostitutes.[27] Now, of course, AIDS is recognized as the result of a viral infection. It concerns every segment of society with enormous social, economic, ethical, and medical consequences. The pathogenesis of the disease begins with alteration and eventual depletion of the T4 cells. This, in turn, leads to an overwhelming immune dysfunction and eventually to opportunistic infections, CNS disease, and malignancies. The search for a retroviral etiology began in our laboratory in 1982.

After the successful in vitro production of several retroviruses, isolates from patients with AIDS and AIDS-related complex (ARC), the cause of AIDS was convincingly demonstrated to be a single retrovirus by the spring of 1984.[28-31] This virus has been called human T-lymphotropic virus-III (HTLV-III), because it was the third type of human T-lymphotropic virus to be discovered, and also lymphodenopathy-associated virus (LAV).

There are lessons to be learned from the early ideas on the origin of AIDS. From 1981 to 1983, speculations outdistanced experiments, and the major ideas included sperm (immunosuppression or autoimmune disease with antibodies to sperm reactive also with T cells), diverse reactions to HLA (exposure to various leukocytes from promiscuous sexual experiences) once again invoking some autoimmunity, amyl nitrite (used by some of the people in risk groups), a fungus, several types of viruses, and (remarkably) multiple and chronic antigenic stimulation without a single specific cause. The idea that AIDS was caused by a new human T-lymphotropic retrovirus was first proposed by Gallo and was discussed in 1982 based on the following considerations: (1) epidemiological data strongly argued that the disease was new, rapidly increasing, and most probably infectious/viral; (2) previously unknown blood transfusions gave rise to AIDS in nonrisk groups, thereby eliminating causes other than a transmissible agent; (3) factor VIII preparations induced AIDS in hemophiliacs (because these preparations are filtered so as to remove bacteria, parasites, and fungi, a virus became the most logical candidate); (4) the disease seemed to specifically involve the T4 cell—such cell specificity is more consistent with a viral than a bacterial or fungal infection; and (5) a human retrovirus was thought to be the most logical candidate based on the earlier experiences with HTLV-I (T4 cell tropism; likely African origin; transmission by blood, sex, and congenital infection; and known capacity to induce some T-cell functional changes)—experiences with an animal retrovirus, the feline leukemia virus (FeLV), reinforced this possibility. FeLV can cause T-cell leukemia, but probably a variant causes an AIDS-like disease. Essex and co-workers[32] noted that immunodeficiency is actually the most frequent outcome of infection by this virus. In contrast, against the idea of a retrovirus were the prevailing feelings that most retroviruses are usually not very cytopathic and a general lack of experience with human retroviral disease.

Retroviruses were detected from lymphocytes of patients with AIDS repeatedly in the United States at the National Institutes of Health as early as November 1982 and throughout 1983. Some of these isolates proved to be HTLV-I, but others were clearly different. The technology to grow and identify HTLV-I provided several well-defined isolates of this virus. This experience was reported[33,34] at the same time as the detection of a retrovirus by Barré-Sinoussi and co-workers from one patient with lymphadenopathy. The extreme and unexpected cytopathogencity of what was later learned to be HTLV-III presented an obstacle to further progress. The infected target T cells died, and the virus could not be characterized or linked to the disease.

The next major advance was the finding that certain clones of human leukemic T4-cell lines, free of any retroviruses, could be productively infected by HTLV-III. This allowed for the first mass production of several isolates and accomplished the following: (1) the first specific reagents (antibodies, antigens, nucleic acid probes) so that all other isolates could be characterized; (2) wide distribution of the virus to other scientists; (3) sufficient viral proteins for specific and wide-scale seroepidemiological studies; (4) initiation of molecular studies and cloning of the virus; and (5) a blood bank assay. With this initial characteristic complete, Popovic,[28] Gallo,[29] Schüpbach,[30] Sarngadharan,[31] and their colleagues, in the spring of 1984, described 48 isolates of HTLV-III and clear epidemiological evidence that this virus was the cause of AIDS. The blood test is based on detection of specific antibodies to HTLV-III envelope and core structural proteins. The assay approach is usually to screen by the ELISA method followed by a confirmatory test. This is usually an immunoblot (Western blot) procedure or an antibody competition assay.

Using virus-specific reagents, the distribution of HTLV-III in cells and tissues of infected individual has been studied. In addition to T4-lymphocytes, the virus has also been found in some B cells, macrophages, and in the brain (probably in microglial cells). The first evidence of infection of the CNS was by Shaw and associates,[35] and is particularly important since neurological abnormalities have been noted in many infected individuals. Free extracellular virus has also been isolated from plasma and virus detected in semen, saliva, tears, and cerebrospinal fluid. These studies have expanded our understanding of the biological basis of diseases associated with HTLV-III infections.

HTLV-III-Associated Diseases

Since HTLV-III infection has been clearly linked to the cause of AIDS, we have begun to focus attention on the etiological agent as a cause of disease. The case definition of AIDS widely used for statistical purposes identifies only the most severely affected patients. This will include approximately 10 to 40% of infected groups. Because it is possible to identify infected individuals using virus-specific reagents, it is possible to describe a more complete clinical spectrum of pathology associated with HTLV-III infection. Several staging classifications based on evidence of retroviral infection, quantitative and qualitative assessment of immune function, and clinical features such as adenopathy, symptoms, infection, and neoplasms have been proposed.[36,37] Once the process is initiated and clinically detectable, it appears to be progressive and rarely, if ever, is long-term spontaneous improvement seen. Since retroviral infection is life-long and the risk of disease appears to be cumulative with time, great emphasis has been placed on primary prevention chemotherapy and vaccine programs. AIDS, like chronic renal failure, is the description of the end-stage disease of a disease process. We use the term HTLV-III-related diseases to unify the pathophysiology, epidemiology, and clinical features by emphasis on the causal agent. Considerable effort over the past 5 years has gone into describing the pathophysiology and clinical manifestations of HTLV-III infection. The characteristic pathological outcome of infection is depletion of the T-helper lymphocyte number and function. As described in the next section, these cells are directly infected by the virus that utilizes the T4 molecule as a viral receptor. Patients are unable to mount an adequate cellular or humoral response to infection. Recurrent severe and dissemenated infection with opportunistic organisms is the hallmark of AIDS. The loss of immunoregulation may also result in autoimmune disease such as thrombocytopenia, neutropenia, and circulating anticoagulants.

The extraordinary frequency of Kaposi's sarcoma in homosexual men is not completely understood. HTLV-III does not seem to be directly involved since viral sequences have not been found in the DNA of the majority of tumor cells. We suspect another virus that transforms endothelial cells in the setting of immunodeficiency. In addition to adenopathy, hypergammaglobulinemia, and polyclonal B-cell activation, there is an increase in high grade, extranodal

B-cell lymphomas.[38] Although EBV-infected B cells may be infected by HTLV-III, so far these tumors have not yielded evidence of retrovirus in the primary tissue. Perhaps the mechanisms are similar to the indirect role described for HTLV-I diseases. Other malignancies such as Hodgkin's lymphoma, T-cell lymphoma, and carcinomas[39] have also been reported in association with HTLV-III infections.

HTLV-III infection causing neurological diseases has been reported by several investigators.[40,41] This very important topic is addressed in several later chapters. Infection of the CNS is most likely in a macrophage or microglial cell. Infection of the lung has been associated with lymphoid interstitial pneumonia. Infection of the macrophage has been demonstrated and may be the primary infected cell in some tissue such as the brain, lung, and perhaps the liver.[42] Further epidemiological data are needed to confirm other associations such as congenital malformations.

Cytopathic Effect of HTLV-III on T4 Cells

Infection of T4 cells by HTLV-III leads to a cytopathic effect, that is, the premature death of these cells. The mechanism is not a direct lytic effect. On the other hand, indirect effects (e.g., mediated by an autoimmune process) need not be postulated since one or more of the cloned genes of HTLV-III lead to T4 cell death upon transfection of the DNA provirus into these cells, and expression of one or more of the viral genes is necessary.[43] It is possible to infect T4 cells in vitro without cell-killing until the T cells are activated by exposure to a mitogen or antigen. The activated infected T cells appear to go through the same process of cell gene expression as uninfected cells, except that the viral genes are eventually expressed. When this occurs, a higher percentage of the cells than normal will terminally differentiate, and the rate of terminal differentiation is faster than in the activated uninfected T cells. This process may involve the *tat*-III gene.[44] Expression of this gene may, in turn, activate an extremely high level of translation of another viral gene or a set of cellular genes augmenting terminal differentiation. If another viral gene is involved in this cell death, it may be the product of the *sor* gene or 3'*orf* gene, whose functions remain unknown. These topics are also taken up in the chapters by Wong-Staal and Haseltine et al.

Heterogeneity of HTLV-III

An early finding in the molecular analysis of various HTLV-III isolates was the variation of nucleotide sequences of certain parts of the genome, especially in the envelope gene.[45] Analysis of more than 30 isolates indicates that there are not different strains of HTLV-III. Instead, there is a continuum—from very closely related isolates (1 to 2% variation) to those that vary by more than 10 to 15%. Variation develops with successive infections, and does not occur during prolonged tissue culture.[46] This suggests that these changes occur during transcription of the viral RNA genome to the DNA form and/or during the integration process when the DNA provirus integrates into the host cell DNA. Reverse transcriptases (RT) and DNA polymerases tend to be error-prone. It is possible that the RT of HTLV-III is particularly error-prone. The recent identification of HTLV-III RT may help to answer this question.[47] Because most of the genomic variation occurs in the envelope, it may be that variation in other parts of the viral genome leads to noninfectious particles or that selective pressure is exerted on the envelope glycoprotein in vivo.

Prevention and Treatment of HTLV-III Infection

Primary prevention that involves avoiding or controlling exposure has become the focus of public health measures to limit the number of infected individuals. The ability to detect viral infection even in asymptomatic individuals by serology should virtually eliminate the risk associated with blood products and tissue donation of any type. Heterosexual transmission is well documented and is the likely route in some populations with a high prevalence of infection.[39] Public health measures that identify infected individuals are likely to provoke controversial, ethical, legal, and social questions.

Protective vaccines have historically provided the best and most economical means of controlling viral infections. There is, however, little experience and almost no success in preventing infection by other retroviruses in animal systems. The exception may be recent vaccines for FeLV. Approaches to developing human retroviral vaccines have been reviewed.[48,49] Neutralizing antibodies to retrovirus have generally been directed to the virus envelop and block viral entry into target cells. Neutralizing antibodies to HTLV-III have been demonstrated.[50] Titers, although low, may be correlated with prognosis. Several special problems must be considered. Since T cells are essential for most immune responses once infection occurs, production of an immune response may be difficult. The viral envelope used for a vaccine may itself be immunosuppressive even without infection. Envelope heterogeneity among different isolates presents a particular challenge. By comparing the nucleotide sequences of several isolates, we hope to be able to identify conserved areas of the envelope protein that are immunogenic. If this concept proves true, a direct approach to prepare a vaccine is feasible based on utilization of these regions to induce protective antibodies. The application of molecular techniques to produce recombinant protein products and recombinant virus or synthetic peptides may provide the appropriate product. Antibody to the virus in some retroviral systems has been associated with more severe disease, presumably by enhancing Fc-mediated uptake of virus.

It is estimated that more than one million Americans and perhaps more Africans are already infected by HTLV-III. Therefore, treatment of infected individuals is urgently needed. A vaccine against the viral envelope could reduce the spread of virus in the infected person and perhaps among individuals. Avoidance of other infections that could activate already infected T cells, promoting both their death and further spread of virus, is important. Additionally, antiviral compounds are urgently needed. Some of the targets are obvious (e.g., reverse transcriptase inhibitors and agents that interact with the viral envelope). Other approaches should come from structural-functional studies of the viral genome (e.g., inhibitors of *tat*-III gene expression or function). Treatment will probably have to be life-long, at least on an intermittant basis. To avoid toxicity and reduce the chances for viral resistance, it may be necessary to use a combination of compounds with different mechanisms of action. Certain concepts related to the development of new therapies for HTLV-III are taken up in the chapter by Yarchoan and Broder.

Summary and Concluding Remarks on HTLV-III

HTLV-III is a new infection of mankind with severe and often fatal consequences. Like HTLV-I (and probably also HTLV-II), it is likely that it or a similar virus was introduced to man from African green monkeys or other primates, either directly or indirectly. In an age of rapid movement, the virus has subsequently spread to other regions. Also similar to HTLV-I is its mode of transmission, T4 tropism, in vitro mimicry of the disease, and presence of a *tat* gene. Unlike HTLV-I or HTLV-II, the virus that causes AIDS contains at least two additional genes, has strong cytopathic effects and greater structural similarities to the lentiretroviruses, and is generally more infectious. We have learned more about human retroviruses, and especially HTLV-III, in a shorter period of time than any microbial agent in the history of biomedical research. Yet, diseases caused by these viruses have outdistanced scientific speed. To avoid still more serious global, medical, and economic problems, we will need even more rapid progress.

References

1. Wong-Staal F, Gallo RC. Human T-lymphotropic retroviruses. Nature 1985; 317:395–403.
2. Gross L. Oncogenic viruses, 3rd ed. Oxford: Pergamon Press, 1983.

3. Krakower JM, Tonick SR, Gallagher RE, Gallo RC, Aaronson SA. Antigenic characterization of a new Gibbon ape leukemia virus isolate: seroepidemiologic assessment of an outbreak of Gibbon leukemia. Int J Cancer 1978; 22:715–720.

4. Jarrett W, Martin B, Crighton W, Dalton R, Stewart M. Leukemia in the cat. Transmission experiments with leukemia (lymphosarcoma) Nature 202:566–567, 1964; 202:566–567.

5. Daniel MD, Letvin NL, King NW, et al. Isolation of T-cell tropic HTLV-III-like retroviruses from macaques. Science 1985; 228:1201.

6. Kanki PJ, Kurth R, Becker W, Dreesman G, McLane M, Essex M. Antibodies to simian T-lymphotropic retrovirus type III in African green monkeys and recognition of STLV-III viral proteins by AIDS and related sera. Lancet 1985; 1:130–132.

7. Temin HM, Mizutani S. RNA-dependent DNA polymerase in virions of Rous sarcoma virus. Nature 1970; 226:1211–1213.

8. Baltimore D. RNA-dependent DNA polymerase in virions of RNA tumour viruses. Nature 1970; 226:1209–1211.

9. Teich N, Wyke J, Mak T, Bernstein A, Hardy W. Pathogenesis of retrovirus-induced disease. In: Weiss R, et al., eds. Molecular biology of tumor viruses, 2nd ed., revised: RNA tumor viruses. Cold Spring Harbor, New York: Cold Spring Harbor Laboratory, 1984:947.

10. Poiesz BJ, Ruscetti FW, Reitz MS, Kalyanaraman VS, Gallo RC. Isolation of a new type C retrovirus (HTLV) in primary uncultured cells of a patient with Sezary T-cell leukemia. Nature 1981; 294:268–271.

11. Sarngadharan MG, Guroff MR, Gallo RC. DNA polymerases of normal and neoplastic mammalian cells. Biochem Biophys Acta 1978; 516:419–487.

12. Morgan DA, Ruscetti FW, Gallo RC. Selective in vitro growth of T-lymphocytes from normal human bone marrows. Science 1976; 193:1007–1008.

13. Volkman DJ, Popovic M, Gallo RC, Fauci AS. Human T cell leukemia/lymphoma virus-infected antigen-specific T cell clones: indiscriminant helper function and lymphokine production. J Immunol 1985; 134:4237–4243.

14. Zagury D, Bernard J, Leonard R, Cheynier R, Feldman M, Sarin PS, Gallo RC. Long-term cultures of HTLV-III-infected T cells: a model of cytopathology of T-cell depletion in AIDS. Science 1986; 231:850–853.

15. Folks TD, Powell M, Lightfoote M, Benn S, Martin MA, Fauci AS. Induction of HTLV-III/LAV from a non-virus producing T-cell line: implications for latency in humans. Science 1986; 231:600–602.

16. Poiesz BJ, Ruscetti FW, Mier JW, Woods AM, Gallo RC. Detection and isolation of type-C retrovirus particles from fresh and cultured lymphocytes of a patient with cutaneous T-cell lymphoma. Proc Natl Acad Sci USA 1980; 77:7415–7419.

17. Gallo RC, Blattner WA. Human T-cell leukemia/lymphoma viruses: ATL and AIDS. In: DeVita VT, Hellman S, Rosenberg SA, eds. Important advances in oncology. 1985: 104–138.

18. Clarke JM, Hahn B, Mann D, et al. Molecular and immunologic analysis of a chronic lymphocytic leukemia case: with antibody against HTLV. Cancer 1985; 56:495–499.

19. Mann D. "HTLV B CLL: A model for indirect retroviral leukemogenesis." (personal communication).

20. Blattner WA, Kalyanaraman VS, Robert-Guroff M, Lister TA, Galton DAG, Sarin PS, Crawford MH, Catovsky D, Greaves M, Gallo RC. The human type-C retrovirus, HTLV, in blacks from the Caribbean region, and relationship to adult T-cell leukemia/lymphoma. Int J Cancer 1982; 30:257–264.
21. Robert-Guroff M, Nakao Y, Notake K, Ito Y, Sliski A, Gallo RC. Natural antibodies to human retrovirus HTLV in a cluster of Japanese patients with adult T cell leukemia. Science 1982; 215:975–978.
22. Gallo RC, Sliski A, Wong-Staal F. Origin of human T-cell leukemia-lymphoma virus. Lancet 1983; ii:962–963.
23. Guo H-G, Wong-Staal F, Gallo RC. Novel viral sequences related to human T-cell leukemia virus in T cells of a seropositive baboon. Science 1984; 223:1195–1197.
24. Gelmann EP, Franchini G, Manzari V, Wong-Staal F, Gallo RC. Molecular cloning of a new unique human T-cell leukemia virus (HTLV-II$_{MO}$). In: Gallo RC, Essex M, Gross L, eds. Human T-cell leukemia/lymphoma virus. Cold Spring Harbor, New York: Cold Spring Harbor Laboratory, 1984:189–195.
25. Gallo RC. The human T-cell leukemia/lymphotropic retroviruses (HTLV) family: past, present, and future. Cancer Res (Suppl) 1985; 45:4524s–4533s.
26. Broder S, Gallo RC. Human T-cell leukemia viruses (HTLV): a unique family of pathogenic retroviruses. Ann Rev Immunol 1985; 3:321–336.
27. Van De Perre P, Carael M, Robert-Guroff M, Freyens P, Gallo RC, Clumeck N, Nzabihimana E, DeMol P, Butzler J-P, Kanyamupira J-B. Female prostitutes: a risk group for infection with human T-cell lymphotropic virus type III. Lancet 1985; ii:524–527.
28. Popovic M, Sarngadharan MG, Read E, Gallo RC. Detection, isolation, and continuous production of cytopathic retroviruses (HTLV-III) from patients with AIDS and pre-AIDS. Science 1984; 224:497–500.
29. Gallo RC, Salahuddin SZ, Popovic M, Shearer GM, Kaplan M, Haynes BF, Palker TJ, Redfield R, Oleske J, Safai B, White, G, Foster P, Markham PD. Frequent detection and isolation of cytopathic retroviruses (HTLV-III) from patients with AIDS and at risk for AIDS. Science 1984; 224:500–503.
30. Schüpbach J, Popovic M, Gilden RV, Gonda MA, Sarngadharan MG, Gallo RC. Serological analysis of a subgroup of human T-lymphotropic retroviruses (HTLV-III) associated with AIDS. Science 1984; 224:503–505.
31. Sarngadharan MG, Popovic M, Bruch L, Schüpbach J, Gallo RC. Antibodies reactive with human T-lymphotropic retroviruses (HTLV-III) in the serum of patients with AIDS. Science 1984; 224:506–508.
32. Essex M, McLane MF, Kanki P, Allan J, Kitchen L, Lee T-H. Retroviruses associated with leukemia and ablative syndromes in animals and human beings. Cancer Res (Suppl) 1985; 45:4534s–4538s.
33. Gallo RC, Sarin PS, Gelmann EP, Robert-Guroff M, Richardson E, Kalyanaraman VS, Mann D, Sidhu GD, Stahl RE, Zolla-Pazner S, Leibowitch J, Popovic M. Isolation of human T-cell leukemia virus in acquired immune deficiency syndrome (AIDS). Science 1983; 220:865–867.
34. Barré-Sinoussi F, Chermann JC, Rey R et al. Isolation of a T-lymphotropic retrovirus from a patient at risk for acquired immune deficiency syndrome (AIDS). Science 1983; 220:868–871.

35. Shaw GM, Harper ME, Hahn BH, Epstein LG, Gajdusek DC, Price RW, Navia BA, Petito CK, O'Hara CJ, Groopman JE, Cho E-S, Oleske JM, Wong-Staal F, Gallo RC. HTLV-III infection in brains of children and adults with AIDS encephalopathy. Science 1985; 227:177–182.
36. Redfield RR, Wright DC, Tramont EC. The Walter Reed staging classification for HTLV-III/LAV infection. N Engl J Med 1986; 314:131–132.
37. Kaplan MH, Pahwa SG, Popovic M, Sarngadharan MG, Gallo RC. A classification of HTLV-III infection based on 75 cases seen in a suburban community. Cancer Res (Suppl) 1985; 45:4655s–4658s.
38. Levine AM, Meyer PB, Begandy MD et al. Development of B-cell lymphoma in homosexual men: Clinical and immunological findings. Annals Int Med 1984; 100:7–13.
39. Redfield RR, Markham PD, Salahuddin SZ, Wright DC, Sarngadharan MG, Gallo RC. Heterosexually acquired HTLV-III/LAV disease (AIDS-related complex and AIDS). JAMA 1985; 254:2094–2096.
40. Resnick L, DiMarzo-Veronese F, Schüpbach J, Tourtellote WW, Ho DD, Muller F, Shapshak P, Vogt M, Groopman J, Markham PD, Gallo RC. Intra-blood-brain-barrier synthesis HTLV-III-specific IgG in patients with neurologic symptoms associated with AIDS or AIDS-related complex. N Engl J Med 1985; 313:1498–1504.
41. Gartner S, Markovits P, Markovitz D, Kaplan M, Gallo RC, Popovic M. Role of monocyte-macrophage in HTLV-III infection. Science (in press).
42. Salahuddin SZ, Rose RM, Groopman JE, Markham PD, Gallo RC. Human T-lymphotropic virus type III (HTLV-III) infection on human alveolar macrophages. Blood (in press).
43. Fisher AG, Collalti E, Ratner L, Gallo RC, Wong-Staal F. A molecular clone of HTLV-III with biological activity. Nature 1985; 316:262–265.
44. Fisher AG, Feinberg MB, Josephs SF, Harper ME, Marselle LM, Reyes G, Gonda MA, Aldovini A, Debouk C, Gallo RC, Wong-Staal F. The trans-activator gene of HTLV-III is essential for virus replication. Nature 1986; 320:367–373.
45. Shaw GM, Hahn BH, Arya SK, Groopman JE, Gallo RC, Wong-Staal F. Molecular characterization of human T-cell leukemia (lymphotropic) virus type III in the acquired immune deficiency syndrome. Science 1984; 226:1165–1171.
46. Wong-Staal F, Shaw GM, Hahn BH, Salahuddin SZ, Popovic M, Markham P, Redfield R, Gallo RC. Genomic diversity of human T-lymphotropic virus type III (HTLV-III). Science 1985; 229:759–762.
47. Veronese F, Di M, Copeland TD, DeVico AL, Rahman R, Oroszian S, Gallo RC, Sarngadharan MG. Characterization of highly immunogenic p66/p51 as the reverse transcriptase of HTLV-III/LAV. Science 1986; 231:1289–1291.
48. Fischinger PJ, Robey WG, Koprowski H, Gallo RC, Bolognesi DP. Current status and strategies for vaccines against diseases induced by human T-cell lymphotropic retroviruses (HTLV-I, -II, -III). Cancer Res (Suppl) 1985; 45:4694s–4699s.
49. Gallo RC, Reitz M, Streicher H. Approaches to a human retroviral vaccine. Cold Spring Harbor, New York: Cold Spring Harbor Laboratory, 1986.
50. Robert-Guroff M, Brown M, Gallo RC. HTLV-III-neutralizing antibodies in patients with AIDS and AIDS-related complex. Nature 1985; 316:72–74.

2

Lymphadenopathy/AIDS Virus: The Prototype Human Lentivirus

Simon Wain-Hobson
Pierre Sonigo
Unité de Recombinaison
et Expression Génétique
Institut Pasteur
Paris, France

Marc Alizon
Luc Montagnier
Oncologie Virale
Institut Pasteur
Paris, France

It is now abundantly clear that AIDS is a relatively recent disease both in developed and developing countries alike, and one that will have a profound impact on our societies. Equally clear is the increasing prevalence and transmission of a novel retrovirus LAV/HTLV-III, the etiological agent of the disease.[1,2] This link between the virus and the disease has been amply described[3,4] and will be only reiterated here as six points:

1. The ability to isolate virus from patients with AIDS, pre-AIDS, as well as from patients in all risk groups
2. A higher seropositivity among people in the risk groups
3. The unfortunate apparent transmission of disease by blood transfusion
4. The apparent coincidental entry of the virus and disease into developed countries

5. The ability of the virus to kill T4 cells
6. The demonstration of a comparable yet distinct retrovirus among macaques with simian AIDS, which can transmit the disease to healthy animals

The virus is, and has been, transmitted by body fluids either by sexual intercourse, the sharing or unsatisfactory sterilization of needles, blood transfusion, and blood-derived products. Virus has been recovered not only from blood and semen,[5] but also from saliva,[6] tears, and urine. The contribution of the latter three sources to the spread of the disease probably constitutes a very minor proportion, if at all. Virus is readily transmitted between homosexuals, to female sex partners of bisexual men, and perinatally to children born to virus-positive mothers.

From the outset, the virus did not declare itself akin, either biologically or biochemically, to the two other extant human retroviruses, human T-cell leukemia viruses types I and II (HTLV-I and HTLV-II)[7] despite one or two apparent common features such as the predominant T4 tropism of all three viruses. The AIDS virus infects and destroys only activated T4$^+$ cells in vitro,[8] which agrees well with the loss of the T4$^+$ cell population in vivo.[9] The cellular receptor for the virus is probably T4 or a protein associated the T4 since viral infection can be blocked by anti-T4$^+$ antibodies.[10,11] (The receptor for HTLV-I is not known; infection is not blocked by anti-T4$^+$ antibodies, indicating that the receptor is not the same.) More recently, it has been shown that the virus can cross the blood-brain barrier,[12] indeed, neurological lesions and disorders seem to be increasingly apparent since the neurotropism of this virus was recognized.[13,14] Lastly the AIDS virus can be cultivated in established monocyte/macrophage cell lines, suggesting that the cell tropism is even wider than hitherto believed.[15] This chapter will concentrate mainly on the virology and the relationship of the AIDS virus to the animal lentiviruses.

Viral Genome

The RNA genome of the AIDS virus is some 9200 bases long, and the integrated provirus 9600 bp.[16-20] The genetic structure of the virus is completely novel for retroviruses (Fig. 1). The greatest surprise is the novel central region separating the *pol* and *env* genes (see below), as well as the extremely large envelope gene. There are at least six genes and perhaps more, the functions of at least two are unknown. (Because retrovirus mRNA transcripts all share the same start and stop, the individual genes are expressed by a complex splicing mechanism. The word gene, that is, a transcription unit, and open reading frame (Fig. 1) are often used interchangeably in retrovirology,

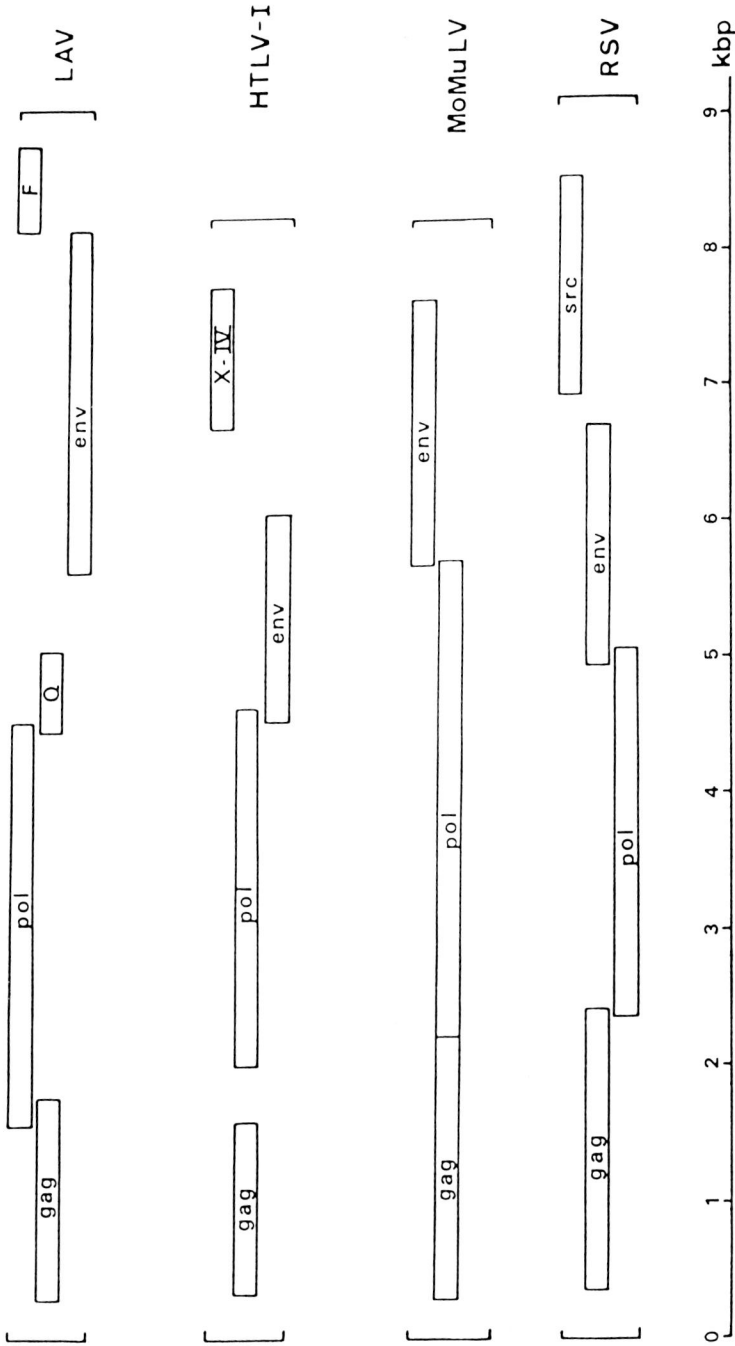

FIGURE 1 Comparison of the genome organization of LAV with those of human T-leukemia/lymphoma virus type I (HTLV-I),[7] Moloney murine leukemia virus (MoMuLV),[58] and Rous sarcoma virus (RSV).[59] The positions and sizes of viral genes are drawn to scale (open boxes) and the viral genomes (RNA forms) are delineated by brackets.

and here we will refer to *orfs* since they correspond most closely to the coding sequences.) Although a detailed transcription map of the virus exists, it seems to be incomplete.

gag: The first *orf* encodes the *gag* polyprotein Pr55 (or Pr53), which is cleaved into three mature *gag* proteins (p18, p25, and p14–16) presumably by the virally encoded protease. We[17] and others[18-20] have sequenced the NH_2 terminus of the p25 and found a perfect match between it and that determined by the DNA sequence. The p25 is the major core protein of the nucleocapsid surrounding the nucleic acid. It is highly immunogenic, and antibodies to p25 are found in more than 50% of patients' sera.[21] Very early on, it was clear that p25 did not ordinarily react with the p24 of the HTLV viruses.[1,22] In contrast, p25 clearly reacts with antibodies to the major core protein of equine infectious anemia virus (EIAV).[23] The p18 molecule is blocked to Edman degradation, which makes it the amino terminus *gag* protein. The p14–16 molecule is the nucleic acid-binding protein (NBP) since a cysteine-rich motif is found repeated within its sequence (this being the hallmark of all retroviral NBPs). Thus, the order of the mature *gag* proteins within the precursor is NH_2-p18-p25-p15-COOH.

pol: The retroviral transcriptase is invariably derived from a *gag–pol* polyprotein precursor. Since *gag* and *pol* are in two different reading frames (Fig. 1), only a splice or a translational frameshift can bring the two together; the latter mechanism is employed by Rous sarcoma virus and is probably the case for the AIDS virus.[24] The calculated molecular weight of such a precursor is in good agreement with a *gag*-related unglycosylated precursor protein Pr160. The polymerase *orf* encodes three functional domains, which are so crucial to the retrovirus that the amino acid sequences are well conserved among all retroviral sequences established to date. The protease domain is responsible for the cleavage of the *gag*-related precursor proteins to mature proteins. The second domain, that of the reverse transcriptase/RNAseH, follows the protease domain. The COOH terminal domain corresponds to the viral endonuclease/integrase protein, which is responsible for cleaving closed circular proviral DNA and integrating it into the host cellular DNA. We will see below that these conserved sequences allow the calculation of a phylogenetic tree for retroviruses.

Q: This *orf* (variably called sor, p', or *orf* 1) can encode a protein of 22.5 kd, and corresponds to the recently described p23. The function of this protein is unknown. Initial reports[17] suggested that *orf* Q was not transcribed in lytically infected cells, but a subsequent study showed that it was.[25]

tat: The *tat* protein is the only AIDS virus protein so far composed of two coding exons.[26,27] This protein is responsible for the *trans*-acting amplification pathway that the virus has for rapid viral replication.[28] The viral target

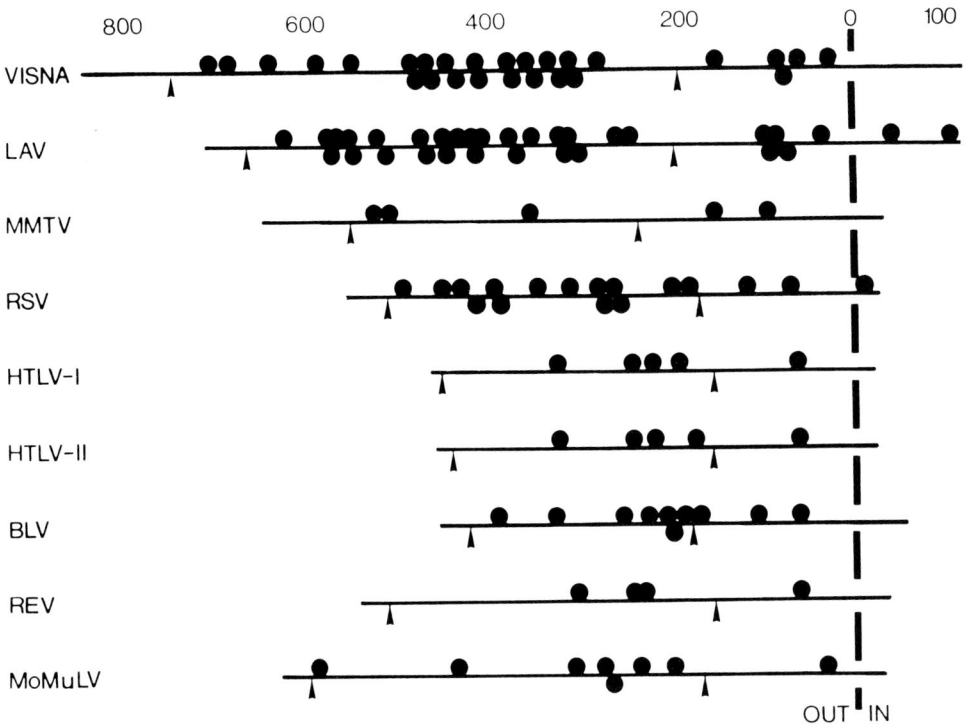

FIGURE 2 Comparison of retroviral envelope glycoprotein sequences. The sequences have been aligned according to their *trans*-membrane segment; those sequences on the outside of the membrane are to the left of the vertical bar (OUT). Arrows represent sites of proteolytic cleavage. The most terminal NH$_2$ eliminates the signal peptide sequence. The second cleavage site splits the precursor protein into the outer and *trans*-membrane proteins (amino and carboxy terminal proteins, respectively). Full circles represent potential N-glycosylation sites. Data are derived from the following reports: visna,[38] LAV,[20] MMTV,[63] RSV,[59] HTLV-I,[7] HTLV-II,[9] BLV,[61] REV,[62] and MoMuLV.[58]

sequences for this protein, or protein induced by *ptat,* map after the *cap* site.[29] It is not yet known if *ptat* acts by activating transcription.

   env: In comparison with other retrovirus *env*^{LAV} is unusually large and heavily glycosylated, there being 32 potential N-linked glycosylation sites (Asn-X-Ser/Thr) in the LAV sequence.[20] The precursor glycoprotein gPr160 can readily be isolated from infected cells and to a lesser extent from virus.[30] These proteins are cleaved into a gp120 (outer membrane protein) and a gp41 (transmembrane protein), which are linked by disulphide bonds.[30] The gp41 is unusual in that it is much larger than any other TMP. This difference lies in the exceedingly long cytoplasmic tail of 150 residues (Fig. 2). The "irony," if that is the appropriate word, is that the TMP of the most immunosuppressive retrovirus we have seen does not have any amino acid sequence homology to the immunosuppressive peptides,[31] which exist in virtually all retroviral TMPs sequenced to date (even xenotopic endogenous retroviruses[32]) and which induce cytostatic effects on T-lymphocytes.[33] Indeed, genetically engineered *env* protein does not exert any cytostatic effect on cultured human lymphocytes.

F: The role of this *orf* (variably called e', *orf* 2, 3'*orf*) is unclear. It is heavily transcribed in lytically infected cells, and a p27 protein has been identified.[34] Yet in certain infectious molecular clones of HTLV-III, a stop codon punctuates the *orf*.[18] It must be concluded that either p27 is unnecessary to the viral life cycle in vitro or that the functional domain occurs 5' to the stop codon. More sequence data from a wide range of viral isolates may clarify this point.

The AIDS Virus Is a Lentivirus

We were intrigued by the similarities between the AIDS virus, both in biology and biochemistry, and what was known of the sheep lentivirus visna.[35,36] Lentiviruses are a subvision of retroviruses, which induce cytopathic effects in vitro and show progressive diseases in vivo. They are not associated with any neoplasms to date. Visna virus is the prototype lentivirus, and was first described in 1949 as being the agent of several diseases that appeared in epidemic form among sheep in Iceland during the period 1930 to 1950.[37] Visna refers to an inflammatory condition of the central nervous system (CNS) that may progress to total paralysis. If unattended, the animals die of inanition, hence the name "visna," which means "wasting" in Icelandic. When helped to obtain food and water, the animals can survive for remarkably long periods of time, sometimes for more than 10 years.[36] Both the AIDS and visna viruses induce cytopathic effects in vitro, induce slow progressive diseases in vivo, and have a similar morphology. Although there is no antigenic cross-reaction between the two viruses, both have at least three *gag* proteins and very large, highly glycosylated envelope proteins. In addition, the proviruses were of comparable length and the base compositions of their RNA genomes so uncannily close that it is worth repeating (LAV/VISNA U 22/22%, C 18/16%, A 36/36%, and G 24/26%).[35] To resolve definitively this curious similitude, we determined the complete genetic structure of the visna provirus.[38] The overall genetic structure of the two viruses is strikingly similar (Fig. 3). Both have the novel central region, the hallmark of the AIDS virus, as well as extremely large envelope glycoprotein genes. By virtue of a very small but

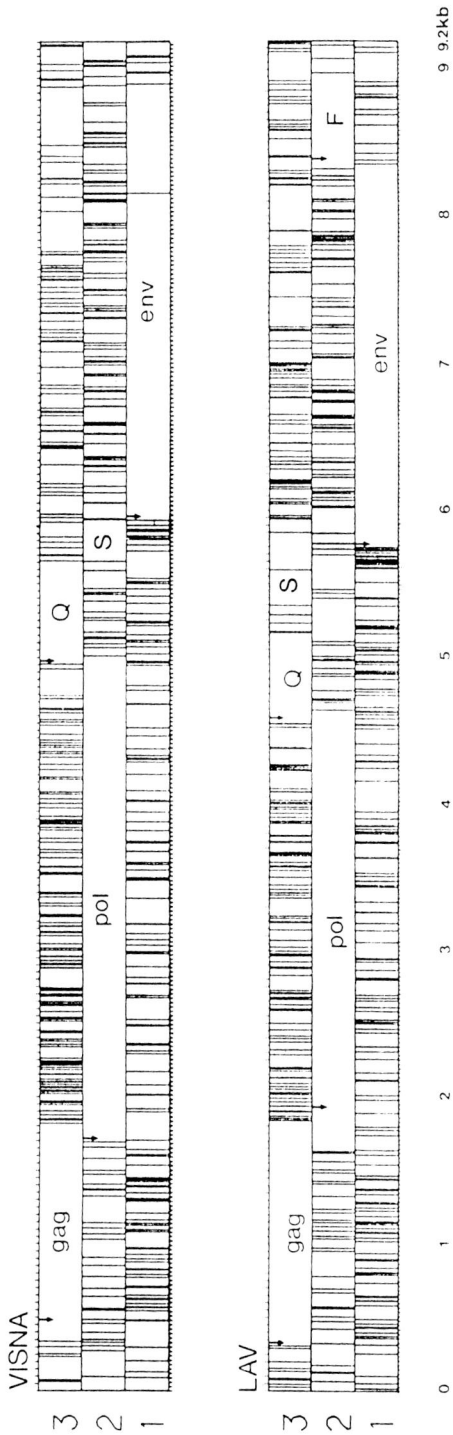

FIGURE 3 Genetic organization of visna virus and lymphadenopathy/AIDS virus (LAV). Stop codons in each phase (1, 2, or 3) are represented as vertical bars. (Regions lacking stop codons correspond to probable genes.) The arrow at the beginning of each orf refers to the first methionine residue.

probably significant amino acid homology between the LAV *tat* exon and visna *orf* S, it is more than likely that *trans*-activation will be soon described for visna virus. The major differences between the two viruses are the absence of an F gene in the visna sequence and a shorter LTR (LAV = 638 bps, visna = 419 bps).

There is extensive amino acid sequence homology between the *pol* sequences of LAV and visna, which we have exploited in order to construct a phylogenetic tree of all retroviral *pol* sequences established to date. The result (Fig. 4) is independent of the method, yet cannot be constructed from other genes (*gag* or *env*) since these amino acid sequences diverge too much. From this, it is clear that among these four families of retrovirus—the HTLV/BLV family of oncogenic viruses, the lentiviruses (LAV and visna), the MoMuLV-like virus, and a broad family encompassing RSV, MMTV, and SMRV—if anything, the HTLV/BLV family is closer to the RSV/MMTV/ SMRV family than it is to the lentiviruses based on an analysis of the endonuclease sequences.

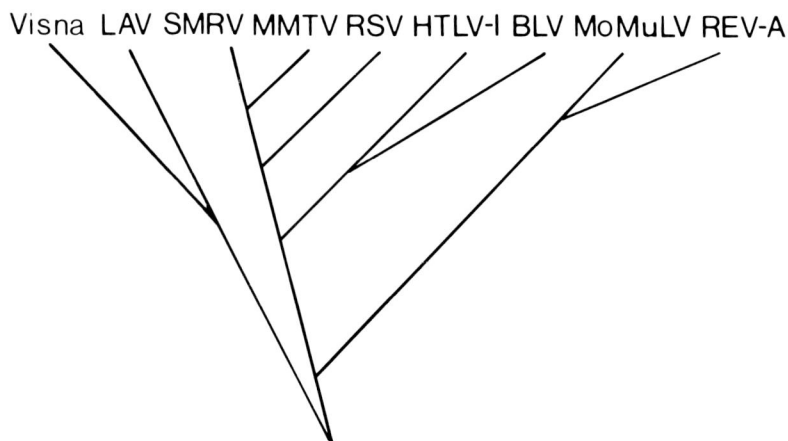

FIGURE 4   Alignment and phylogenetic tree of retroviral endonuclease/integrase protein sequences. The eight sequences known to date are aligned, the boundaries being set to the SMRV and MMTV sequences. The sequences are: LAV 3775-4288,[20] squirrel monkey retroviruses (SMRV),[60] mouse mammary tumour virus (MMTV),[60] Rous sarcoma virus (RSV) 4210-4746,[59] human T-cell leukemia virus type I (HTLV-I) 4307-4846,[7] bovine leukemia virus (BLV) 3979-4503,[61] Moloney murine leukemia virus (MoMuLV) 4746-5327,[58] and reticuloendotheliosis virus A (REV-A) 349-928.[62] Only the positions of the branch points are meaningful.

Relevance of Visna to AIDS

Viruses of the visna group, maedi virus, progressive pneumonia virus, and zwoegerziekte virus,[36] in contrast to LAV, are not immunosuppressive. They are the inciting agents for an immunopathological process in the lungs and CNS of the infected animal. This group of agents may nonetheless be relevant to AIDS—first as a nonprimate model in which the neurological complications of disease can be studied, and second as a model of latent infection of leukocytes.

The spread of visna virus in blood and tissue fluids such as cerebrospinal fluid continues unabated in the presence of neutralizing antibodies.[39] Two explanations relevant to AIDS can be advanced to account for the ability of lentiviruses to survive under these conditions: antigenic variation and a "Trojan horse" mechanism.

Antigenic variants of visna virus can be isolated in many instances from animals. Since these variants are not neutralized by antibodies to the inoculum strain, they could, in principle, provide a mechanism for temporary escape from immune surveillance.[39,40] These variants are generated by point mutations in the *env* gene, whose product elicits neutralizing antibodies[41] and may correspond to hypervariable regions in the env gene of LAV.[42] If this analogy holds, there would be good reason to be concerned about the efficacy of vaccination programs to provide protection from infections by variant viruses that differ from viruses or viral subcomponents used for vaccinations. However, in the case of visna, there is increasing evidence that emergence of antigenic variants plays little, if any, role in pathogenesis.[43,44]

We think the most likely explanation of virus spread and persistence in the face of the host's immune response is the covert infection of mobile cells, designated the "Trojan horse" mechanism. This hypothesis links the explanation of spread and persistence to a common theme of restricted gene expression[45] supported by recent analysis of leukocytes by in situ hybridization. Geballe and co-workers[46] and Peluso and associates (unpublished data) have shown that monocytes in lung and cerebrospinal fluids harbor the visna genome and have the same low level of viral RNA previously documented in epithelial cells[45,47] and glial cells.[48] The maturation of monocytes latently infected with visna virus to macrophages seems to provoke the disease by including viral expression,[49] and the pathological changes in visna develop in response and proportion to the presentation of viral antigens.[48]

In developing an analogous model for LAV, we have to consider the T4-lymphocytes, which are the main target of the virus and whose destruction characterizes AIDS.[8] These cells represent mainly the helper/inducer subset of lymphocytes and play a key role in the immune response, during which they are usually stimulated and proliferate in response to antigens. It is thus possible that antigenic stimulation of a "Trojan horse" T4-lymphocyte, harboring LAV in a latent form, modifies RNA splicing and induces viral expression, resulting in the destruction of this cell, probably as a consequence of a second immune response directed against viral antigen(s). Such a control of viral expression would explain the long incubation period between LAV infection and the occurrence of AIDS, as well as the role of antigenic load already suggested by two arguments. One argument is that LAV production in vitro requires lymphocyte stimulation and proliferation, which can be obtained by mitogens, soluble bacterial or viral antigens, or alloantigens. The other is that multiple infections are frequently observed in populations in which AIDS is epidemic. Finally, repeated antigenic stimulation may induce viral expression in latently infected lymphocytes, and subsequent destruction of cells expressing viral antigens may explain the passage from minor pathologies to frank AIDS. Thus, immunodeficiency appears to be a consequence of immunostimulation in a virally infected host, and specific immunosuppression might paradoxically be a treatment of AIDS.

Prospects of Handling Lentiviral Diseases

The handling of AIDS represents an enormous scientific and public health problem—the sheer numbers of people infected and the high attendant mortality mean that we need animal models for this disease to determine experimentally how the virus destroys the immune system. In this sense, the isolation and characterization of a lentivirus from macaques closely resembling the human AIDS virus[50,51] is of paramount importance and will constitute the most pertinent animal model. In addition, we believe that a wealth of data including long-term studies (i.e., of 10 years duration) of experimentally induced visna infections should not be overlooked. We will examine the three areas of diagnostics, therapy, and vaccination with visna in mind.

env Variation

The most variable region in the AIDS virus at both nucleic and amino acid sequence levels is that of the env gene. Within this region, there are some hypervariable domains as well as conserved sequence. The latter may explain why most but not all of antisera against different AIDS virus isolates react with original LAV isolate. It is conceivable that as more and more isolates are established, greater and greater antigenic variation will be found. It has been known for a number of years that visna viral isolates differ essentially in their *env* genes/proteins. Furthermore, it is known that visna virus can evolve in vivo,[43,44] i.e., after a number of years, serologically distinct isolates in addition to the inoculum strain can be isolated. It is not clear if this represents mutation or the selection of a minor form present in the inoculum strain that is, however, no more or less cytopathic in vitro than the initial viral stock.

Antiviral Therapy

While it appears that in AIDS, the immunosuppression is probably the result of the immunostimulation of a virally infected host, there are already examples where immunosuppression can lead to disastrous consequences as a result of opportunistic infections. Specific antiviral drugs have shown initial promise, but much more work is needed.[52-54] With visna in mind, it has been experimentally established that immunostimulants aggravate the disease while immunosuppresants, although not blocking viral replication, reduce the immune-mediated lysis of infected cells.[55] Little or no antiviral therapy by way of drugs has been attempted.

Vaccination

The development of an effective vaccine represents an enormous challenge not simply because of the antigenic variation of the virus, but due to the very poor (if at all) titers of neutralizing antibody. The record of making antiretroviral vaccines is not a good one, and it may be associated with the way in which the antigens presented. Ultraviolet-inactivated or heat-denatured visna virus in conjunction with Freund's complete adjuvant did not protect inoculated sheep against a live virus challenge. Perhaps we should concentrate on the induction of cell-mediated immunity since, even in the presence of neutralizing antibodies, the spread of visna virus in blood and tissues continues unabated.

Conclusion

Lentiviral infection in animals is associated with ubiquitous pathologies: CNS and lung infection (visna group), arthritis and encephalitis (caprine arthritis and encephalitis virus),[56] and blood cell infection (equine infectious anemia virus).[57] That LAV is clearly the first described human lentivirus, suggesting that there could also be a lentiviral etiology for some human neurological, pulmonary, hematological, or arthritic disorders. In this sense, acquisition of the T4 tropism by the highly variable envelope protein of an ancestral lentivirus could explain the recent apparition of AIDS.

References

1. Barré-Sinoussi F, Chermann J, Rey F, et al. Isolation of a T-lymphotropic retrovirus from a patient at risk of acquired immune deficiency syndrome (AIDS). Science 1983; 220:868–870.

2. Popovic M, Sarngadharan MG, Read E, Gallo RC. Detection, isolation and continuous production of cytopathic retroviruses (HTLV-III) from patients with AIDS and pre-AIDS. Science 1984; 224:497–500.

3. Montagnier L, Chermann JC, Barré-Sinoussi F, et al. A new human T-lymphotropic retrovirus: characterization and possible role in lymphadenopathy and acquired immune deficiency syndromes. In: Gallo RC, Essex M, Gross L, eds. Human T-cell leukemia/lymphoma virus. Cold Spring Harbor, New York: Cold Spring Harbor Laboratory, 1984:363–370.

4. Curran JW, Morgan WM, Hardy AM, et al. The epidemiology of AIDS: current status and future prospects. Science 1985; 229:1352–1357.

5. Zagury D, Bernard D, Leibowitch J, et al. HTLV-III in cells cultured from semen of two patients with AIDS. Science 1984; 226:449–451.

6. Groopman JG, Salahuddin SZ, Sarngadharan MG, et al. HTLV-III in saliva of people with AIDS-related complex and healthy homosexual men at risk for AIDS. Science 1984; 226:447–449.

7. Seiki M, Hattori S, Hirayama Y, Yoshida M. Human adult T-cell leukemia virus: complete nucleotide sequence of the provirus genome integrated in leukemia cell DNA. Proc Natl Acad Sci USA 1983; 80:3618–3622.

8. Klatzman D, Barré-Sinoussi F, Nugeyre MT, et al. Selective tropism of lymphadenopathy associated virus (LAV) for helper-inducer T-lymphocytes. Science 1984; 225:59–63.

9. Shimotohno K, Takahashi Y, Shimizu N, et al. Complete nucleotide sequence of an infectious molecular clone of human T-cell leukemia virus type II: an open reading frame for the protease gene. Proc Natl Acad Sci USA 1985; 81:3101–3105.

10. Dalgleish AG, Beverley PCL, Clapham PR, Crawford DH, Greaves MF, Weiss RA. The CD4 (T4) antigen is an essential component of the receptor for the AIDS retrovirus. Nature 1984; 312:763–767.

11. Klatzmann D, Champagne E, Chamaret S, et al. T-lymphocyte T4 molecules behaves as the receptor for human retrovirus LAV. Nature 1984; 312:767–768.

12. Shaw GM, Harper ME, Hahn BM, et al. HTLV-III infection in brains of children and adults with AIDS encephalopathy. Science 1985; 227:177–182.

13. Ho DD, Rota TR, Schooley RT, et al. Isolation of HTLV-III from cerebrospinal fluid and neural tissues of patients with neurologic syndromes related to the acquired immunodeficiency syndrome. N Engl J Med 1985; 313:1493–1497.

14. Resnick L, diMarzo-Veronese F, Schüpbach J, et al. Intra-blood-brain barrier synthesis of HTLV-III specific IgG in patients with neurologic symptoms associated with AIDS or AIDS-related complex. N Engl J Med 1985; 313:1498–1504.

15. Levy JA, Kaminsky LS, Morrow WJW, et al. Infection by the retrovirus associated with the acquired immunodeficiency syndrome: clinical, biological and molecular features. Ann Intern Med 1985; 103:94–99.

16. Alizon M, Sonigo P, Barré-Sinoussi F, et al. Molecular cloning of lymphadenopathy-associated virus. Nature 1984; 312:757–760.
17. Muesing MA, Smith DM, Cabradilla CD, et al. Nucleic acid structure and expression of the human AIDS/lymphadenopathy retroviruses. Nature 1985; 313:450–458.
18. Ratner L, Haseltine W, Patarca R, et al. Complete nucleotide sequence of the AIDS virus, HTLV-III. Nature 1985; 313:277–284.
19. Sanchez-Pescador R, Power MD, Barr PJ, et al. Nucleotide sequence and expression of an AIDS-associated retrovirus (ARV-2). Science 1985; 227:484–492.
20. Wain-Hobson S, Sonigo P, Danos O, Cole S, Alizon M. Nucleotide sequence of AIDS virus, LAV. Cell 1985; 40:9–17.
21. Brun-Vézinet F, Rouzioux C., Barré-Sinoussi F, et al. Detection of IgG antibodies to lymphadenopathy associated virus (LAV) by ELISA, in patients with acquired immuno-deficiency syndrome of lymphadenopathy syndrome. Lancet 1984; i:1253–1256.
22. Carey SM, Kim Y, Andersen PR, et al. Human T-cell lymphotropic virus type III: immunologic characterization and primary structure analysis of the major internal protein p24. J Virol 1985; 55:417–423.
23. Montagnier L, Dauguet C, Axler C, et al. A new type of retrovirus isolated from patients presenting with lymphadenopathy and AIDS: structural and antigenic relatedness with equine infectious anemia virus. Ann Virol (Institut Pasteur) 1984; 135E:119–134.
24. Jacks T, Varmus HE. Expression of the Rous sarcoma virus pol gene by ribosome frameshifting. Science 1985; 230:1237–1242.
25. Rabson AB, Daugherty DF, Venkalesan S, et al. Transcription of novel open reading frames of AIDS retrovirus during infection of lymphocytes. Science 1985; 229:1388–1390.
26. Arya SK, Guo C, Josephs SF, Wong-Staal F. Trans-activater gene of human T-lymphotropic virus type III (HTLV-III). Science 1985; 229:69–73.
27. Sodroski J, Patarca R, Rosen C, Haseltine W. Location of the trans-acting region on the genome of human T-cell lymphotropic virus type III. Science 1985; 229:74–77.
28. Sodroski J, Rosen C, Wong-Staal F, et al. Trans-acting transcriptional regulation of human T-cell leukemia virus type III long terminal repeat. Science 1985; 227:171–173.
29. Rosen CA, Sodroski J, Haseltine WA. The location of cis-acting regulatory sequences in the human T-cell lymphotropic virus type III (HTLV-III/LVA) long terminal repeat. Cell 1985; 41:813–823.
30. Kitchen LW, Barin F, Sulivan JL, et al. Aetiology of AIDS-antibodies to human T-cell leukemia virus (type III) in hemophiliacs. Nature 1984; 312:367–369.
31. Cianciolo GJ, Kipnis RJ, Snyderman R. Similarity between p15E of murine and feline viruses and p21 of HTLV. Nature 1984; 311:515.
32. Copeland TD, Tsai WP, Oroszlan S. Antibody to a synthetic peptide detects a conserved region of retrovirus trans-membrane proteins. Biochem Biophys Res Commun 1985; 126:672–677.
33. Cianciolo GJ, Copeland TD, Oroszlan S, Snyderman R. Inhibition of lymphocyte

proliferation by a synthetic peptide homologous to retroviral envelope proteins. Science 1985; 230:453–455.

34. Allan JS, Coligan JE, Lee TH, et al. A new HTLV III/LAV encoded antigen detected by antibodies from AIDS patients. Science 1985; 230:810–813.

35. Wain-Hobson S, Alizon M, Montagnier L. Relationship of AIDS to other retroviruses. Nature 1985; 313:743.

36. Brahic M, Haase AT. Lentivirinae: maedi/visna virus group infections. Comparative aspects and diagnosis. Comp Diag Viral Dis 1981; 4 (part B):619–643.

37. Sigurdsson B, Palsson PA, Grimsson M. Visna, a demyelinating transmissible disease of sheep. J Neuropathol Exp Neurol 1957; 16:389–403.

38. Sonigo P, Alizon M, Staskus K, et al. Nucleotide sequence of the visna lentivirus: relationship to the AIDS virus. Cell 1985; 42:369–382.

39. Petursson F, Nathanson N, Georgsson G, Panitch H, Palsson P. Pathogenesis of visna. I. Sequential virologic, serologic, and pathologic studies. Lab Invest 1976; 35:402–412.

40. Clements JE, Narayan O, Griffin DE, Johnsson RT. Genomic changes associated with antigenic variation of visna virus during persistent infection. Proc Natl Acad Sci USA 1980; 77:4454–4458.

41. Scott JV, Stowring L, Haase AT, Narayan O, Vigne R. Antigenic variation in visna virus. Cell 1979; 18:321–327.

42. Rabson AB, Martin MA. Molecular organization of the AIDS retrovirus. Cell 1985; 40:477–480.

43. Lutley A, Petursson G, Palsson PA, Georgsson G, Klein J, Nathanson N. Antigenic drift in visna: virus variation during long term infection of Icelandic sheep. J Gen Virol 1983; 64:1433–1440.

44. Thormar H, Barshatsky MR, Arnesen K, Kozlowski PB. The emergence of antigenic variants is a rare event in long term visna virus infection in vivo. J Gen Virol 1983; 64:1427–1432.

45. Haase AT, Stowring L, Narayan O, Griffin D, Price D. Slow persistent infection caused by visna virus: role of host restriction. Science 1977; 195:175–177.

46. Geballe AP, Ventura P, Stowring L, Haase AT. Quantitative analysis of visna virus replication in vivo. Virology 1985; 141:148–154.

47. Brahic M, Stowring L, Ventura P, Haase AT. Gene expression in visna virus infection. Nature 1981; 292:240–242.

48. Stowring L, Haase AT, Petursson G. Detection of visna virus antigens and RNA in glial cells in foci of demyelination. Virology 1985; 141:311–318.

49. Narayan O, Kennedy-Sfoskopf S, Sheffer D, Griffin DE, Clements J. Activation of caprine arthritis-encephalitis virus expression during maturation of monocytes to macrophages. Infect Immunol 1983; 41:67–73.

50. Daniel MD, Letvin NK, King NW, et al. Isolation of T-cell tropic HTLV-III like retroviruses from macaques. Science 1985; 228:1201–1204.

51. Kanki PJ, Mc Lane MF, King NW. Serologic identification and characterization of a macaque T-lymphotropic retrovirus closely related to HTLV-III. Science 1985; 228:1199–1201.

52. Rozenbaum W, Dormont D, Spine B, et al. Antimoniotungstate (HPA23) treatment of three patients with AIDS and one with prodrome. Lancet 1985; i:450–451.

53. Mitsuya H, Popovic M, Yarchoan R, Matsushita S, Gallo RC, Broder S. Suramin protection of T cells in vitro against infectivity and cytopathic effect of HTLV-III. Science 1984; 226:172–174.
54. Sarin PS, Gallo RC, Scheer DI, et al. Effects of a novel compound (AL 721) on HTLV-III infectivity in vitro. N Engl J Med 1985; 313:1289–1290.
55. Nathanson N, Panitch H, Palsson PA, Petursson G, Georgsson G. Pathogenesis of visna. II. Effect of immunosuppression upon early central nervous system lesions. Lab Invest 1976; 35:444–451.
56. Crawford TB, Adams DS, Cheevers WP, Cork LC. Chronic arthritis in goats caused by a retrovirus. Science 1980; 207:997–999.
57. Nakajima H, Tanaka S, Ushime C. Physicochemical studies of equine infectious anemia virus. IV. Determination of nucleic acid type in the virus. Arch Ges Virusforsch 1970; 31:273–280.
58. Shinnick TM, Lerner RA, Sutcliffe JG. Nucleotide sequence of Moloney murine leukemia virus. Nature 1981; 293:543–548.
59. Schwartz DE, Tizard R, Gilbert W. Nucleotide sequence of Rous sarcoma virus. Cell 1983; 32:853–869.
60. Chiu IM, Callahan R, Tronick SR, Scholm J, Aaronson SA. Major pol gene progenitors in the evolution of oncornaviruses. Science 1984; 223:364–370.
61. Sagata N, Yasunaga T, Tsuzuku-Kawamura J, Ohishi K, Ogawa Y, Ikawa Y. Complete nucleotide sequence of the genome of bovine leukemia virus: its evolutionary relationship to other retroviruses. Proc Natl Acad Sci USA 1985; 82:677–681.
62. Wilhemsen KC, Eggleton K, Temin H. Nucleic acid sequences of the oncogen v-rel in reticuloendotheliosis virus strain T and its cellular homolog, the proto-oncogene c-rel. J Virol 1984; 52:172–182.
63. Majors JE, Varmus HE. Nucleotide sequencing of an apparent proviral copy of env mRNA defines determinants of expression of the mouse mammary tumor virus env gene. J Virol 1983; 47:495–504.

3

Molecular Biology of the HTLV Family

Flossie Wong-Staal
Laboratory of Tumor Cell Biology
National Cancer Institute
National Institutes of Health
Bethesda, Maryland

Introduction

The discovery of the human T-lymphotropic retroviruses has not only facilitated our understanding of the pathogenesis of the diseases associated with them and our efforts to control these diseases, it has also revolutionized our concepts of virus-cell interactions. HTLV-I and HTLV-II, both associated with leukemias, transform T cells in vitro via a mechanism distinct from those of any previously characterized transforming viruses. HTLV-III, the causative agent of AIDS, kills T4 cells via a mechanism we still do not fully understand. The unusual biological properties of these viruses can, in part, be explained by their complex genetic structures. In this chapter, I will attempt to summarize our current understanding of the structure and function of the HTLV genomes in relation to their transforming or cytopathic activities. Because of the clinical impact of HTLV-III and AIDS, there was also an urgency to apply our knowledge and reagents toward disease control, and some of these efforts in the realm of molecular biology will also be described here.

Genetic Structures of HTLV-I, HTLV-II, and HTLV-III

All nondefective retroviruses contain three structural genes coding for the core antigens (*gag*), the polymerase (*pol*), also called reverse transcriptase, and the envelope glycoprotein (*env*). These are bounded by the long terminal repeat (LTR) sequences, which house the regulatory elements for transcription and translation. Most retroviruses contain only these genes (see Fig. 1, MoMuLV as an example). A minority of retroviruses are the so-called acutely transforming viruses, which have acquired a cellular gene by recombination somewhere in their evolutionary past, and frequently in so doing, have lost, in exchange, part of their replicative genes and become defective (see Fig. 1, SSV as an example). All the HTLVs contain gene(s) in addition to *gag, pol,* and *env* that have no counterparts in normal chromosomal DNA. HTLV-I and HTLV-II contain an extra gene located between the *env* gene and 3'LTR (Fig. 1).[1,2] The protein product of this gene, which is highly conserved between the two viruses, has been shown to mediate transcriptional activation of the viral LTR and genes linked to it.[3-5] The target nucleotide sequences for the transactivation have been identified and found to overlap with the enhancer and promo-

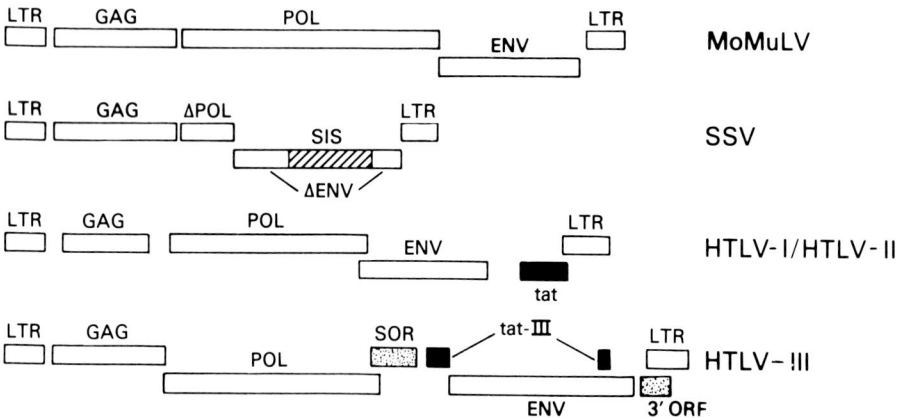

FIGURE 1   Genetic structures of retroviruses MoMuLV = Moloney murine leukemia virus; SSV = simian sarcoma virus; *gag* = group-specific core antigens; *pol* = DNA polymerase; *env* = envelope; LTR = long terminal repeat; *sis* = the oncogene of SSV; *tat* = transactivator; SOR = short open reading frame; 3'*orf* = 3' open reading frame.

tor sequences for transcription.[6] The presence of this gene, now named *tat*-I and *tat*-II for transactivator, is critical for virus replication.[7] HTLV-III also encodes a transactivator gene (*tat*-III) that is specific for its LTR.[8-11] However, the basis for this activation is still not clear. Since the target sequences for *tat*-III map to the start site of viral RNA,[12] it is possible that the enhanced gene expression can be explained at least in part at the level of mRNA stabilization and translational efficiency. In addition to *tat*-III, the nucleotide sequence of HTLV-III revealed two additional potential coding regions (*sor* and *3'orf*) (Fig. 1).[13-15] Although there is now evidence that these are real genes coding for proteins that are immunoreactive with patients' sera,[16-18] their functions are as yet unknown.

Putting Together the Genes for Transactivation

Although most cellular genes are transcribed from multiple coding regions (exons) that are discontiguous, mRNA of retroviruses are usually derived from one (unspliced) or at most two (single-spliced) exons. The *tat* genes of HTLV are unusual in that they are generated by two splicing events (Fig. 2). *Tat*-I and *tat*-II genes encode protein products of relative molecular mass of 42,000 (42kD) and 38kD, respectively.[19-21] A 2.0 kilobase (kb) *tat* mRNA is generated by bringing together three exons, using a donor splice site located in the LTR, an acceptor splice site upstream of the *env* gene, followed by a donor 190 nucleotides apart and a second acceptor splice site that marks the beginning of the major *tat* coding region.[22-24] The middle short exon contributes an initia-

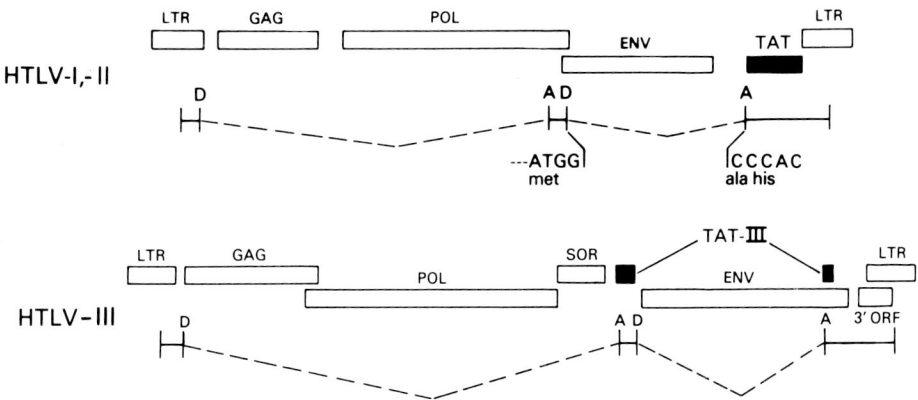

FIGURE 2   The double-splice processing of *tat* mRNA. D = donor splice site; A = acceptor splice site.

tor ATG codon, which is also the initiator codon for the *env* gene. The 42kD *tat*-I protein is immunoreactive against sera of some adult T-cell leukemia (ATL) patients and healthy carriers, and has been shown to be a nuclear protein.[5,25]

The *tat* gene of HTLV-III is also transcribed into a doubly spliced 2.0 kb mRNA.[8] The relatively small *tat* coding region of 86 amino acids is split between the second and third exons (Fig. 2), with the major and critical functional domain residing in the second exon. Within this domain is a stretch of highly basic residues (8/9 are lysine or arginine) that may be responsible for nucleic acid binding.[9-11]

Transcriptional Regulation of Cellular Genes by HTLV-I and HTLV-II: The Way to Immortality

HTLV-I, the causative agent of adult T-cell leukemia (ATL), is unique among leukemia viruses not containing oncogenes in that it can transform the same target cell in vitro and in vivo. Cells transformed in vitro by both HTLV-I and HTLV-II resemble ATL leukemic cells in their expression of specific T-cell markers (predominantly OKT4$^+$, TAC$^+$, Ia$^+$), morphology (formation of multinucleated syncytial cells), and growth properties (reviewed in Ref. 26). Although both the in vivo and in vitro transformed cells contain HTLV provirus and the infected cells are of clonal (ATL cells) or oligoclonal (in vitro transformed cells) origin, there is no conserved site of provirus integration, suggesting that viral transformation is via a *trans* mechanism. In other words, a diffusible viral product must be the effector of transformation. Discovery of extra coding sequences at the 3′ end (originally called x or lor, subsequently identified to encode the trans-activator protein *tat*) of HTLV-I and HTLV-II immediately called attention to this gene as the candidate transforming gene of these viruses. This speculation is strengthened by the fact that the presence and expression of this gene are the one constant element in all HTLV-transformed cells, including those that contained only defective proviruses and those not expressing some or all of the other viral proteins.[24] One proposal for the mechanism of transformation via *tat* was drawn from analogies with the transforming proteins of DNA tumor viruses, which are also frequently transcriptional activators. These proteins (e.g., *E1a* of adenovirus) regulate expression of both viral and cellular genes.[27] It is feasible that similarly the *tat* protein could regulate expression not only of viral genes, but also cellular genes involved in T-cell proliferation. This proposal would also provide a unifying mechanism for retrovirus leukemogenesis, that is, activation of a growth-promoting gene (e.g., an oncogene or proto-oncogene in the case of the acute leukemia and chronic leukemia virus, respectively) (Fig. 3).

Acute
Leukemia
Viruses

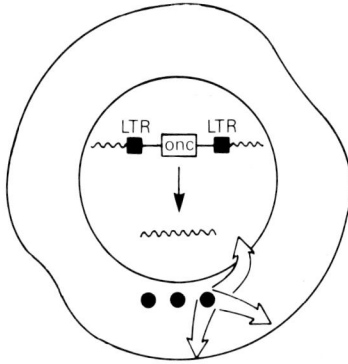

*trans*acting
oncogene
protein

random integration

Chronic
Leukemia
Viruses

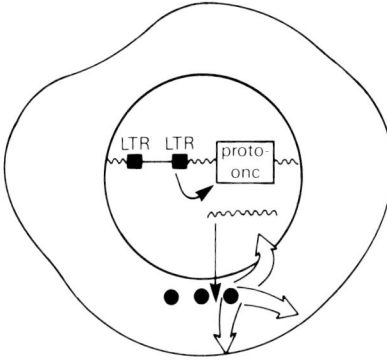

cis activation
of cellular
(proto-onc) genes

conserved site(s)
of integration

HTLV/STLV/BLV

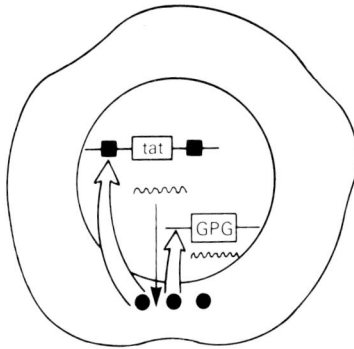

*trans*acting
transcriptional
regulation

random integration

FIGURE 3 Mechanisms of leukemogenesis. Acute leukemia viruses have captured cell-derived genes (*onc* genes), which encode transformation-specific proteins. Some of these proteins are growth-promoting proteins, and may be localized to the membrane (e.g., growth factor receptors), cytoplasm (e.g., growth factors), or nucleus (e.g., DNA-binding proteins). These possible sites of action are shown by arrows. Because these viral proteins are *trans*acting, no conserved site of provirus integration is necessary. Chronic leukemia viruses activate cellular genes by proximal integration of the provirus. The activated cellular genes may be proto-*onc* genes. The mechanism of *cis* activation requires conserved site(s) of integration. The HTLV/STLV/BLV family of viruses makes a nuclear protein (*tat*), which activates transcription in *trans*. Therefore, a conserved integration site for the provirus is not necessary.

One of the hallmarks of HTLV-I and HTLV-II–transformed cells as well as the ATL cells is the constitutive expression of high levels of the receptor for interleukin-2 (IL-2R).[28,29] Recent work from W. Greene's laboratory suggests that tat-II directly activates the expression of IL-2R in certain T cells (W. Greene, personal communication), and this may well be the initiating event for transformation.

Several observations suggest that a complex sequence of events must take place before frank leukemic conversion by HTLV-I. First, although HTLV-I immortalizes and "transforms" T-lymphocytes efficiently in vitro, development of ATL requires a long latency period. Second, ATL cells usually contain clonal karyotypic abnormalities. Third, most fresh ATL cells do not express any viral mRNA, including that for tat-I,[30] suggesting that virus infection has set in motion a chain of events such that its continued expression is not

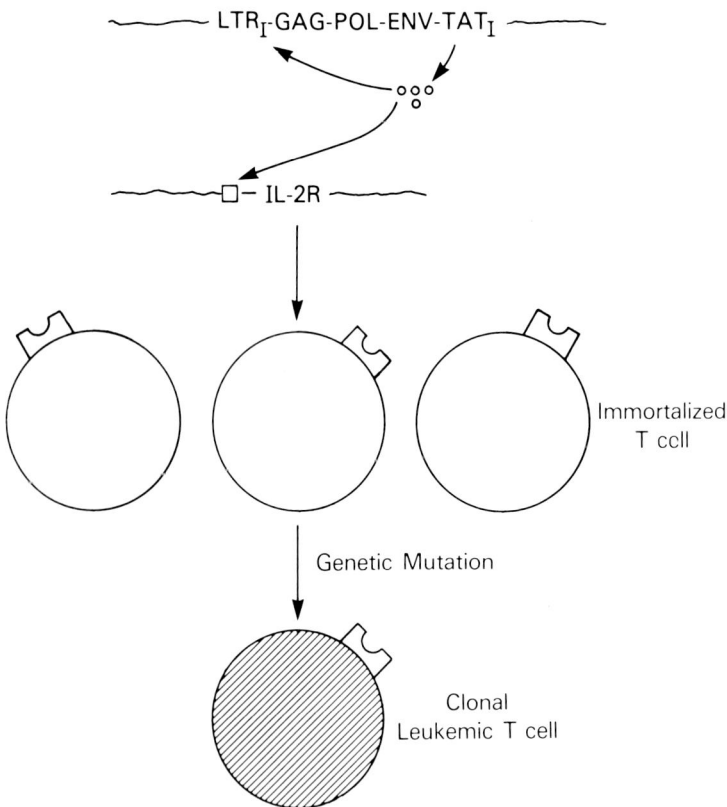

FIGURE 4   Two-stage leukemogenesis by HTLV-I. See text for details.

necessary to maintain the leukemic state. We speculate that expression of *tat*-I early after infection activates the IL-2 receptor and possibly other growth-promoting genes specific for T cells. Consequently, the cells are immortalized and continuously proliferating. This in turn increases the chance of mutations or gene rearrangements. A pivotal event for leukemogenesis may require the appropriate gene rearrangements. Once that occurs, continued function of *tat*-I is no longer necessary (Fig. 4).

HTLV-III and Cytopathicity: Viral and Cellular Factors

HTLV-III infects and kills the T4 cell in vivo and in vitro. As a first step to dissect the genetic determinants of the cytopathic activity of HTLV-III, we have obtained a cloned virus genome that directs the synthesis of infectious and cytopathic virions.[31] Normal cord-blood T cells transfected with this clone contained viral DNA and expressed p15 and p24, extracellular reverse transcriptase, and complete virions with the characteristic cylindrical cores as detected by electron microscopy. The percentage of virus-infected cells increased steadily up to 18 days post-transfection, suggesting that infectious virus was being produced. However, after 20 days, there was a dramatic decrease in cell viability, rapidly leading to depletion of the infected cells. At 30 days, the culture consisted only of uninfected cells. Furthermore, while more than half the cells were OKT4+ at day 0, more than 90% of cells were of the OKT8 phenotype at day 30, indicating selective killing of the OKT4+ cells (A. Fisher et al., unpublished observations). Therefore, the HTLV-III genome alone contains all the essential information for inducing the primary defect in AIDS (i.e., depletion of the T4+-helper cells). It is now possible to systematically manipulate this genome to localize the genes responsible for the cytopathic activity of the virus.

There is also evidence for cellular determinants for the cytopathic response. We have superinfected HTLV-I-transformed cell clones with HTLV-III.[32] Although most of these cell clones were OKT4+, one cell clone expressed the OKT8 phenotype. HTLV-III replicates efficiently in all these cell clones. However, the OKT4+ cells were susceptible to the cytopathic effect, but the OKT8+ cell clone was completely resistant. This was not due to an adaptation of the virus since virus produced by the T8 line retained its tropism and cytopathic activity for T4 cells. This result indicates that virus replication alone is not sufficient for cytopathicity. The mechanism by which HTLV-III exerts its cytopathic effect is still unclear. At least two hypotheses can be envisioned. One is that the *tat*-III gene may facilitate expression of cellular genes that lead to terminal differentiation. If so, such genes would have to be specific for the T4 lineage. Alternatively, a viral gene product may directly function in the cell-killing. This then would also be highly specific for the T4 target cell. Cells that are infectable by HTLV-III, but not killed by it, can potentially serve as reservoirs for virus replication.

Development of Immunodiagnostic Reagents for AIDS by Recombinant DNA Technology

Once the etiological agent of AIDS has been identified, there is an urgent need to develop a blood bank assay to remove the hazards of blood transfusion. Although such assays with whole disrupted virus are available, increased sensitivity, economy, and safety in implementation of these assays can be achieved through recombinant DNA technology. Now all six genes of HTLV-III have been expressed in bacteria, and peptides derived from these regions have been tested for their immunoreactivity against patients' sera.[16-18,33-35] The results showed that all peptides were recognized by some but not all infected individuals, and there was no apparent correlation between seropositivity against specific proteins and the clinical status of the sera donors. One exception may be reactivity against the major *gag* protein (p24), which was much higher among healthy carriers than among patients with ARC and AIDS as defined by the Centers for Disease Control.[36] The most immunogenic antigen appeared to be the transmembrane envelope protein (gp41), which detected close to 100% of infected individuals in all disease categories. A bacterially expressed peptide derived from the gp41-coding region has been purified and adapted to a solid phase immunoassay system.[34] The sensitivity of this assay far surpassed that using whole disrupted virus, and has not yielded any false-positives after screening over 500 normal samples. General application of this or analogous assays should be available soon as second generation tests.

Genetic Polymorphism of HTLV-III and the Prospects for a Vaccine

Genomic variation of different HTLV-III isolates was first recognized by restriction endonuclease analysis of a few proviruses.[37] As more and more isolates were subjected to restriction enzymes, heteroduplex mapping, and nucleotide sequence analyses, the picture that emerged was one of a family of related but distinct viruses evolving through time. (Ref. 38 and unpublished data.) A significant observation from the analyses of genomic diversity is that the greatest divergence is localized to the extracellular envelope protein (gp120).[39,40] Since this is expected to be the most antigenic viral protein and the one to contain the epitopes for eliciting neutralizing antibodies in the infected individuals, this finding raises concern for the feasibility of developing a broadly cross-reactive vaccine for AIDS. Further justification for this concern lies in the finding of increasing parallels between HTLV-III and the ungulate lentiviruses (visna, equine infectious anemia virus, or EIAV, for examples).[41] (See the chapter by Gallo and Streicher in this book.) Both visna and EIAV are known to undergo changes in their envelope proteins, and this "chameleon" may be one of the strategies that these viruses utilize to escape immunosurveillance of the host.[42,43] To further scrutinize this issue, we have examined the amino acid sequence of the envelope of several divergent HTLV-III isolates, using a computer program that predicts the secondary structure of proteins superimposed with values for hydrophilicity.[44] Similar analysis of other proteins, including viral envelopes, has shown that continuous antigenic epitopes are often associated with hydrophilic domains containing β-turns. Continuous epitopes are defined as those peptides whose antigenicity is reflected in the secondary structure of the primary amino acid sequence, whereas discontinuous epitopes are antigenic loci formed by the tertiary folds of the native protein. Such analysis showed that among the exterior envelope proteins of the four retroviruses (HTLV-III RF, HTLV-III BH10, LAV, and ARV), each contains sites that are likely to be antigenic based on the previously mentioned criteria. Most of these coincide with hypervariable regions that exhibit differences in hydrophilicity, secondary structure, and potential glycosylation patterns. Because of this variability, it is likely that the antigenicity of the corresponding envelope proteins of these viruses could differ considerably. This finding also suggests that these changes result at least in part from selective pressures present in vivo and that they are biologically meaningful.

Interspersed with the variable regions of the exterior envelope protein were highly conserved areas. One of these corresponded to a stretch of 45 amino acid residues immediately adjacent to the processing site of the envelope precursor, was hydrophilic, and contained numerous β-turns. Therefore, this region of the exterior envelope glycoprotein would be expected to be both immunogenic and cross-reactive among isolates. Other conserved antigenic epitopes (e.g., the discontinuous epitopes) not predicted by this analysis may also be present in the native protein. All these conserved epitopes may possess important biological functions (e.g., for interaction with the cellular receptor) and, furthermore, serve as targets for recombinant DNA-based vaccines.

Summary and Perspectives

The human lymphotropic retroviruses HTLV-I, HTLV-II, and HTLV-III are the prototypes of a new category of retroviruses linked together not only by their common target cell tropism, but also by a novel regulatory mechanism for virus expression, which is dependent on transactivation by a viral protein (*tat*). Specific interaction between the *tat* protein and *tat* responsive sequences in the LTR of these viruses leads to two or three logs increase in gene expression. The implications of this finding are manifold. First, identification of a protein that is critical for viral expression provides yet another handle to limit replication of these viruses. This is particularly pertinent in the case of HTLV-III, in which continual virus synthesis and recruitment of newly infected cells appear to be important for pathogenesis. Second, this very efficient gene expression system can be utilized for overproduction of any protein desired. This should have wide applications in the field of biotechnology. Third, there is evidence that the *tat* genes of HTLV-I and HTLV-II are the critical transforming genes of these viruses and that they may directly activate expression of cellular genes involved in T-cell proliferation. The fact that cellular genes can respond to the *tat* proteins would also imply that the strategy of transactivation may be used by the cell to turn on genes at specific stages of differentiation and/or development.

HTLV-III offers a challenge all its own. Two of its genes are still looking for a function. For a virus with all the ingredients for efficient replication, it is unusually elusive—with only a minor fraction of T4 cells infected in any given lymphoid tissue, and a further subset of the infected cells actually expressing virus. Virus expression is held in check until the infected cell is triggered by a series of events linked to immune activation, and the basis of this latency is not at all understood. It is possible that one of the HTLV-III-specific genes is involved in a negative regulatory mechanism. The greatest challenge that HTLV-III offers, of course, is a clinical one. The urgency exists not only to understand every intricacy of its gene structure and function, but also to contain virus infection and spread of disease. In this regard, molecular biological approaches have facilitated development of second generation diagnostic reagents, which are projected to be much more sensitive and economical than currently available tests. Development of a vaccine is also being pursued by many research groups. Our studies on the genomic diversity of the HTLV-III genome indicate that although the major envelope glycoprotein is highly variable overall, there are conserved regions that may contribute antigenic sites which are group-specific. These analyses will be valuable guides for devising recombinant DNA-based vaccines.

Acknowledgments

I am grateful to Dr. R. C. Gallo for his collaboration and support in many of these studies, all my colleagues at the Laboratory of Tumor Cell Biology for their contributions, and, in particular, Drs. A. Fisher, G. Franchini, B. Hahn, G. Shaw, L. Ratner, A. Aldovini, B. Starchich, and S. Josephs. I also thank Ms. Dee Goodrich for editorial assistance.

References

1. Seiki M, Hattori T, Hirayama Y, Yoshida M. Human adult T-cell leukemia virus: complete nucleotide sequence of the provirus genome integrated in leukemia cell DNA. Proc Natl Acad Sci USA 1983; 80:3618–3622.
2. Shaw G, Gonda M, Flickinger G, Hahn BH, Gallo RC, Wong-Staal F. Genomes of evolutionarily divergent members of the human T-cell leukemia virus family (HTLV-I and HTLV-II) are highly conserved, especially in pX. Proc Natl Acad Sci USA 1984; 81:4544–4548.
3. Haseltine WA, Sodroski J, Patarca R, Briggs D, Perkins D, Wong-Staal F. Structure of 3′ terminal region of type II human T lymphotropic virus: evidence for new coding region. Science 1984; 225:419–421.
4. Sodroski JG, Rosen CA, Haseltine WA. Transacting transcriptional activation of the long terminal repeat of human T-lymphotropic viruses in infected cells. Science 1984; 225:381–383.
5. Felber BK, Paskalis H, Kleinman-Ewing C, Wong-Staal F, Pavlakis GN. The pX protein of human T-cell leukemia virus-I is a transcriptional activity of its long terminal repeats. Science 1985; 229:675–679.
6. Rosen CA, Sodroski JG, Haseltine WA. Location of cis-acting regulatory sequences in the human T-cell leukemia virus Type I long terminal repeat. Proc Natl Acad Sci USA 1985; 82:6502–6506.
7. Chen ISY, Slamon DJ, Rosenblatt JD, Shah NP, Ouan S, Wachman W. The x gene is essential for HTLV replication. Science 1985; 229:54–57.
8. Sodroski J, Rosen C, Wong-Staal F, Salahuddin SZ, Popovic M, Arya SK, Gallo RC, Haseltine WA. Trans-acting transcriptional regulation of human T-cell leukemia virus type III long terminal repeat. Science 1985; 227:171–173.
9. Arya SK, Chan G, Josephs SF, Wong-Staal F. Transactivator gene of human T-cell leukemia (lymphotropic) virus type II (HTLV-III). Science 1985; 229:69–73.
10. Sodroski J, Patarca R, Rosen C, Wong-Staal F, Haseltine WA. Location of the trans-activating region of the genome of HTLV-III/LAV. Science 1985; 229:74–77.
11. Seigel LJ, Ratner L, Josephs SF, Derse D, Feinberg MB, Reyes BR, O'Brien SJ, Wong-Staal F. Transactivation induced by human T-lymphotropic virus Type III (HTLV-III) maps to a viral sequence encoding 58 amino acids and lacks tissue specificity. Virology 1986; 148:226–231.
12. Rosen CA, Sodroski JG, Haseltine WA. The location of cis-acting regulatory sequences in the human T-cell lymphotropic virus type III (HTLV-III/LAV) long terminal repeat. Cell 1985; 41:813–823.
13. Ratner L, Haseltine W, Patarca R, Livak K, Starcich B, Josephs S, Doran ER, Rafalski JA, Whitehorn EA, Baumeister K, Ivanoff L, Petteway SR Jr, Pearson ML, Lauten-

berger JA, Papas TS, Ghrayeb J, Chang NT, Gallo RC, Wong-Staal F. Complete nucleotide sequence of the AIDS virus, HTLV-III. Nature 1985; 313:277–284.

14. Sanchez-Pescador R, Power MD, Barr PJ, Steinmer KS, Stempien MM, Brown-Shimer SL, Gee WW, Renard A, Randolph A, Levy JA, Dina D, Luciw PA. Nucleotide sequence and expression of an AIDS-associated retrovirus (ARV-2). Science 1985; 227:484–492.

15. Wain-Hobson S, Sonigo P, Danos O, Cole S, Alizon M. Nucleotide sequence of the AIDS virus. LAV. Cell 1985; 40:9–17.

16. Kan NC, Franchini G, Wong-Staal F, DuBois GC, Robey WG, Lautenberger JA, Papas TS. A novel protein (sor) of HTLV-III expressed in bacteria is immunoreactive with sera from infected individuals. Science 1986; 231:1553–1554.

17. Arya SK, Gallo RC. Three novel genes of human T-lymphotropic retrovirus-III (HTLV-III): immune reactivity of their products with sera from acquired immune deficiency syndrome patients. Proc Natl Acad Sci 1986; 83:2209–2213.

18. Franchini G, Robert-Guroff M, Wong-Staal F, Ghrayeb J, Kato N, Chang N. Expression of the 3′ open reading frame of the HTLV-III in bacteria: demonstration of its immunoreactivity with human sera. Proc Natl Acad Sci USA (in press).

19. Lee TH, Coligan JE, Sodroski JG, Haseltine WA, Salahuddin SZ, Wong-Staal F, Gallo RC, Essex M. Antigens encoded by 3′-terminal region of human T-cell leukemia virus: evidence for a functional gene. Science 1984; 226:57–61.

20. Kigokawa T, Seike M, Imagawa R, Shimigu F, Yoshida M. Identification of a protein (p40ˣ) encoded by a unique sequence pX of human T-cell leukemia virus type I. Gann 1984; 75:747–751.

21. Slamon DJ, Shimotohao K, Cline MJ, Golde DW, Chen ISY. Identification of the putative transforming protein of the human T-cell leukemia viruses HTLV-I and II. Science 1984; 226:61–64.

22. Seiki M, Hikikoshi A, Taniguchi T, Yoshida M. Expression of the pX gene of HTLV-I general splicing mechanism in the HTLV family. Science 1985; 228:1532–1534.

23. Okamoto T, Josephs SF, Kawanishi M, Wong-Staal F. Determination of a splice acceptor site of pX gene in HTLV-I infected cells. Virology 1985; 143:636–639.

24. Aldovini A, DeRossi A, Feinberg M, Wong-Staal F, Franchini G. Molecular analysis from HTLV-I deleting mutant provirus: evidence for a double spliced x-lor mRNA. Proc Natl Acad Sci USA (in press).

25. Goh WC, et al. Subcellular localization of the product of the long open reading frame of human T-cell leukemia virus type I. Science 1985; 227:1227–1228.

26. Wong-Staal F, Gallo RC. Human T-lymphotropic retroviruses. Nature 1985; 317:395–403.

27. Nevins JR. Induction of the synthesis of a 70,000 dalton mammalian heatshock protein by the adenovirus EIA gene product. Cell 1982; 29:913–923.

28. Poiesz BJ, Ruscetti FW, Mier JW, Woods AM, Gallo RC. T-cell lines established from human T-lymphocytic neoplasias by direct response to T-cell growth factor. Proc Natl Acad Sci USA 1980; 77:6815–6819.

29. Waldmann T, Broder S, Greene W, Sarin PS, Saxinger C, Blayney DW, Blattner WA, Goldman C, Frost K, Sharrow S, Depper J, Leonard W, Michiyama T, Gallo

RC. A comparison of the function and phenotype of Sezary T-cells with human T-cell leukemia/lymphoma virus (HTLV)-associated adult T-cell leukemia. Clin Res 1983; 31:5474–5475.

30. Franchini G, Wong-Staal F, Gallo RC. Human T-cell leukemia virus (HTLV-I) transcripts in fresh and cultured cells of patients with adult T-cell leukemia. Proc Natl Acad Sci USA 1984; 81:6207–6211.

31. Fisher AM, Collalti E, Ratner L, Gallo RC, Wong-Staal F. A molecular clone of HTLV-III with biological activity. Nature 1985; 316:262–265.

32. De Rossi A, Franchini G, Aldovini A, Del Mistro A, Chieco-Bianchi L, Gallo RC, Wong-Staal F. Differential response to the cytophatic effects of HTLV-III superinfection in IKT4 and OKT8 cell clones transformed by HTLV-I. Proc Natl Acad Sci USA (in press).

33. Chang NT, Chandra PK, Barne AD, McKinney S, Rhodes DP, Tam SH, Shearman C, Huang J, Chang TW, Gallo RC, Wong-Staal F. Expression of E. coli of open reading frame gene segments of type III human T-cell lymphotropic virus. Science 1985; 228:93–96.

34. Chang TW, Kato I, McKinney S, Chanda P, Barone AD, Wong-Staal F, Gallo RC, Chang NT. Detection of human T-cell lymphotropic virus (HTLV-II) infection with a sensitive and specific immunoassay employing a recombinant E. coli derived viral antigenic peptide. Biotech 1985; 3:905–909.

35. Crowl R, Ganguly K, Gordon K, Conroy R, Schaber M, Kramer R, Shaw G, Wong-Staal F, Reddy EP. HTLV-III env gene products synthesized E. coli are recognized by antibodies present in the sera of AIDS patients. Cell 1985; 41:979–986.

36. Franchini G, Robert-Guroff M, Aldovini A, Kan N, DeBouck C, Wong-Staal F. Spectrum of natural antibodies against five HTLV-III antigens in infected individuals: correlation of immunoresponse with clinical status. Blood (submitted).

37. Shaw GM, Hahn BH, Arya SK, Groopman JE, Gallo RC, Wong-Staal F. Molecular characterization of human T-cell leukemia (lymphoma) virus type III in the acquired immune deficiency syndrome. Science 1984; 226:1165–1170.

38. Wong-Staal F, Shaw GM, Hahn BH, Salahuddin SZ, Popovic M, Markham PD, Redfield R, Gallo RC. Genomic diversity of human T-lymphotropic virus type III (HTLV-III). Science 1985; 229:759–762.

39. Ratner L, Gallo RC, Wong-Staal F. HTLV-III, LAV and ARV are variants of the same AIDS virus. Nature 1985; 313:636–637.

40. Hahn BH, Gonda MA, Shaw GM, Popovic M, Hoxie J, Gallo RC, Wong-Staal F. Genomic diversity of the AIDS virus HTLV-III: different viruses exhibit greatest divergence in their envelope genes. Proc Natl Acad Sci USA 1985; 82:4813–4817.

41. Gonda MA, Wong-Staal F, Gallo RC, Clements JE, Narayan O, Gilden RV. Sequence homology and morphologic similarities of HTLV-III and visna virus, a pathogenic lentivirus. Science 1985; 227:173.

42. Clements JE, Pedersen FS, Narayan O, Haseltine WA. Genomic changes associated with antigenic variation of visna virus during persistent infection. Proc. Natl Acad Sci USA 1980; 77:4454–4458.

43. Montelaro RC, Parekh B, Orrego A, Issel CJ. Antigenic variation during persistent

infection by equine infections anemia virus, a retrovirus. J Biol Chem 1984;
259:10539–10544.

44. Starcich B, Hahn B, Shaw GM, Modrow S, Josephs SF, Wolf H, Gallo RC, Wong-
Staal F. Identification and characterization of conserved and divergent regions in
the envelope gene of AIDS viruses. Cell (in press).

4

Progress and Puzzles: Molecular Biology of HTLV-III

William A. Haseltine
Dana-Farber Cancer Institute
Harvard Medical School
and Harvard School of Public Health
Boston, Massachusetts

Joseph G. Sodroski
Craig A. Rosen
Dana-Farber Cancer Institute
and Harvard Medical School
Boston, Massachusetts

The human T-lymphotropic virus type III (HTLV-III/LAV) is the etiological agent of a complex disease that includes destruction of the immune system (AIDS)[1-4] and degeneration of the central and peripheral nervous systems.[5] Infection by HTLV-III also results in a high incidence of a number of neoplasias.[6,7] A long latent period between the time of infection and the appearance of severe symptoms is typical.[8,9] The fraction of people infected who become symptomatic is not known with precision, but is likely to be greater than 30 to 50% over a prolonged period.[8,51]

The complex disease manifestations as well as the variable latent period raise important questions about the biology of the causative agent HTLV-III.

- How does the virus infection lead to the loss of immune function?
- How does infection lead to central and peripheral nervous system damage?

53

- What accounts for the long and variable latent period?
- How is the virus transmitted, and are all infected persons active or potential carriers of infection?
- In short, how can the transmission and pathogenesis of the disease be understood in terms of what we know about the virus?

The task of explaining pathogenesis based on virology is a formidable one, not only because this disease is itself complex, but because the virus that is responsible for the disease represents a new type of infectious agent. Although similar in many respects to retroviruses that have been previously studied, the full complexity of the HTLV-III virus is now only beginning to be appreciated. It appears as if there are no convenient analogies that can be drawn between the life cycle of other and more thoroughly studied animal retroviruses (which provide convenient points of reference) and that of HTLV-III.

What follows is a brief description of the molecular biology of HTLV-III. The progress that has been made as well as the puzzles that remain will be summarized.

gag, pol and *env* Genes: Analogy Prevails

The virus HTLV-III is a retrovirus.[1-4] As such, it shows features common to all well-studied members of this family of viruses. The basic features of the virus that are common to all retroviruses have been identified. The complete nucleotide sequence of several strains of the virus has been determined.[10-13] The size of the major virion capsid and envelope proteins has been analyzed, and the progress toward definition of the nonstructural genes required for replication, the protease, the reverse transcriptase, and the integrase has also proceeded smoothly.[4,14-19] The major classes of messenger RNAs that encode the individual proteins have also been defined.[13,20] This information is summarized in several figures. Figure 1 gives the life cycle of the retrovirus. Figure 2 presents a schematic diagram of a genome of HTLV-III, depicting the mRNAs and major proteins synthesized. Figure 3 presents a schematic diagram of HTLV-III-encoded proteins.

In large measure, this information tells us that the *gag, pol,* and *env* genes resemble, in overall structure and function, similar genes of other retroviruses. Some notable points of difference from other well-studied retroviruses, such as the Moloney murine leukemia virus and the avian leukosis virus, include:

1. The *gag* gene contains a somewhat different capsid structure from the other retroviruses. There is no protein interposed between the amino

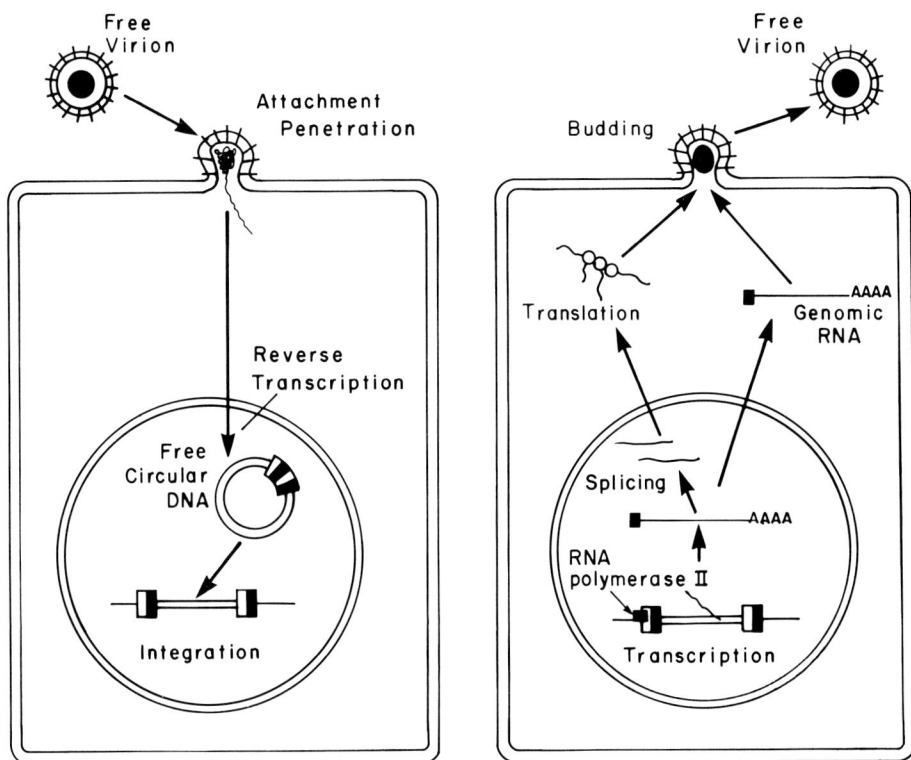

FIGURE 1 The life cycle of a retrovirus.

terminus and major capsid proteins for the HTLV-III virus as there is for most of the other retroviruses.[10-13]

2. Two small proteins rather than one small protein are derived from the carboxy terminal end of the *gag* gene precursor.[10-13]

3. A long overlap exists between the reading frames of the *gag* and *pol* gene, in contrast to the shorter overlap in this region for most of the other retroviruses.[10-13] The *gag* gene precursor is found to be associated with the nucleus or the perinuclear space for HTLV-III, in contrast to most other retroviruses (W.C. Goh et al., unpublished observations).

4. In the *pol* gene, the reverse transcriptase enzyme is shorter than that of most retroviruses. It appears to be comprised of two subunits, 66kD and 51kD.[10-13]

5. The reverse transcriptase enzyme exhibits a preference for the divalent magnesium rather than manganese.[2]

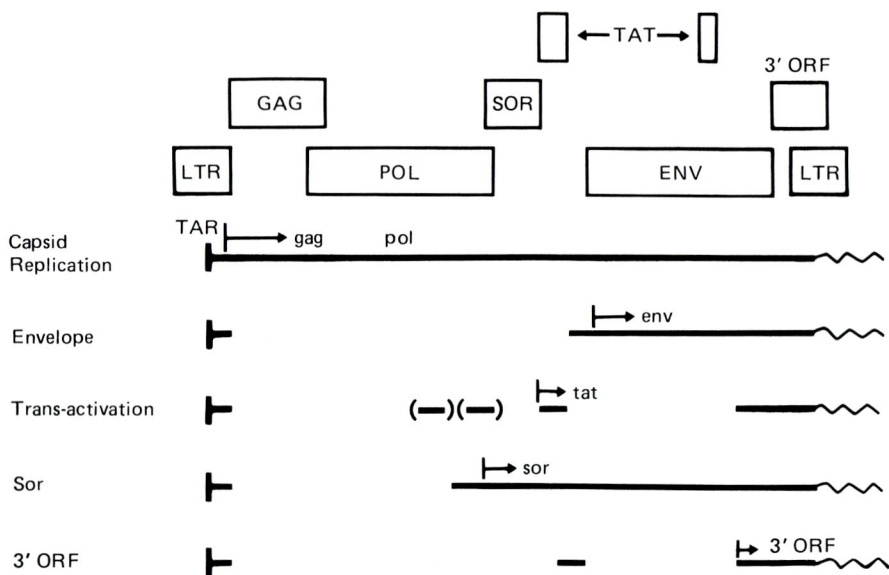

FIGURE 2   The genome of HTLV-III, with a depiction of mRNAs and major proteins.

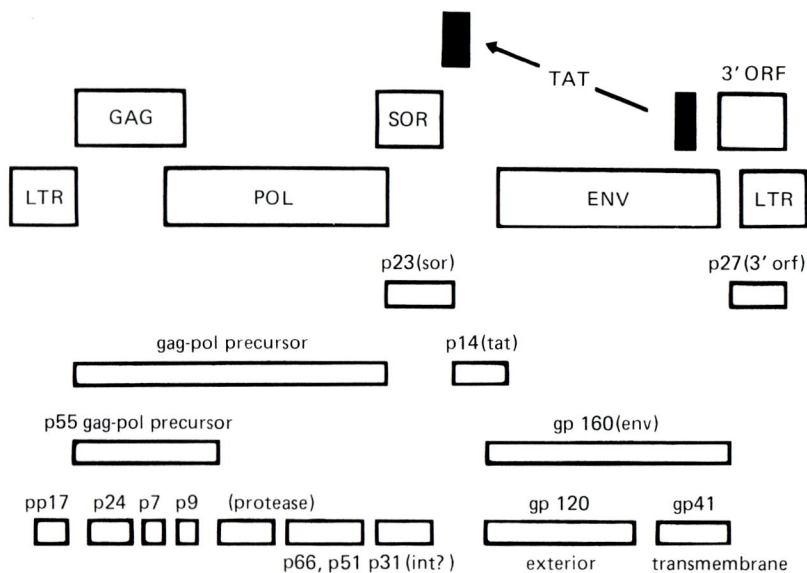

FIGURE 3   HTLV-III-encoded proteins.

env Genes

The external portion of the envelope glycoprotein of the HTLV-III envelope gene is extensively glycosylated.[14,18,19] Almost 50% of the weight of this protein is accounted for by sugar residues.

Strain-dependent hypervariability exists in the sequence of certain regions of the exterior glycoprotein of the HTLV-III envelope gene.[21] The transmembrane protein of the HTLV-III envelope gene is unusually long, almost twice the length of the transmembrane proteins of other retroviruses.[10-13,17] The majority of the additional molecular weight is derived from what is presumed to be the cytoplasmic face of the transmembrane protein.[10-13,17]

How Might These Features Account for Some of the Unusual Features of the Virus Life Cycle and Disease?

A mature virion capsid structure of HTLV-III is highly condensed and cylindrical in shape.[2] This is a different structure from that usually seen for retroviruses. This feature is most likely the consequence of assembly of the capsid components. The unusual structure of the individual proteins undoubtedly contributes to the unusual capsid structure. It is unknown whether this peculiar capsid structure, abnormally rich in reverse transcriptase and integrase, is relatively more resistant to inactivation. If so, this structure may play an important role in transmission of the disease.

An unusual feature of infection by HTLV-III is a high number of unintegrated provirus DNA copies.[22-23] To what extent the activity of the integrase determines the ratio of unintegrated to integrated proviral forms is unknown.

It is known that the integrase functions in HTLV-III infections. As expected, integrated proviral forms can be observed upon infection of some cell lines with HTLV-III.

It is very likely that the envelope gene plays a major role in the tissue tropism and possibly cytopathic effects of the virus.

There is a marked, but apparently not absolute, requirement for a subset of T4+ epitopes for infection by HTLV-III or even by HTLV-III envelope VSV pseudotypes.[24-25] A physical association of the HTLV-III envelope gene product with the T4+ molecule has been reported.[26] Selective infection and consequent destruction of T4+ cells may be in large measure a consequence of the specificity of the envelope gene. Additionally, it is likely that syncytia formation and possibly cell death are the result of high levels of expression of the *env* gene-determinants on the cell surface.

Recent reports indicate that both monocytes and macrophages can be infected by HTLV-III (M. Popovic, personal communication; R. Rose, personal communication). Infection of such cells would provide an explanation of how the virus enters the central nervous system. It may also explain how infection occurs in body cavities such as the oral pharynx or vagina. The nature of the receptors for HTLV-III on the surface of monocytes and macrophages is still a puzzle, but may also depend on surface expression of T4-related epitopes (Wigzell, personal communication).

Molecular mechanisms of cell death, possibly involving cell lysis via syncytial formation, remain a puzzle.

The structure of the *env* gene may also explain several of the unusual antigenic reactivities observed for this molecule. Typically, the titer of antibodies that bind to the envelope gene is very high in the sera of infected persons. However, the titer of neutralizing antibodies is usually either undetectable or very low.[27] In fact, human sera do not, in general, neutralize HTLV-III envelope VSV pseudotypes, despite the fact that such pseudotypes display T4$^+$-dependence for infection (R. Weiss, personal communication).[24]

In this respect, the HTLV-III virus resembles the caprine arthritis and encephalitis virus (CAEV), for which high ratios of binding to neutralizing antibodies are found, rather than the visna or equine infectious anemia retroviruses, for which good neutralizing titers are detected in infected animals.[29-33] The exterior glycoproteins of both the HTLV-III and CAEV are both highly glycosylated, whereas the envelope glycoproteins of visna and equine encephalitis virus are only moderately glycosylated.[10-13,15,18,32-36] It is possible that the highly glycosylated protein serves as an antigenic screen for critical epitopes involved in neutralizing activity.

The extent to which hypervariability of the envelope gene is an important pathogenic determinant remains a puzzle. Questions include:

- To what extent does variability of the envelope gene reflect changes in neutralizing phenotype?
- Do *env* gene variants differ in tissue tropism? For example, are some HTLV-III variants better able to infect the CNS (central nervous system) than are others?
- Do different variants of the *env* gene differ with respect to cytopathic effect?
- Does variation of the *env* gene play a role in chronic aspects of HTLV-III infection? For example, does the prolonged course of HTLV-III-induced disease reflect successive waves of growth of antigenic variants, as appears to be the case for infections with the equine infectious anemia virus.[33]

sor, tat, and 3'*orf* Genes: Analogy Fails

Although the genome of HTLV-III is not much longer than that of most other retroviruses, it encodes at least three genes not described heretofore. These include the *sor* gene located 3' to the *pol* gene, the *tat* gene comprised of two coding exons, and the 3'*orf* gene.[10-13,38-41] All three open reading frames produce proteins, the 23kD *sor* gene product, the 14kD *tat* gene product, and the 27kD 3'*orf* gene product.[38-41] These proteins are made at least in the course of some infections because antibodies to these proteins can be detected in some patient sera.[38-41]

Indications that these three proteins play an important role in the HTLV-III life cycle are that they are present in all the variant strains sequenced to date, and that similar polypeptides are made by the STLV-III viruses as judged by antigenic cross-reactivity.[10-13,42,43]

What Role Might These Proteins Play in the Virus Life Cycle?

The effects of deletions on the ability of mutant HTLV-III virus to grow and to kill T4$^+$ cells provide some insight regarding their function. Viruses deleted for the *sor* and 3'*orf* genes replicate in and kill T4$^+$-lymphocytes.[39,44] On the contrary, viruses deleted for the amino terminal domain of the *tat* gene are replication-deficient.[45] The defect in *tat*-deleted viruses can be complemented in cells that are designed to express constitutively the *tat* gene product.[45]

Analysis of the defect in replication of *tat*-deleted viruses reveals that viral RNA but not viral protein accumulates.[46] Evidently, the *tat* gene product is required for efficient utilization of *gag* and *env* messenger RNAs.

A separate series of experiments revealed that a sequence located between nucleotides +1 and +80 of the viral messenger RNA is required for response to the transactivator (*tat*) product.[46,47] Efficiency of translation of heterologous mRNA such as dihydrofolate reductase is greatly increased (greater than 500-fold) in transient assays by tagging of the heterologous messenger RNA at the 5' end with the HTLV-III +1 to +80 sequences.[46,47] It is a curiosity that whereas heterologous mRNAs that contain the HTLV-III +1 to +80 5' sequences demonstrate a low but detectable level of activity in the absence of the *tat* product, no capsid or envelope proteins can be detected in the absence of the *tat*-III gene product.[45,46]

What Role Might These Genes Play in HTLV-III-Induced Pathogenesis?

The *tat*-III gene is clearly needed for virus expression.[45] Virion production cannot occur in the absence of the *tat* product, even if the corresponding mRNAs are present.[45,46] The *tat* gene may play an important role in maintenance of the latent state. Inhibition of *tat* gene activity by cellular and/or viral mechanisms would interfere with productive infection. A cellular latent state of virus infection could explain some of the disease manifestations. Prolonged asymptomatic infection might reflect virus latency at the cellular level. Intermittent activation of virus replication by external stimuli could trigger a progressive degenerative disease. In this regard, work in several laboratories including those of Zagury and Gallo, Hoxie, and Fauci indicates that the HTLV-III virus can latently infect T4+ cells.[48-50] Antigenic stimulation of T4+ cells may be a signal that releases the HTLV-III virus from latency.[50] At present, one can only speculate regarding the role of the *tat* product in this process. One obvious possibility is that the *tat* gene function is inhibited in resting T4+ cells. T-cell activation may release *tat* inhibition, thereby facilitating viral growth. It is unlikely that the *tat* gene alone is responsible for the cytopathic effects of infection in T4+ cells. T4+ cell lines that express high levels of the functional *tat* protein have been constructed. Such cell lines are viable. However, transfection of such cell lines with an HTLV-III provirus deleted for the *tat* gene leads to cell death.[45] Evidently, at least one other viral component is needed to kill T4+ cells in culture.

How Might the *sor* and 3′*orf* Genes Fit into This Picture?

The assays used to examine the effect of *sor* and 3′*orf* deletions measured only the effect on the growth and cytopathic activity in T4+ cells.[39] Neither gene was found to be necessary.[39]

Two very different roles for these genes may be imagined. They may be involved in either the establishment or maintenance of the latent state or in the reactivation from the latent state. Establishment and/or maintenance of the latent state may require the concerted action of multiple gene products. Alternatively, the growth of the virus in other cell types, such as monocytes and macrophages, or in cells of the nervous system may require gene functions not required for growth in activated in T4+ cells. Tests of these and other possibilities remain for the future.

Other Puzzles and Prospects

Still other major unresolved problems remain. At the molecular level, these include the role of the integrated forms of viral DNA in the life cycle of the virus, and the requirement (or lack thereof) of the T4+ epitopes for infection. At the systemic level, the major mechanisms of pathogenesis remain unclear. Do T cells in patients die because they are killed by the virus itself or because virus infection triggers systemic factors that kill such cells? What accounts for the brain pathology? Are neurons killed directly/indirectly or do they die because supporting cells have been eliminated? What accounts for the peculiar spectrum of cancers associated with HTLV-III infection? Are they all consequent to immune suppression or does the virus itself play a more direct role in the disease? The answers to these questions will require a felicitous blend of virology, cell biology, molecular biology, and astute clinical observation. Fortunately, much of the ground work for answering these questions has been laid. The prospects now appear to be bright, both for understanding the pathogenesis and for controlling it.

Recent progress in controlling the disease includes:

1. Development of reverse transcriptase inhibitors suitable for use in humans, such as azidothymidine, a member of the dideoxy nucleotide family of compounds that appear to show some clinical efficacy without major toxicity (S. Broder, personal communication).
2. Tests of immunoreactivity of the envelope glycoprotein in animals preparative to vaccine trials.
3. Identification of new potential targets for antiviral therapies, such as the *tat* gene product.
4. Resolution of the current puzzles will not only speed intervention strategies, but will also illuminate fundamental questions in gene regulation and immune cell function.

Summary

HTLV is an unusual retrovirus that induces a new and unusual disease. The descriptions of the virus and the disease it causes have progressed rapidly. Puzzles remain regarding mechanisms of virus growth and latency, and there is much to learn regarding the mechanisms of pathogenesis as well. If progress continues to be rapid, as is expected, prospects are bright for control of this disease.

References

1. Gallo RC, et al. Science 1984; 224:500.
2. Popovic M, Sarngadharan MG, Read E, Gallo RC. Science 1984; 224:497.
3. Barré-Sinnousi F, et al. Science 1983; 220:868.
4. Sarngadharan MG, Popovic M, Bruch L, Shupbach J, Gallo RC. Science 1984; 224:506.
5. Shaw GM, et al. Science 1985; 227:177.
6. Friedman-Kien AE, et al. Ann Intern Med 1982; 96:693.
7. Seligman M, et al. N Engl J Med 1984; 311:1286.

8. Curran J, et al. Science 1985; 229:1352.
9. Centers for Disease Control. MMWR 1982; 31:365.
10. Ratner L, et al. Nature 1985; 313:277.
11. Wain-Hobson S, et al. Cell 1985; 40:9.
12. Sanchez-Pescador R, et al. Science 1985; 227:484.
13. Muesing MA, et al. Nature 1985; 313:450.
14. Robey WG, et al. Science 1985; 228:593.
15. Shupbach J, et al. Science 1985; 224:503.
16. Sarngadharan MG, Bruch L, Popovic M, Gallo RC. Proc Natl Acad Sci USA 1985;
    82:3481.
17. Veronese FD, et al. Science 1985; 229:1402.
18. Allan JS, et al. Science 1985; 228:1091.
19. Kitchen L, et al. Nature 1984; 312:367.
20. Arya S, Guo C, Josephs S, Wong-Staal F. Science 1985; 229:69.
21. Wong-Staal F, et al. Science 1985; 229:759.
22. Hahn B, et al. Nature 1984; 312:166.
23. Luciw P, et al. Nature 1984; 312:760.
24. Dalgleish A, et al. Nature 1984; 312:763.
25. Klatzmann D, et al. Nature 1984; 312:767.
26. McDougal JS, et al. Science 1986; 231:382.
27. Ho DD, Rota TR, Hirsch M. N Engl J Med 1985; 312:649.
28. Sodroski J. et al. Science 1985; 229:74.
29. Narayan O, Griffen D, Chase E. Science 1977; 197:376.
30. Haase A, et al. Science 1977; 195:175.
31. Narayan O, et al. J Virol 1984; 49:349.
32. Kleujer-Anderson P, McGuire T. Infec Immunol 1982; 38:455.
33. Montelaro R, et al. J Biol Chem 1984; 259:10529.
34. Sonigo P, et al. Cell 1985; 42:369.
35. Vigne R, et al. J Virol 1982; 42:1046.
36. Bruns M, Frenzel B. Virology 1979; 97:207.
37. Johnson GC, et al. Infect Immunol 1983; 41:657.
38. Allan JS, et al. Science 1985; 230:810.
39. Sodroski J, et al. Science (in press).
40. Goh WC, et al. J Virol (in press).
41. Lee TH, et al. Science (in press).
42. Kanki P, et al. Science 1985; 230:954.
43. Kanki P, et al. Science 1985; 228:1199.
44. Terwilliger E, Sodroski J, Rosen C, Haseltine WA. Submitted.
45. Dayton A, et al. Cell (in press).
46. Rosen C, et al. Nature 1986; 319:555.
47. Rosen C, Sodroski J, Haseltine WA. Cell 1985; 41:813.
48. Hoxie JA, et al. Science 1985; 229:1400.
49. Folks T, et al. Science 1986; 231:600.
50. Zagury D, et al. Science 1986; 231:850.
51. Golder J, et al. Science 1986; 231:992.

5

Animal Models of HTLV-III/LAV Infection and AIDS

Phyllis J. Kanki
Max Essex
Harvard School of Public Health
Boston, Massachusetts

Introduction

Research on retroviruses infecting a wide variety of animal species has provided much of the background and direction for the studies of human retroviruses and the pathogenesis of leukemia and immunosuppressive disease. It is from these various animal models that we have begun to understand some of the complexities of these viruses and, particularly, the virus-host interactions that ultimately lead to disease. The retroviruses of cats, monkeys, and humans all have in common the ability to infect and alter T cells. In many cases, these viral infections lead to similar clinical and pathological syndromes in their respective hosts. This has allowed researchers to study the pathogenesis of HTLV infection in closely paralleled animal systems. Various vaccine and therapy modalities are being devised and tested in these animal systems, paving the way for the development of future human retrovirus vaccines and therapy. HTLV-III/LAV infection and AIDS are rapidly emerging as a major worldwide public health problem. Therefore, the study of these animal retroviruses becomes increasingly important for the basic understanding of this general group of pathogens as well as directing the rationale for effective immunoprophylaxis.

Feline Leukemia Viruses

T-lymphotropic retroviruses of cats, known as feline leukemia viruses (FeLV), cause T-cell tumors as well as other forms of lymphoma and leukemia.[1,2] However, among naturally and persistently infected cats, only a small proportion will develop neoplasia. In fact, more FeLV-infected cats will die of the immunosuppressive effects of these viruses, representing the most common cause of death in this species.[3] FeLV causes lymphopenia, depressed cell-mediated immune response, thymic atrophy, and depressed humoral responses to T cell-dependent antigens despite the presence of hypergammaglobulinemia.[4-7] As a result, cats will develop a variety of lethal opportunistic infections including coronavirus-induced peritonitis, pneumonia, and septicemia of other viral, bacterial, fungal, or protozoal origin.[3] Many of these same clinical and pathological findings are also seen in human AIDS.

Infection with FeLVs is characterized by a prolonged induction period that can last several years. The virus shows extreme variation from one isolate to another, and many cats are infected with more than one type of virus.[8] Major variation occurs in the *env* gene, but all types appear to show some degree of cross-neutralization. A vaccine is now available for field use to prevent infection with FeLV. Although the antibody titers it induces are low, they appear sufficient to provide protection in the majority of cats that become exposed to virus.

While some strains of FeLV appear to have a major propensity for causing thymic lymphoma after only 4 to 5 months, other strains appear to lack the ability to cause leukemia but still cause immunosuppression.[9] Differences have also been observed between strains that are highly immunosuppressive and those that are not.[10] However, the apparent absence in FeLV of several genes that are present in HTLV/LAV (i.e., *sor, tat* and 3'*orf*) suggests that the mechanism by which these agents cause immunosuppression may be quite different.

Simian T-Lymphotropic Viruses

In recent times, a new group of exogenous type C retroviruses has been described in a variety of primate species. These retroviruses have been designated simian T-lymphotropic viruses (STLV) because of the many properties they share with members of the human T-lymphotropic virus (HTLV) family. These properties include the affinity for growth in T4-lymphocyte populations, similarities in in vitro growth characteristics, cross-reactive viral proteins of similar sizes, and association with similar diseases. There are two known members of the STLV family. The first, STLV-type I (STLV-I), is the simian counterpart of HTLV-I, the etiological agent of adult T-cell leukemia/lymphoma (ATLL). The remarkable similarities between STLV-I and HTLV-I most probably indicate a common origin. These similarities also illustrate the availability of an excellent animal model to study the biological effects of these viruses in vivo. The second, STLV-type III (STLV-III), is the simian counterpart of HTLV-III/LAV, the etiological agent of AIDS, and has been described in captive rhesus macaques with an immunodeficiency syndrome similar to human AIDS, and in a significant proportion of apparently healthy wild-caught African green monkeys. The similarities between STLV-III and its human counterpart provide an important model system for the study of many aspects of HTLV-III/LAV and the pathogenesis of AIDS.

STLV-I

STLV-I is known to naturally infect most Asian and African Old World primates and Great Apes.[11-18] Similar to HTLV-I, this simian virus is capable of in vitro immortalization of T lymphocytes, with the production of C-type retrovirus particles similar to HTLV-I.[19,20] The major viral proteins of STLV-I are similar in size and cross-reactive with the major antigens of HTLV-I.[21]

Molecular studies[22,23] indicate that STLV-I and HTLV-I are closely related, with 90% sequence homology in the *env*, pX, and LTR regions. We have previously reported on the association of spontaneous lymphoma or lymphoproliferative disorder with the possession of STLV-I antibodies in three species of captive macaques.[21] Tsujimoto and co-workers[24] have described a case of ATL-like disease in a captive African green monkey, and tumor cells from this animal demonstrated monoclonal integration of STLV-I sequences. Thus, it appears that STLV-I may have similar biological features to HTLV-I in vivo, representing an important animal model of viral leukemogenesis.

The immunosuppressive properties of lymphotropic retroviruses have been well recognized in the feline leukemia virus system. Seroepidemiological studies conducted in this laboratory[25] demonstrated that HTLV-I infection in people significantly increased the risk for infectious diseases other than AIDS. In similar studies of macaques with clinical or pathological manifestations of tumors or an immunodeficiency syndrome, we also noted a high correlation with exposure to STLV-I (unpublished data). Although the immunosuppressive properties of HTLV-I/STLV-I are certainly less pronounced than those of the type III viruses, further studies are necessary to fully understand the spectrum of HTLV-I/STLV-I-associated disease.

STLV-III

There is now strong evidence for an etiological relationship of HTLV-III/LAV and AIDS.[26-30] This member of the HTLV family is characterized by its cytopathic effect and T4 tropism. However, there are many features of this virus, such as its unique genetic structure and its apparent rapid mutation rate, that are distinct. To our knowledge, there have been no previous reports of a similar agent found naturally in animals. We previously described the identification and preliminary characterization of a related agent of subhuman primates (simian T-lymphotropic virus type III [STLV-III]) from three immunodeficient macaques and one macaque with malignant lymphoma.[31,32] STLV-III was isolated by co-cultivation of simian peripheral blood lymphocytes, splenic lymphocytes, or cell-free serum samples on Hut-78, a well-characterized mature human T-cell line. Analysis of cell-free supernatants for reverse transcriptase yielded positive results for Mg^{++}-dependent activity 12 to 18 days after initiation of co-cultivation. Maximum reverse transcriptase levels were detected approximately 10 days later, and maintained for over 4 months in culture. STLV-III-infected Hut-78 cells demonstrated a characteristic cytopathic effect with the formation of pleomorphic, multinucleated giant cells.

Filtered cell-free supernatants from cells infected with STLV-III could efficiently infect fresh human T-lymphocytes grown in the presence of T-cell growth factor. STLV-III demonstrated an affinity for growth in T4-lymphocyte populations. Retroviral particles were observed budding from and aggregated around infected cells. Mature, extracellular viral particles had a cylindrical-shaped nucleoid, similar to HTLV-III/LAV.

We have serologically identified and characterized STLV-III of macaques and African green monkeys by radioimmunoprecipitation and sodium dodecyl sulfate polyacrylamide gel electrophoresis (RIP-SDS/PAGE) techniques.[31,33] Virus-specific proteins of approximately 160, 120, 64, 55, 53, 32, 24, and 15 kilodaltons (kD) were identified, all similar in size to the major *gag-*, *env-*, and *pol*-encoded proteins of HTLV-III/LAV.[31,33,34] These protein species were similarly recognized by select simian serum samples and human reference serum samples from HTLV-III/LAV antibody-positive individuals. Monoclonal antibodies directed to the major core protein of HTLV-III/LAV p24 also recognized a protein species with slightly slower electrophoretic mobility in the STLV-III-infected cell lysate, therefore designated p24. Select monkey sera with antibodies to STLV-III were also capable of immunoprecipitating the major *gag*-encoded proteins of HTLV-III/LAV, p55, and p24. These showed minimal cross-reactivity with the gp120 and gp160 of HTLV-III/LAV, thus demonstrating the apparent type immunoreactivity of the *env*-encoded glycoproteins, consistent with observations in other retrovirus systems. The similarities and cross-reactivity of STLV-III viral proteins to the major antigens of HTLV-III/LAV indicate a probable close relationship of these viruses.

An immunodeficiency syndrome of macaque monkeys has been described at various primate centers, and is characterized by infection with a variety of opportunistic infections, impaired T-cell function, and lymphoproliferative disorders.[35,36] Type D retroviruses have been isolated at these primate colonies, but their definitive role in this spontaneous disease syndrome is not yet clear.[36,37] However, most of the macaques in our study were apparently free of type D retrovirus based on repeated unsuccessful isolation attempts and negative serology.[32]

Future studies on the seroepidemiology of STLV-III in the macaque (STLV-III$_{mac}$) are still needed to further characterize its association with spontaneous disease or neoplasia. It is quite likely that multiple exogenous retroviruses of primates may play a role in naturally occurring disease, which by analogy may also occur in humans. At present, our serological data compiled from three different primate centers indicate that STLV-III$_{mac}$ is not a highly prevalent virus in these populations. In addition, all seropositive macaques to date have been described with some clinical or pathological evidence of disease. Of over 100 samples tested from apparently healthy macaques, both wild-caught and captive, we have no serological evidence of exposure to STLV-III$_{mac}$ (unpublished observations). Future studies will determine if STLV-III$_{mac}$ represents a virus that naturally infects macaque species or if it is possible that it has been artifically introduced to these species in captive situations.

We have previously described the high prevalence of antibodies to STLV-III in healthy wild-caught African green monkeys (*Cercopithecus sp.*), but not in other African primates such as the chimpanzee (*P. troglodytes*), baboon (*Papio sp.*), Patas monkey (*Erthrocebus patas*), or colobus monkey (*Colobus polykomos*).[38] We were successful in isolating infectious virus from seven of eight antibody-positive African green monkeys.[33] Characteristics of STLV-III of African green monkeys (STLV-III$_{AGM}$) were similar to those already described for STLV-III$_{mac}$.

Investigators at the New England Regional Primate Research Center have reported on the inoculation of STLV-III$_{mac}$ into six juvenile rhesus macaques. Four of six macaques died within 160 days of STLV-III$_{mac}$ inoculation, with a wasting syndrome, opportunistic infections, encephalitis, and immunological abnormalities including a decrease in T4$^+$ peripheral blood lymphocytes.[39] All six inoculated macaques seroconverted to STLV-III$_{mac}$ viral antigens by 32 days postinoculation (unpublished observations). The gp160/120 of STLV-III$_{mac}$ was the first and most consistently recognized viral antigen in the inoculated macaques. In two of the six macaques, recognition of the presumed gag-encoded antigens of STLV-III$_{mac}$, p55, p24, and p17, was also demonstrated, but followed the antibody response to the gp160/120. Four of the six macaques died of an immunodeficiency syndrome, and in all four cases, these animals had lost detectable antibody to all viral antigens of STLV-III$_{mac}$ by MIF and RIP-SDS/PAGE techniques prior to death. In contrast, the two macaques that are still alive postinoculation have consistently demonstrated the best antibody response to STLV-III$_{mac}$, both by apparent titer and reactivity to presumed env- and gag-encoded antigens. These results extend our previous observations that the gp160/120 are the most immunogenic antigens of STLV-III. Further, it appears that disease induction was accompanied by loss of antibody reactivity to STLV-III$_{mac}$. Loss of antibody reactivity may have occurred secondary to primary helper lymphocyte loss and dysfunction. Alternatively, antibodies to portions of certain viral antigens may be virus-neutralizing and, hence, protective to the host; this is supported by the fact that the two macaques that remain virus-positive and apparently healthy continue to demonstrate a strong antibody response to all the STLV-III$_{mac}$ antigens.

From a biological standpoint, the STLV-IIIs of macaque and African green monkey represent two important model systems for the study of AIDS. Virus isolation, serology, and inoculation studies of STLV-III in the macaque host indicate that this related virus is closely associated with an immunodeficiency syndrome that has similar features to human AIDS. Preliminary data on inoculation of STLV-III$_{AGM}$ in the macaque host also indicate that this species may be particularly sensitive to the pathogenic effects of this simian virus (unpublished observations), thus providing a useful system in which to test various antivirals and other therapeutic regimes for HTLV-III/LAV. In contrast, the African green monkey system is most interesting because of the apparent lack of disease in this primate host. Detailed comparative studies in the pathogenesis of STLV-III$_{AGM}$ infection may indicate whether this represents a unique virus or virus-host adaptation, such that the monkeys can mount an effective immune response that protects against disease development.

The similarities and cross-reactivity of STLV-III with the env-, gag-, pol-, and 3'orf-encoded products of HTLV-III/LAV indicate that these are related members of the family of T-lymphotropic viruses. The existence of cross-reactive epitopes in the env-related antigens of these related viruses would suggest that despite a high degree of genetic variation in this region, conserved sequences between these viruses may be identified, expressed, and evaluated as potential vaccine immunogens. STLV-III of primates are also similar to HTLV-III/LAV in their propensity for growth in T4-lymphocyte populations. Recent evidence indicates that the mature envelope protein of HTLV-III/LAV directly interacts with the T4 molecule present on the target cell.[40] This would indirectly imply that conserved epitopes of the *env* proteins of STLV-III and HTLV-III/LAV are critical to virus infection and can potentially be useful in vaccine development.

Our serological studies have indicated that a significant proportion of wild-caught African green monkeys have been exposed to STLV-III$_{AGM}$. These species are widely prevalent in most regions of tropical Africa. We postulated early on that this simian virus may have been transmitted to human populations during the evolution of these viruses. It would, therefore, be likely that human retroviruses in Africa might exist that would be more closely related to STLV-III than to the prototype AIDS virus, HTLV-III/LAV. Most recently, we have described the serological evidence for a virus similar to STLV-III$_{AGM}$ infecting apparently healthy people in West Africa and the isolation of virus from these individuals.[34,41] A new human T-lymphotropic virus (termed HTLV-IV) isolated from these people has shown retroviral type particles, in vitro growth characteristics, and major viral proteins similar to those of the STLV-III/HTLV-III/LAV group of retroviruses. The serological data suggest that this virus shares more common epitopes with STLV-III$_{AGM}$ than with the prototype HTLV-III/LAV that infects people in the United States and Europe. Further studies on these related viruses may help us better understand how the unique pathogenicity of this family of viruses has evolved and how we can better approach the development of an effective vaccine.

Experimental Infection of HTLV-III/LAV in Chimpanzees

Experimental inoculation and infection with HTLV-III/LAV in an animal species represent another type of model system that can be useful for AIDS studies. Obviously, the development of such an animal model system can be utilized for vaccine studies and therapy trials. A variety of animal species have been experimentally inoculated with AIDS materials or HTLV-III/LAV virus preparations. Based on these studies, it appears that the chimpanzee (*Pan troglodytes*) is the only animal species that can reproducibly be persistently infected with this agent.[42-44]

Chimpanzees have been infected with plasma, blood, and brain tissue from AIDS patients. In later studies, cell-free virus preparations or autologous-infected lymphocytes were also capable of infecting this primate species. Seroconversion to HTLV-III/LAV antigens was demonstrated by ELISA and/or Western blot analysis. In many cases, infectious virus was reisolated from these animals. Although the data demonstrate persistent infection with HTLV-III/LAV in this primate, an AIDS-like disease has not been shown. Some animals did demonstrate lymphadenopathy with some alterations in T4 and/or T8 levels; however, these signs did not progress or persist.[42,43]

The chimpanzee model system will no doubt provide an important model for HTLV-III/LAV infection. It has been amply demonstrated that these species can be reproducibly infected with a variety of virus preparations, and that viremia is persistent. Further studies on the humoral and cell-mediated response to virus infection will have obvious significance to our understanding of human infection. In addition, molecular characterization of chimpanzee-passaged virus may determine the role of the immune system in the recognized genetic variability of HTLV-III/LAV in people. Most importantly, this animal model will be useful in the testing of potential HTLV-III/LAV vaccines for the prevention of HTLV-III/LAV viremia.

Conclusions

AIDS is caused by a human T-lymphotropic virus, HTLV-III/LAV, which has many characteristics that appear unique to this class of retroviruses. This devastating disease can only be effectively prevented or cured with a better understanding of the pathobiology of this complex virus. Many retroviruses found in outbred mammal systems provide valuable model systems for the study of AIDS. The T-lymphotropic retrovirus of cats causes lymphopenia and immunosuppression as well as leukemia. The study of this particular system may provide important parallels for the understanding of these viruses, which may be capable of a spectrum of disease. The STLV-III viruses appear to be closely related to HTLV-III/LAV, with common epitopes in all the major antigens of this virus. The further identification and characterization of these cross-reactive epitopes may be directly applicable to vaccine development. The availability of a primate species infected with a related virus that either resists disease development (African green monkey) or succumbs to an AIDS-like syndrome (rhesus monkey) provides two models that should aid in our understanding of the pathobiology of these viruses and the development of an AIDS vaccine.

References

1. Jarrett W, Mackey L, Jarrett O, Laird HM, Hood C. Antibody response and virus survival in cats vaccinated against feline leukemia. Nature (Lond) 1974; 248:230–232.
2. Jarrett WFH, Martin WB, Crighton GW, Dalton RG, Stewart MF. Leukemia in the cat: transmission experiments with leukemia (lymphosarcoma). Nature (Lond) 1964; 202:566–567.
3. Essex M. Horizontally and vertically transmitted oncornavirus of cats. Adv Cancer Res 1975; 21:175–248.

4. Essex M, Hardy WD Jr, Cotter SM, Jakowski RM, Sliski A. Naturally occurring persistent feline oncornavirus infections in the absence of disease. Infect Immunol 1975; 11:470–475.

5. Perryman LE, Hoover EA, Yohn DS. Immunological reactivity of the cat: immunosuppression in experimental feline leukemia. J Natl Cancer Inst 1972; 49:1357–1365.

6. Hoover EA, Perryman LE, Kociba GI. Early lesions in cats inoculated with feline leukemia virus. Cancer Res 1973; 33:145–152.

7. Trainin Z, Wernicke D, Essex M, Ungar-Waron H. Suppression of the humoral antibody response in natural retrovirus infections. Science 1983; 220:858–859.

8. Russell PH, Jarrett O. The occurrence of feline leukemia virus neutralizing antibodies in cats. Int J Cancer 1978; 22:351–357.

9. Hoover EA, Olsen RG, Hardy WD, Schaller JP, Mathes LE. Feline leukemia virus infection: age-related variation in susceptibility of cats to experimental infection. J Natl Cancer Inst 1976; 58:365–369.

10. Mullins JM, Chen CS, Hoover EA. Disease-specific and tissue-specific production of unintegrated feline leukemia virus variant DNA in feline AIDS. Nature (Lond) 1986; 319:333–336.

11. Miyoshi I, Ohtsuki Y, Fujishita M, et al. Natural adult T-cell leukemia virus infection in Japanese monkeys. Lancet 1982; ii:658.

12. Hayami M, Oshikawa K, Kommuro A, et al. ATLV antibody in cynomologus monkeys in the wild. Lancet 1983; ii:620.

13. Hunsmann G, Schneider J, Schmitt J, et al. Detection of serum antibodies to adult T-cell leukemia virus in non-human primates and in people from Africa. Int J Cancer 1983; 32:329–332.

14. Ishida T, Yamamoto K, Kaneko R, et al. Seroepidemiological study of antibodies to adult T-cell leukemia virus-associated antigen (ATLA) in free-ranging Japanese monkeys (Macaca fuscata). Microbiol Immunol 1983; 27:297–301.

15. Yamamoto N, Hinuma Y, Zur Hausen H, et al. African green monkeys are infected with adult T-cell leukemia virus or a closely related agent. Lancet 1983; i:240.

16. Miyoshi I, Fujishita M, Taguchi H, et al. Natural infection in non-human primates with adult T-cell leukemia virus or a closely related agent. Int J Cancer 1983; 32:333.

17. Hayami M, Komuro A, Nozawa K, et al. Prevalence of antibody to adult T-cell leukemia virus-associated antigens (ATLA) in Japanese monkeys and other nonhuman primates. Int J Cancer 1984; 33:179–183.

18. Saxinger WC, Linge-Wantzin G, Thomsen K, et al. Human T-cell leukemia virus: a diverse family of related exogenous viruses of humans and Old World primates. In: Gallo RC, Essex M, Gross L, eds. Human T-cell leukemia viruses. Cold Spring Harbor, New York: Cold Spring Harbor Press, 1984:323–330.

19. Miyoshi I, Taguchi H, Fujishita M, et al. Transformation of monkey lymphocytes with adult T-cell leukemia virus. Lancet 1981; i:1016.

20. Miyoshi I, Taguchi S, Yoshimoto M, et al. Transmission of Japanese monkey type C virus to human lymphocytes. Lancet 1983; ii:166.

21. Homma T, Kanki PJ, King JW Jr, et al. Lymphoma in macaques: association with exposure to virus of human T-lymphotropic family. Science 1984; 225:716–718.

22. Guo H-G, Wong-Staal F, Gallo RC. Novel viral sequences related to human T-cell leukemia virus in T-cells of a seropositive baboon. Science 1984; 223:1195–1197.
23. Komuro A, Watanabe T, Miyoshi I, et al. Detection and characterization of provirus genomes of simian retroviruses homologous to human T-cell leukemia virus. Virology 1984; 138:373–378.
24. Tsujimoto H, Seiki M, Nakamura H, et al. Adult T-cell leukemia-like disease in monkey naturally infected with simian retrovirus related to human T-cell leukemia virus type I. Jpn J Cancer Res 1985; 76:911–914.
25. Essex M, McLane MF, Tachibana N, et al. Seroepidemiology of human T-cell leukemia virus in relation to immunosuppression and the acquired immunodeficiency syndrome. In: Gallo RC, Essex M, Gross L, eds. Human T-cell leukemia viruses. Cold Spring Harbor, New York: Cold Spring Harbor Press, 1984:355–361.
26. Popovic M, Sarngadharan M, Read E, et al. Detection, isolation, and continuous production of cytopathic retroviruses (HTLV-III) from patients with AIDS and pre-AIDS. Science 1984; 224:497–500.
27. Gallo R, Salahuddin S, Popovic M, et al. Frequent detection and isolation of cytopathic retroviruses (HTLV-III) from patients with AIDS and at risk for AIDS. Science 1984; 224:500–503.
28. Schüpbach J, Popovic M, Gilden RV, et al. Serological analysis of a subgroup of human T-lymphotropic retroviruses (HTLV-III) associated with AIDS. Science 1984; 224:503–506.
29. Sarngadharan M, Popovic M, Bruch L, et al. Antibodies reactive with human T-lymphotropic retroviruses (HTLV-III) in the serum of patients with AIDS. Science 1984; 224:506.
30. Barré-Sinoussi F, Chermann JC, Rey F, et al. Isolation of a T-lymphotropic retrovirus from a patient at risk for acquired immune deficiency syndrome (AIDS). Science 1983; 220:868–871.
31. Kanki PJ, McLane MF, King NW, et al. Serologic identification and characterization of a macaque T-lymphotropic retrovirus closely related to human T-lymphotropic retroviruses (HTLV) type III. Science 1985; 228:1199–1201.
32. Daniel MD, Letvin NL, King NW, et al. Isolation of a T-cell tropic HTLV-III-like retrovirus from macaques. Science 1985; 228:1201–1204.
33. Kanki PJ, Alroy J, Essex M. Isolation of T-lymphotropic retrovirus related to HTLV-III/LAV from wild-caught African green monkeys. Science 1985; 230:951–954.
34. Barin F, M'Boup S, Denis F, et al. Serological evidence for virus related to simian T-lymphotropic retrovirus III in residents of West Africa. Lancet 1985; ii:1387–1389.
35. King NW, Hunt RD, Letvin NL. Histopathologic changes in macaque monkeys with an acquired immune deficiency syndrome (AIDS). Am J Pathol 1983; 113:382–388.
36. Marx PA, Maul DH, Osborn KG, et al. Simian AIDS: isolation of a type D retrovirus and transmission of the disease. Science 1984; 223:1083–1086.
37. Daniel MD, King NW, Letvin NL, et al. A new type D retrovirus isolated from macaques with an immunodeficiency syndrome. Science 1984; 223:602–605.
38. Kanki PJ, Kurth R, Becker W, et al. Antibodies to simian T-lymphotropic retrovirus type III in African green monkeys and recognition of STLV-III viral proteins by AIDS and related sera. Lancet 1985; i:1330–1332.

39. Letvin NL, Daniel MD, Sehgal PK, et al. Induction of AIDS-like disease in macaque monkeys with T-cell tropic retrovirus STLV-III. Science 1985; 230:71–73.
40. McDougal JS, Kennedy MS, Sligh JM, et al. Binding of HTLV-III/LAV to T4+ T-cells by a complex of the 110K viral protein and the T4 molecule. Science 1986; 231:382–385.
41. Kanki PJ, Barin F, M'Boup S, et al. New human T-lymphotropic retrovirus related to simian T-lymphotropic virus type III (STLV-III$_{AGM}$). Science 1986; 232:238–243.
42. Alter HJ, Eichberg JW, Masur H, et al. Transmission of HTLV-III infection from human plasma to chimpanzees: an animal model for AIDS. Science 1984; 226:549–552.
43. Francis DP, Feorino PM, Broderson JR, et al. Infection of chimpanzees with lymphadenopathy-associated virus. Lancet 1984; ii:1276–1277.
44. Gajdusek DC, Gibbs CJ Jr, Rodgers-Johnson P, et al. Infection of chimpanzees by human T-lymphotropic retroviruses in brain and other tissues from AIDS patients. Lancet 1985; i:55–56.

6

AIDS: A New Kind of Epidemic Immunodeficiency

Ann M. Hardy
James W. Curran
AIDS Program
Center for Infectious Diseases
Centers for Disease Control
Atlanta, Georgia

Background

In the spring of 1981, physicians in Los Angeles reported five young, previously healthy, homosexual men with biopsy-confirmed *Pneumocystis carinii* pneumonia (PCP) diagnosed at three different hospitals.[1] This was an important observation since PCP previously had occurred primarily in immunocompromised individuals. Shortly thereafter, 26 cases of Kaposi's sarcoma (KS), a rare type of skin cancer, were reported in homosexual men in New York City and California.[2] Seven of these men also had serious opportunistic infections, including four with PCP.

Because of the unusual and severe nature of these illnesses, the Centers for Disease Control (CDC) organized a task force to conduct an investigation shortly after the initial reports were received. The task force initially set out to determine if this was a new phenomenon and to search for additional cases.

Physicians in 18 major metropolitan areas were surveyed, tumor registries were reviewed, and requests to CDC for pentamidine isethionate (a drug used to treat PCP, available only from CDC at that time) were examined. An additional 125 cases were identified; the earliest first appeared in the late 1970s.[3] By June 9, 1986, more than 21,000 people in the United States had been reported with what was later termed acquired immunodeficiency syndrome (AIDS), and over half of them had died.

Search for a Cause

The observation that persons with AIDS were more sexually active than healthy controls and the finding of a large cluster of cases linked by sexual contact suggested that AIDS was caused by an infectious agent.[4-6] This theory became more widely accepted by early 1983 with the documentation of the syndrome in persons with hemophilia and in blood transfusion recipients.[7,8] The consistent finding of the depletion of lymphocytes bearing the OKT-4 marker in patients with AIDS seemed to indicate that this cell was the target of the AIDS agent. Because of this, attention was focused on viruses. The known tropism of human T-cell leukemia virus type I, the first retrovirus known to infect humans, for OKT-4 cells suggested that the etiological agent might belong to the retrovirus family.

During 1983 and 1984, several reports[9-12] documented the isolation of a retrovirus from the blood of patients with AIDS and AIDS-related conditions. The retrovirus was variously termed lymphadenopathy-associated virus (LAV), human T-lymphotropic virus type III (HTLV-III), and AIDS-associated retrovirus (ARV). The development of a cell line that permits growth of this virus facilitated large-scale virus and antigen production and the development of serological tests to detect antibodies to HTLV-III/LAV.[13]

Epidemiological studies using these antibody tests and culture techniques have produced convincing evidence that this virus causes AIDS. Almost all patients with AIDS who have been tested have been shown to be infected;[10,12,14] this compares with an infection rate of less than 1% in persons with no known risk for AIDS.[15] In one longitudinal study,[16] antibodies to HTLV-III/LAV were detected in all the patients who developed AIDS before there was clinical evidence of disease. Studies of transfusion-associated AIDS[11] have documented the isolation of virus in both the implicated blood donor and the recipient.

AIDS Surveillance

CDC established a prospective surveillance system for AIDS shortly after receiving the reports of the first cases. An early observation was that patients

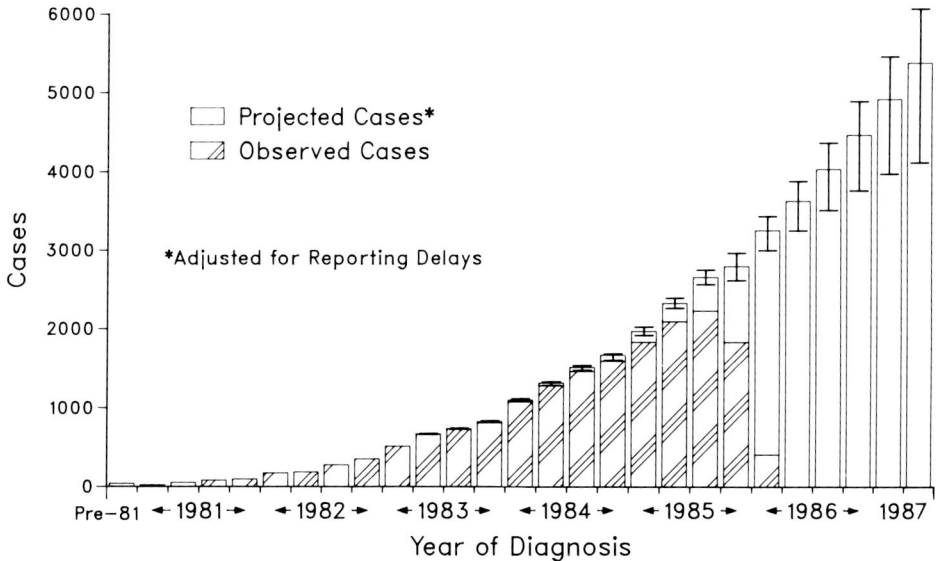

FIGURE 1 Incidence of AIDS in the United States by quarter of diagnosis projected from cases reported as of February 28, 1986.

with AIDS had similar patterns of cell-mediated immune impairment and developed diseases consistent with this defect.[17-19] This observation was used to formulate the first surveillance case definition for AIDS based on the presence of certain reliably diagnosed diseases in patients without a known cause of immunosuppression.[20] This surveillance definition has recently been modified to include other serious diseases as indicative of AIDS-associated immunodeficiency if a patient also has evidence of AIDS virus infection.[21]

As of June 9, 1986, 21,517 cases of AIDS, including 304 in children, had been reported to CDC. Of these, 11,713 (54% of the adults and 61% of the children) are reported to have died. The number of cases reported each half-year continues to increase (Fig. 1). Using an ad hoc polynomial model, it is estimated that cases will continue to increase into 1987, and that the current number of cases will double in 12–15 months.[22] Cases have been reported from all 50 states, the District of Columbia, and three U.S. territories. Approximately 73% of the cases have been reported from five states: New York, California, Florida, New Jersey, and Texas.

AIDS in Adults

Among adult patients with AIDS, 90% are between the ages of 20 and 49 years old; 93% are men. Fifty-nine percent are white, 25% are black, 14% are

Hispanic, and 2% are of other or unreported races. There has been little change over time in the distribution of cases by age, sex, and race.

Seventy-three percent of adult cases were in homosexual or bisexual men (12% of whom also used drugs intravenously), and 17% occurred in heterosexual men and women who used intravenous (IV) drugs. Two percent were patients who had received a transfusion of whole blood or one of its components within the 5 years before diagnosis, and 1% were persons with hemophilia. Heterosexual partners of AIDS patients or persons at increased risk for AIDS accounted for 2% of the cases. The remaining 6% of the cases could not be classified by recognized risk factors for AIDS. This group includes persons born in countries where AIDS has not been associated with known risk factors (about 3% of the total); most of these are from Haiti. The other 714 cases include 393 cases still under investigation, 134 cases in persons for whom no risk could be identified in follow-up interview, and persons for whom sexual and drug histories were unobtainable because of severe illness or death (n=153), refusal of patients to be interviewed (n=25), or loss to follow-up (n=9).

Reported cases have increased in all patient groups. There has been no change over time in the proportion of cases categorized as homosexual or bisexual men, intravenous (IV) drug users, or persons with hemophilia (Table 1). There has been a slight but significant increase in the proportion of cases occurring in blood transfusion recipients and heterosexual contacts of risk group members. Because of the long incubation period of AIDS, persons exposed through transfusion before donor self-deferral and HTLV-III/LAV antibody screening of donated blood remain at risk for developing AIDS, and cases of transfusion-associated AIDS will continue to occur. The slight increase in heterosexually acquired cases is of interest and warrants continued close monitoring. There has also been a significant decrease in the proportion of cases in the other/unknown risk group. This decrease is solely a result of a slower growth in numbers of cases in persons born in countries where heterosexual transmission is thought to play a major role (e.g., Haiti). The reasons for this slower growth among the latter cases are not clear.

Pneumocystis pneumonia has been diagnosed in 64% of the patients with AIDS; 23% have had Kaposi's sarcoma (KS); 14% have had *Candida* esophagitis. The other opportunistic diseases have been diagnosed in less than 10% of patients. The rates of opportunistic diseases vary by patient group. Kaposi's sarcoma has been reported in 32% of AIDS cases in homosexual men, but in only 6% of patients in all other groups. Toxoplasmosis is more common in Haitian patients than in others, while PCP accounts for a higher proportion of diseases in IV drug users, transfusion recipients, and persons with hemophilia than in other groups. The reasons for all these differences are not completely understood. It is possible that for some diseases, such as toxoplasmosis, the organism is more prevalent in some groups than in others.

TABLE 1   Distribution of Cases of AIDS by Patient Category and Date of Report

	Report date			
	Before June 1, 1984	June 1, 1984– May 31, 1985	June 1, 1985– June 9, 1986	Total
Adult	n=4,983	n=6,145	n=10,085	n=21,213
Homosexual/bisexual men	73%	74%	73%	73%
IV drug user	17%	17%	17%	17%
Hemophilia/coag. disorder	0.7%	0.6%	0.9%	0.8%
Heterosexual contact	1.0%	1.5%	1.8%	1.5%
Transfusion recipient	1.1%	1.7%	1.9%	1.7%
Other/unknown	7%	5%	5%	6%
Pediatric	n=79	n=65	n=160	n=304
Parent at risk	74%	82%	75%	77%
Hemophilia	5%	8%	2%	4%
Transfusion recipient	15%	11%	16%	15%
Other/unknown	6%	0%	4%	4%

A significant change has been noted in the proportion of reported opportunistic diseases over time. The proportion of KS cases has decreased from 24 to 14% of reported AIDS-associated diseases. PCP has accounted for an increasing proportion of diseases (from 32 to 54%), while the other opportunistic diseases have remained stable. This proportional decrease in KS and increase in PCP may be a reporting artifact or an actual trend. If it is real trend, it may be due to a change in factors, as yet unrecognized, associated with the development of these two opportunistic diseases in persons infected with HTLV-III/LAV.

AIDS in Children

Among the 304 AIDS patients less than 13 years of age, 55% are male. Eighteen percent are white, 60% black, and 22% Hispanic. Two hundred thirty-five (77%) were born to a parent who has AIDS or who is in a group at increased risk for AIDS, 45 (15%) had received transfusions, 12 (4%) had hemophilia, and 12 (4%) could not be placed into a risk group because risk factor information on the parents was incomplete (Table 1). *Pneumocystis* pneumonia has been diagnosed in 58%, disseminated cytomegalovirus in 19%,

Candida esophagitis in 15%, cryptosporidiosis in 6%, KS in 4%, and other opportunistic diseases in 21%. Pediatric cases have been reported from 23 states, the District of Columbia, and Puerto Rico.

Incidence Rates and Premature Mortality

Estimates of group-specific incidence rates illustrate the relative importance of AIDS in certain population groups (Table 2). Single men in Manhattan and San Francisco, intravenous drug users in New York City and New Jersey, and hemophilia A patients have extremely high rates of disease (>250 per 100,000 in 1984).[23,24] These rates are similar to 1973–1977 U.S. average annual incidence rates for all cancers (331.5 per 100,000).[24] Blood transfusion recipients and female sexual partners of men who use intravenous drugs had much lower estimated rates of AIDS. However, their rates were still 6 to 60 times higher than the estimated rate of 0.1 per 100,000 for those not in any of these groups.[23,24]

Because AIDS has a high case fatality rate and affects a relatively young

TABLE 2 Estimated Incidence Rates of AIDS in Selected Population Groups in 1984

Group	Rate per 100,000
Single men	
United States	14.3
Manhattan	263.2
San Francisco	339.8
IV drug users	
United States	167.7
New York City	261.1
New Jersey	350.0
Persons with hemophilia	
Type A	345.7
Type B	34.5
Female contacts of male IV drug users	6.0
Transfusion recipients	
Adults	0.6
Children	2.8

population, it has a substantial effect of premature mortality in areas and groups with a high incidence of disease. One measure of premature mortality is years of potential life lost before age 65 (YPLL), which takes into account age at death in addition to number of deaths for specific causes. By 1984, AIDS had become the sixth leading cause of YPLL for women in New York City and the fourth leading cause for men, accounting for 4 and 10% of premature mortality, respectively, in New York City.[25] In single men 25 to 44 years old in the United States, YPLL due to AIDS in 1984 was only slightly less than YPLL attributable to cancer. For this same group in Manhattan and San Francisco, AIDS-related YPLL ranked above other causes and may increase YPLL due to all causes by as much as 50%.[24]

Other Manifestations of Infection with the AIDS Virus

It became apparent early that cases of AIDS represented only the tip of the disease spectrum iceberg for persons found to be infected with the AIDS virus. Other medical problems reported in this group include unexplained generalized lymphadenopathy, idiopathic thrombocytopenia purpura, and other less serious opportunistic infections.[26-28] Serological tests for HTLV-III/LAV have shown that many of the persons with these conditions who are in high risk groups are infected with the virus.[29] It is hoped that these tests will allow researchers to better define the entire spectrum of illness associated with HTLV-III/LAV infection.

Infection rates among high risk group members vary, depending on geographic location and the characteristics of the populations tested. Of homosexual men tested in large cities in the United States and Europe, 22 to 73% have been reported to have antibodies to HTLV-III/LAV.[15,28-30] For intravenous drug users, rates have ranged from 50 to 87% in New York and New Jersey.[31,32] Seroprevalence rates of 72 to 85% have been reported in persons with hemophilia A who had been treated with clotting factor concentrates.[33,34] A study of blood donors carried out by CDC and the Atlanta Region of the American Red Cross found that 0.07% had a repeatedly reactive enzyme immunoassay confirmed by Western blot analysis.[35]

Infection with HTLV-III/LAV is much more common than the clinical occurrence of AIDS in all groups. One report[24] estimates that between 500,-000 and 1,000,000 Americans had been infected with the AIDS virus by late 1985. The number of cases projected to be diagnosed and reported in the next 12 months would represent an annual attack rate of between 1 and 3% of those currently infected.

An acute mononucleosis-like illness characterized by fever, malaise, sore throat, diarrhea, myalgia, and lymphadenopathy has been described in 11 homosexual men within days to weeks after exposure to HTLV-III/LAV.[36] In three of these patients, seroconversion occurred after the onset of clinical manifestations. These observations indicate that an acute, transient clinical illness may occur as an initial result of infection with HTLV-III/LAV.

The San Francisco City Health Department and CDC have conducted studies involving a cohort of homosexual male patients from clinics in San Francisco. These studies have provided information about the frequency of various manifestations of infection with HTLV-III/LAV in this population. In a representative sample of 435 men first seen between 1978 and 1980 and enrolled in a follow-up study in 1984, 293 (67%) were found to be seropositive. Of the positive subjects, 10 (3%) had AIDS, 93 (32%) had generalized lymphadenopathy or other symptoms of the AIDS-related complex (ARC), 10 (3%) had hematologic abnormalities, and 180 (62%) had no signs of illness.[37]

Several prospective studies of persons with persistent, generalized lymphadenopathy due to HTLV-III/LAV infection have been conducted. During 2 years of follow-up, 6 to 22% of patients have subsequently developed AIDS.[16,38,39] One of these follow-up studies[38] indicated that patients who had low T-helper cell counts, anemia, lymphopenia, and symptoms in addition to lymphadenopathy upon enrollment were more likely to later develop AIDS than those without these characteristics.

Modes of Transmission

In this country, AIDS is transmitted primarily in four ways: through sexual contact, among intravenous drug users through sharing contaminated needles or equipment, through administrations of infected blood or blood products, and perinatally from infected mothers to their fetuses or newborns. HTLV-III/LAV has been isolated from a variety of body fluids, including blood, saliva, semen, urine, and tears[40-43] and is likely to be isolated from other fluids containing lymphocytes or blood, such as cervical or vaginal secretions. However, HTLV-III/LAV is isolated infrequently and in small quantities from saliva, so contact with this substance is not felt to be an important mode of transmission.[44]

The most consistent risk factor for AIDS and HTLV-III/LAV infection in homosexual men is a large number of male sexual partners or sexual contact with a person known to be infected.[4,5,16] In addition, receptive anal intercourse and other potentially traumatic sexual practices have been associated with AIDS or infection in many studies.[5,16,45] Heterosexual transmission has most often been associated with being the steady partner of a person with AIDS or in a risk group for AIDS.[46] Contact with female prostitutes in Rwanda has been suggested as a risk factor, and antibody prevalence among prostitutes in that country has been noted to be high.[47] In two studies in the United States, 5% of prostitutes in Seattle, Washington and 40% in Miami, Florida were found to be seropositive.[48]

Needle sharing and frequent drug injection have been reported to be risk factors for AIDS and HTLV-III/LAV infection in intravenous drug users.[32,49]

The reports of AIDS in persons with hemophilia and in blood transfusion recipients led to the recognition that this disease could be transmitted by contaminated blood or blood products. Persons with hemophilia had acquired the infection through pooled plasma products, especially clotting-factor concentrates. HTLV-III/LAV seropositivity increases with the increased use of clotting factor caused by increased severity of hemophilia. In addition, the use of cryoprecipitate has also been implicated in the transmission of HTLV-III/LAV.[50] Among recipients of single donor transfusion products, patients with transfusion-associated AIDS had received components from larger numbers of donors than had the average transfusion recipient;[23] the receipt of a larger number of units presumably increased their chance of virus exposure.

Approximately 75% of the pediatric AIDS patients were born to parents who have AIDS or who are in one of the high risk groups. The virus is believed to be transmitted from infected mothers to their fetuses or offspring during pregnancy or perhaps during or shortly after birth. Two AIDS cases have occurred in children separated at birth from their biological mothers; one of these was delivered by Cesarean section.[51,52] Transmission after birth has been suggested by the occurrence of HTLV-III/LAV seroconversion in an infant born to a mother who acquired her infection from a postpartum blood transfusion. Since this child was breastfed for 6 weeks, researchers theorized that the virus was transmitted through breastfeeding.[53]

As of June 9, 1986, there have been no reports of cases of AIDS definitely linked to occupational exposure. Approximately 3% of AIDS cases have occurred in health-care workers, but over 90% of these belonged to known risk groups. In completed investigations of cases outside risk groups, no specific occupational exposures could be identified.

The development of HTLV-III/LAV antibodies was reported to have occurred in a nurse from England 27 to 49 days after her exposure by accidental needlestick to the blood of an AIDS patient.[54] In the United States, CDC researchers and others have studied over 1700 health-care workers involved in the care of AIDS patients. Many of these workers had been exposed by a parenteral or mucous membrane route to blood or other body fluids of these patients. Four workers were found to have antibodies to HTLV-III/LAV without evidence of any other risk factors for AIDS.[55,70,71] For three workers, seroconversion could not be demonstrated because sera were not drawn until 8–9 months after the presumed exposure.[55,70] In the fourth case, seroconversion after the exposure was demonstrated and an investigation failed to reveal any other possible source of infection.[71] The risk of developing HTLV-III/LAV infection following a needlestick involving an infected source patient is less than 1%.[56]

According to information gathered on AIDS cases for 5 years, there is no evidence of transmission of HTLV-III/LAV through air, food, water, or fomites, or by arthropods or casual contact.

Prevention Efforts

Without a vaccine or effective antiviral chemotherapy, prevention of HTLV-III/LAV transmission is the best strategy for controlling the AIDS epidemic. Much progress has been made in reducing the risk of transmission through transfusion of blood products. In March 1983, the U.S. Public Health Service recommended that members of high risk groups voluntarily refrain from donating blood or plasma.[57] Serological tests for HTLV-III/LAV were licensed in March 1985 and are currently used to screen donated blood and plasma in all centers in this country. Heat-treated clotting-factor concentrates are now available and are recommended for hemophilia patients. Since HTLV-III/LAV is sensitive to heat in vitro, this treatment should make factor concentrates much less likely to transmit infection.[58]

Prevention efforts also include educating the public about known risk factors to decrease the chance of exposure to HTLV-III/LAV. The U.S. Public Health Service has recommended that members of high risk groups reduce their number of sexual partners to avoid acquiring or transmitting AIDS[57] and that seropositive persons avoid infecting others by preventing their contact with potentially infectious body fluids.[59] There are several indications that changes in sexual behavior are occurring among homosexual men. Several cities have reported substantial decreases in the rates of rectal and pharyngeal gonorrhea in homosexual men.[60,61] Other reports[62,63] have documented decreases in the number of partners and other behavioral changes in this population. However, the increasing HTLV-III/LAV seroprevalence means that the risk of exposure to HTLV-III/LAV for homosexual men from a single casual sexual encounter is much greater now than it was in the early 1980s. To reduce the risk of exposure to HTLV-III/LAV, persons should avoid any sexual activity that involves the exchange of body fluids with persons known or suspected of being infected. Preventive measures, such as condoms, should reduce but may not entirely eliminate the risk of infection.

The risk of transmission of HTLV-III/LAV from infected mother to infants is well recognized, but not yet quantified. In one study,[64] 13 (65%) of 20 infants born to infected mothers who had already delivered one infant with

AIDS had serological and/or clinical evidence of HTLV-III/LAV infection several months after birth. This may overestimate the risk of transmission for all infected pregnant women since the women in the study were selected because they had previously transmitted HTLV-III/LAV perinatally. There is also evidence that perinatal transmission from an infected mother is not inevitable. Of three children born to women infected by artificial insemination from one infected donor, all were seronegative and clinically well more than 1 year after birth.[65]

Recommendations to assist in preventing perinatal transmission have been published.[66] Counselling and, when indicated, testing for antibody to HTLV-III/LAV for all women who are at increased risk of infection and who may become, or who are, pregnant are recommended.

Persons with clinical, epidemiological, or serological evidence of HTLV-III/LAV infection should avoid transmission to others through sexual contact or sharing needles and should not donate blood or plasma.[59] They should also not donate tissues, body organs, or sperm[59] because of the reports of women becoming infected through artificial insemination, and graft recipients becoming infected after receiving organs from infected donors.[65,67] Additionally, donors of organs, tissue, or sperm should be tested for antibodies to HTLV-III/LAV to prevent transmission through these routes.[67]

Outlook for the Future

High priorities in AIDS research include the development of a vaccine and effective antiviral therapy and research to further our understanding of the natural history of HTLV-III/LAV infection and AIDS. In the interim, current strategies for controlling the epidemic depend primarily on education, testing, and counselling to prevent sexual transmission, transmission among IV drug users, and transmission from infected mothers to their infants. These efforts must be able to constantly assimilate new information about AIDS and its transmission as it is uncovered. Thus, prevention programs must involve the cooperation of the scientific community, public health agencies, and community groups.

Even if the incidence of new infections can be decreased, the incidence of AIDS in the United States is likely to continue to increase in the next few years since large numbers of persons have already been infected. Because of the wide-ranging effect of HTLV-III/LAV on the immune system, infection with this agent may affect the course and prognosis of other diseases. Studies suggesting that HTLV-III/LAV may cause neurological complications indicate that we may have not yet recognized all the clinical manifestations of infection with this virus.[68] Co-factors that may determine clinical outcome among those infected remain to be identified.

The modes of transmission outlined in this chapter have remained stable over the course of the epidemic and will likely remain so in the future. It is unlikely that casual contact will ever play a significant role in the transmission of HTLV-III/LAV. Sexual transmission will continue to account for the majority of cases in this country. Homosexual men and IV drug abusers will remain at extremely high risk for AIDS; the disease may well become the leading cause of death in these populations.

In addition to the medical and epidemiological aspects of AIDS, there are also economic aspects that must be recognized and addressed. A CDC report[69] estimated that the first 10,000 patients with AIDS would require 1.6 million hospital days at a cost of over $1.4 billion in expenditures. Losses incurred from the disability and premature death of these patients were estimated to be over $4.8 billion. These estimates did not include expenditures for out-of-hospital treatment and care, nor did they consider costs for patients with ARC or other manifestations of HTLV-III/LAV infection. As the number of AIDS cases increases, so will the resources being used and being lost as a result of this disease. The economic burden also underscores the need to develop and implement effective methods of disease prevention.

In the 5 years since AIDS was recognized, research has resulted in an understanding of the etiology and pathogenesis of this disease and has identified the major modes of transmission of the virus causing it. Continued efforts are needed to better define the natural history of HTLV-III/LAV infection and to develop a vaccine and therapy. In the meantime, community groups and health professionals must work together and use the tools currently available to them to prevent the spread of AIDS and care for those affected.

References

1. Centers for Disease Control. *Pneumocystis* pneumonia—Los Angeles. MMWR 1981; 30:250.
2. Centers for Disease Control. Kaposi's sarcoma and *Pneumocystis* pneumonia among homosexual men—New York City and California. MMWR 1981; 30:305–308.
3. Centers for Disease Control. Centers for Disease Control Task Force on Kaposi's Sarcoma and Opportunistic Infections. N Engl J Med 1982; 306:248–252.
4. Jaffe HW, Choi K, Thomas PA, et al. National case-control study of Kaposi's sarcoma and *Pneumocystis carinni* pneumonia in homosexual men: part 1, epidemiologic results. Ann Intern Med 1983; 99:145–151.
5. Marmor M, Friedman-Kien AE, Zolla-Pazner S, et al. Kaposi's sarcoma in homosexual men: a seroepidemiologic case-control study. Ann Intern Med 1984; 100:809–815.

6. Auerbach DM, Darrow WW, Jaffe HW, et al. Cluster of cases of the acquired immune deficiency syndrome: patients linked by sexual contact. Am J Med 1984; 76:487–492.
7. Centers for Disease Control. Pneumocystis carinii pneumonia among persons with hemophilia A. MMWR 1982; 31:365–367.
8. Curran JW, Lawrence DN, Jaffe HW, et al. Acquired immunodeficiency syndrome (AIDS) associated with transfusions. N Engl J Med 1984; 310:69–75.
9. Barré-Sinoussi F, Chermann JC, Rey F, et al. Isolation of a T-lymphotropic retrovirus from a patient at risk for acquired immunodeficiency syndrome (AIDS). Science 1983; 220:868–871.
10. Gallo RC, Salahuddin SZ, Popovic M, et al. Frequent detection and isolation of cytopathic retroviruses (HTLV-III) from patients with AIDS and at risk for AIDS. Science 1984; 224:500–503.
11. Feorino PM, Kalyanaraman VS, Haverkos HW, et al. Lymphadenopathy associated virus infection of a blood donor-recipient pair with acquired immunodeficiency syndrome. Science 1984; 225:69–72.
12. Levy JA, Hoffman AD, Kramer AD, et al. Isolation of lymphocytopathic retrovirus from San Francisco patients with AIDS. Science 1984; 225:840–842.
13. Popovic M, Sarngadharan MG, Read E, et al. Detection, isolation, and continuous production of cytopathic retroviruses (HTLV-III) from patients with AIDS. Science 1984; 224:497–500.
14. Safai B, Sarngadharan MG, Groopman JE, et al. Seroepidemiological studies of human T-lymphotropic retrovirus type III in acquired immunodeficiency syndrome. Lancet 1984; i:1438–1440.
15. Weiss SH, Goedert JJ, Sarngadharan MB, et al. Screening test for HTLV-III (AIDS agent) antibodies: specificity, sensitivity, and applications. JAMA 1985; 253:221–225.
16. Goedert JJ, Sarngadharan MG, Biggar RJ, et al. Determinants of retrovirus (HTLV-III) antibody and immunodeficiency conditions in homosexual men. Lancet 1984; ii:711–716.
17. Masur H, Michelis MA, Greene JB, et al. An outbreak of community-acquired Pneumocystis carinii pneumonia: initial manifestation of cellular immune dysfunction. N Engl J Med 1981; 305:1431–1438.
18. Gottlieb MS, Schroff R, Schanker HM, et al. Pneumocystis carinii pneumonia and mucosal candidiasis in previously healthy homosexual men. N Engl J Med 1981; 305:1425–1431.
19. Siegal FP, Lopez C, Hammer GS, et al. Severe acquired immunodeficiency in male homosexuals manifested by chronic perianal ulcerative herpes simplex lesions. N Engl J Med 1981; 305:1439–1444.
20. Centers for Disease Control. Update on acquired immune deficiency syndrome (AIDS)—United States. MMWR 1982; 31:507–514.
21. Centers for Disease Control. Revision of the case definition of acquired immunodeficiency syndrome (AIDS) for national reporting—United States. MMWR 1985; 34:373–375.
22. Morgan WM, Selik RM, Hardy AM, et al. Current trends of AIDS in the United

States. Presented at the International Conference on Acquired Immunodeficiency Syndrome (AIDS), Atlanta, April 1985.

23. Hardy AM, Allen JR, Morgan WM, et al. The incidence rate of acquired immunodeficiency syndrome in selected populations. JAMA 1985; 253:215–220.

24. Curran JW, Morgan WM, Hardy AM, et al. The epidemiology of AIDS: current status and future prospects. Science 1985; 229:1352–1357.

25. Centers for Disease Control. Changes in premature mortality—New York City. MMWR 1985; 34:669–671.

26. Miller B, Stansfield SF, Zack MM, et al. The syndrome of unexplained generalized lymphadenopathy in young men in New York City. JAMA 1984; 251:242–244.

27. Klein RS, Harris CA, Small CB, et al. Oral candidiasis in high-risk patients as the initial manifestation of the acquired immunodeficiency syndrome. N Engl J Med 1984; 311:354–358.

28. Morris L, Distenfeld A, Amorosi E, et al. Autoimmune thrombocytopenic purpura in homosexual men. Ann Intern Med 1982; 96:714–717.

29. Centers for Disease Control. Antibodies to a retrovirus etiologically associated with acquired immunodeficiency syndrome (AIDS) in populations with increased incidences of the syndrome. MMWR 1984; 33:377–379.

30. Centers for Disease Control. Update: acquired immunodeficiency syndrome in the San Francisco cohort study, 1978–1985. MMWR 1985; 34:573–575.

31. Spira TJ, Des Jarlais DC, Marmor M, et al. Prevalence of antibody to lymphadenopathy-associated virus among drug-detoxification patients in New York. N Engl J Med 1984; 311:467–468.

32. Weiss SH, Ginzburg HM, Goedert JJ, et al. Risk for HTLV-III exposure and AIDS among parenteral drug abusers in New Jersey. Presented at the International Conference on Acquired Immunodeficiency Syndrome (AIDS), Atlanta, April 1985.

33. Ramsey RB, Palmer EL, McDougal JS, et al. Antibody to lymphadenopathy-associated virus in hemophiliacs with and without AIDS. Lancet 1984; ii:397–398.

34. Evatt BL, Gomperts ED, McDougal JS, et al. Coincidental appearance of LAV/HTLV-III antibodies in hemophiliacs and the onset of the AIDS epidemic. N Engl J Med 312:483–486, 1985; 312:483–486.

35. Ward JW, Grindon AJ, Feorino PM, et al. Laboratory and epidemiologic evaluation of an enzyme immunoassay for antibodies to human T-lymphotropic virus, type III. (submitted)

36. Cooper DA, Gold J, MacLean P, et al. Acute AIDS retrovirus infection: definition of a clinical illness associated with seroconversion. Lancet 1985; i:537–540.

37. Jaffe HW, Darrow WW, Echenberg DF, et al. The acquired immunodeficiency syndrome in a cohort of homosexual men: a six year follow-up study. Ann Intern Med 1985; 103:210–214.

38. Fishbein DB, Kaplan JE, Spira TJ, et al. Unexplained lymphadenopathy in homosexual men: a longitudinal study. JAMA 1985; 254:930–935.

39. Abrams DI, Lewis BS, Beckstead JH, et al. Persistent diffuse lymphadenopathy in homosexual men: end point or prodrome? Ann Intern Med 1984; 100:801–808.

40. Jaffe HW, Feorino PM, Darrow WW, et al. Persistent infection with human T-lymphotropic virus type III/lymphadenopathy-associated virus in apparently healthy homosexual men. Ann Intern Med 1985; 102:627–628.

41. Groopman JE, Salahuddin SZ, Sarnagadharan MG, et al. HTLV-III/LAV in saliva of people with AIDS related complex and healthy homosexual men at risk for AIDS. Science 1984; 226:447–449.

42. Zagury D, Bernard J, Leibowitch J, et al. HTLV-III in cells cultured from semen of two patients with AIDS. Science 1984; 226:449–451.

43. Fujikawa LS, Salahuddin SZ, Palestine AG, et al. Isolation of human T-cell leukemia/lymphotropic virus type III (HTLV-III) from the tears of a patient with acquired immunodeficiency syndrome (AIDS). Lancet 1985; ii:529.

44. Ho DD, Byington RE, Schooley RT, et al. Infrequency of isolation of HTLV-III virus from saliva in AIDS. N Engl J Med 1985; 313:1606.

45. Darrow WW, O'Malley P, Jaffe HW, et al. Risk factors for HTLV-III/LAV seroconversion in a cohort of homosexual male clinic patients. Presented at the International Conference on Acquired Immunodeficiency Syndrome (AIDS), Atlanta, April 1985.

46. Harris C, Cabridilla C, Robert-Guroff M, et al. Immunodeficiency and HTLV-III/LAV serology in heterosexual partners (HP) of AIDS patients (pts.) Presented at the International Conference on Acquired Immunodeficiency Syndrome (AIDS), Atlanta, April 1985.

47. Van de Perre P, Clumeck N, Carael M, et al. Female prostitutes: a risk group for infection with human T-lymphotropic virus type III. Lancet 1985; ii:524–526.

48. Centers for Disease Control. Heterosexual transmission of human T-lymphotropic virus type III/lymphadenopathy-associated virus. MMWR 561–563, 1985; 34:561–563.

49. Harris CA, Small CB, Klein RS, et al. Needle sharing as a route of transmission of the acquired immune deficiency syndrome. Presented at the Twenty-third Interscience Conference on Antimicrobial Agents and Chemotherapy, Las Vegas, October 1983.

50. McGrady G, Gjerset G, Kennedy S. Risk of exposure to HTLV-III/LAV and type of clotting factor used in hemophilia. Presented at the International Conference on Acquired Immunodeficiency Syndrome (AIDS), Atlanta, April 1985.

51. LaPointe N, Michaud J, Pekovic D, Chausseau JP, Dupuy JM. Transplacental transfusion of HTLV-III virus. N Engl J Med 1985; 312:1325–1326.

52. Cowan MJ, Hellmann D, Chuchwin D, et al. Maternal transmission of acquired immune deficiency syndrome. Pediatrics 1984; 73:382–386.

53. Ziegler JB, Cooper DA, Johnson RO, et al. Postnatal transmission of AIDS-associated retrovirus from mother to infant. Lancet 1985; i:896–898.

54. Anonymous. Needlestick transmission of HTLV-III from a patient infected in Africa. Lancet 1984; ii:1376–1377.

55. Centers for Disease Control. Update: evaluation of HTLV-III/LAV infection in health-care personnel—United States. MMWR 1985; 38:575–578.

56. Centers for Disease Control. Recommendations for preventing transmission of infection with human T-lymphotropic virus type III/lymphadenopathy-associated virus in the work place. MMWR 1985; 34:682–695.

57. Centers for Disease Control. Prevention of acquired immunodeficiency syndrome (AIDS): report of inter-agency recommendations. MMWR 1983; 32:101–104.

58. Rouzioux C, Chamaret S, Montagnier L, et al. Absence of antibodies to AIDS virus

in haemophilics treated with heat-treated factor VIII concentrate. Lancet 1985; i:271–272.

59. Centers for Disease Control. Provisional public health service inter-agency recommendations for screening donated blood and plasma for antibody to the virus causing acquired immunodeficiency syndrome. MMWR 1985; 34:1–5.

60. Centers for Disease Control. Declining rates of rectal and pharyngeal gonorrhea among males—New York City. MMWR 1984; 33:295–297.

61. Judson FN, Lemaster FI. Fear of AIDS and rates of gonorrhea in Denver, Colorado. Presented at the International Conference on Acquired Immunodeficiency Syndrome (AIDS), Atlanta, April 1985.

62. McKusik L, Horstman W, Coates TJ. AIDS and sexual behavior reported by gay men in San Francisco. Am J Public Health 1985; 75:493–496.

63. Cohn DL, Muldrou MA, Root CJ, et al. AIDS awareness and changes in sexual activity of patients in a metropolitan STD clinic. Presented at the Twenty-fifth Interscience Conference on Antimicrobial Agents and Chemotherapy, September 1985.

64. Scott GM, Fischl MA, Khmas N, et al. Mothers of infants with the acquired immunodeficiency syndrome: evidence for both symptomatic and asymptomatic carriers. JAMA 1985; 253:363–366.

65. Stewart GJ, Tyler JPP, Cunningham AL, et al. Transmission of human T-lymphotropic virus type-III (HTLV-III) virus by artificial insemination by donor. Lancet 1985; ii:581–584.

66. Centers for Disease Control. Recommendations for assisting in the prevention of perinatal transmission of human T-lymphotropic virus type III/lymphadenopathy-associated virus and acquired immunodeficiency syndrome. MMWR 1985; 34:721–732.

67. Centers for Disease Control. Testing donors of organs, tissues, and semen for antibodies to T-lymphotropic virus type III/lymphadenopathy-associated virus. MMWR 1985; 34:294.

68. Ho DD, Rota TR, Schooley RT, et al. Isolation of HTLV-III from cerebrospinal fluid and neural tissues of patients with neurologic syndromes related to the acquired immunodeficiency syndrome. N Engl J Med 1985; 313:1493–1497.

69. Hardy AM, Rauch K, Echenberg D, et al. The economic impact of the first 10,000 cases of acquired immunodeficiency syndrome in the United States. JAMA 1986; 255:209–211.

70. Weiss SH, Saxinger WC, Rechtman D, et al. HTLV-III infection among health care workers: association with needle-stick injuries. JAMA 1985; 254:2089–2093.

71. McCray E. Occupational risk of the acquired immunodeficiency syndrome among health care workers. N Engl J Med 1986; 314:1127–1132.

Epidemiology of Human Retroviruses and Related Clinical Conditions

Robert J. Biggar
International AIDS Epidemiology
Environmental Epidemiology Branch
National Cancer Institute
National Institutes of Health
Bethesda, Maryland

Retroviruses are a class of RNA viruses first identified in animals early in this century. For a variety of reasons, it proved difficult to identify retroviruses in humans. In 1980, however, following a methodological breakthrough in culture techniques for T-lymphocytes, the first human retrovirus was reported by Poiesz and his co-workers.[1] Shortly thereafter, a second agent, similar but not identical, was found.[2] But it was not until 1984 that the scope and importance of human retroviruses became dramatically emphasized with the establishment that a human retrovirus was responsible for the acquired immunodeficiency syndrome (AIDS).[3]

History and Nomenclature

The first human retrovirus to be discovered was called the human T-cell leukemia/lymphoma virus (HTLV) because it was isolated from a subject with this condition and because it was tropic for T-lymphocytes.[1] Epidemiological observations continue to show an association between this agent and adult T-cell lymphoma/leukemia (ATL), a malignancy rare in the United States but more common in parts of southern Japan and the Caribbean.[4] Recently, it has been suggested that the spectrum of illnesses following infection with this agent may include a tropical neurological illness, idiopathic tropical spastic hemiplegia or paraplegia,[5] but the evidence to support this association needs confirmation. Both ATL and tropical paraplegia are rare even among those with evidence of exposure to the infection, and it appears that most seropositive subjects have no evidence of clinical abnormality.

With the discovery of the second human retrovirus in 1980, the nomenclature was modified to indicate their sequence of discovery, HTLV-I representing the first virus, and HTLV-II the new virus. It was still appropriate to consider these as human T-leukemia/lymphoma viruses because the second agent, virologically distinct but related to HTLV-I, was isolated from a patient with hairy cell leukemia of the T-cell type.[2] However, there is no disease, malignant or otherwise, that has been formally established as being related to this virus. In part, the disease association and natural history of HTLV-II have been difficult to establish because of the cross-reactivity in the antibody to this agent with that from the apparently more common HTLV-I antibody.

The third human retrovirus was described by French workers in 1983.[6] Since it was first isolated from a homosexual man with a lymphadenopathy syndrome thought to be related to AIDS, they named the virus "lymphadenopathy-associated virus" (LAV) and speculated that it could be the cause of AIDS. Soon, repeated isolations of what proved to be an almost identical virus emerged, and technological advances facilitated the continuous production of the agent, enabling the development of sensitive serological techniques that clearly established the causal role of the virus in AIDS in 1984.[7,8] This agent was also T-lymphotropic, but was not thought to be a cause of leukemia/lymphoma per se. To accommodate the existing abbreviation, the name given by the National Cancer Institute for this agent was the human T-lymphotropic virus type III, HTLV-III.[3] In addition, it was independently isolated by workers in San Francisco and named AIDS-related virus (ARV).[9]

This trail of discoveries indicates that there are likely to be other human retroviruses discovered in the near future. The HTLV-III genome, for example, is quite different from HTLV-I and HTLV-II, but shares some distant homology with other animal retroviruses, including visna, a lentivirus of sheep.[10] Retroviruses similar but not identical with those of humans have also been isolated from nonhuman primates.[11-13] These agents, called simian T-lymphotropic viruses type I (STLV-I) and III (STLV-III) in analogy to their human counterparts, share considerable molecular similarity with HTLV-I and HTLV-III, as well as T-cell tropism. STLV-III appears to be widespread among the green monkeys of Africa, but is not known to cause illness among them.[14] In some primate species (i.e., rhesus) not naturally infected in the wild but capable of becoming infected when colony-housed, infection may result in an immunological abnormality and secondary opportunistic infections in a manner similar to that of AIDS in humans.[15] Emerging studies suggest that STLV-III itself may be a composite of variants. Among humans, antibody against STLV-III isolates is said to be common in parts of Africa, but it is unclear if these antibodies reflect true infection or cross-reactivities to other unknown agents or other factors. Recently, a variant quite similar to STLV-III has been isolated from humans in Africa (P. Kanki, personal communication). Aspects of this virus (HTLV-IV) are discussed in other chapters of this book.

Serology

A general profile of the virology and immunology of these agents is presented in the chapter by Gallo and Streicher. However, epidemiology and natural history studies depend heavily on the technical considerations, especially with respect to serology, and it will be necessary to review some aspects of the testing systems.

The most commonly used test for the presence of antibodies against the HTLVs has been the enzyme-linked immunosorbant assay (ELISA). However, methodological problems can introduce variation into the results by different tests. The antigen preparation may vary in its concentration, especially since there are no widely available tools for measuring the number of infectious units per unit volume. Also, there may be variation introduced by the methods of culture such that the extracts may vary in the amount of subcomponent polypeptides recovered to become the antigen. Finally, the plate system itself may introduce variation because the plastics used may have some capability of retaining antibody nonspecifically.

Despite these potential problems, ELISA screening has proven to be a very useful screening mechanism for detecting antibodies against these retroviruses. Among its many advantages are the sensitivity of the assay, the speed of obtaining results, the capability of being automated for large-scale screening programs, and the economy in terms of requiring only minute amounts of reagents, including antigen. However, it remains a screening assay that will require confirmation by other tests before definitive results can be applied to the assessment of the exposure status of any individual.

The degree of error depends on two factors: the type of test used and the population to be studied. The test itself is capable of being loaded with antigen in such a way as to be extraordinarily sensitive to any suggestion of antibody. Such a test is required for the screening of blood donors, for example, in which there should be, as nearly as possible, no chance of an infected unit entering the blood supply. The drawback of such a test is that it will also have a higher proportion of nonspecific positive results. Among nonrisk group blood donors, for example, less than one-third of those repeatedly positive in the sensitive screening ELISA will be confirmed by more specific tests.[16] Since positive screening results are relatively rare among nonrisk group donors, however, this "loss" from exclusion of positive screening bloods is acceptable, as is the cost of conducting further confirmation assays on such results. However, in AIDS-risk populations, reactivity in this assay is usually confirmed.[17]

In some populations living in areas such as Africa and northern South America where malaria and other parasitic diseases are endemic, there are nonspecific reactivities in very sensitive assays that create serious problems with interpreting the results.[18-20] These appear to be more common in persons with high antibody titers against malaria.[18] The cause is unknown because there is no cross-reactivity between malaria antibodies and HTLV-III, but recurrent malaria induces formation of multiple autoantibodies as well as hypergammaglobulinemia, and one or more of these may be contributing. It is also possible that cross-reactive retroviruses may be prevalent in some of these areas as well. The reactivity can be recognized as nonspecific by a variety of confirmation assays. The newer ELISA systems are able to discriminate accurately between reactivity of this type and HTLV-III-specific reactivity.

Confirmation tests are intended to be specific, even at the expense of sensitivity. Most widely used of these are the Western blot, a method in which virus polypeptides are applied to a gel, electrophoresed to separate them by migration properties (principally molecular weight), transferred to paper strips, and exposed to serum with possible antibody.[21] The pattern of adherence between the antibody and band of polypeptide allows recognition of the reactivity profile of the antibody being produced. This method has been particularly good for visualizing reactivity against the lower molecular weight polypeptides.

The general pattern of Western blot reactivity is that gag proteins (p24 and p55) are seen earliest after seroconversion, to be followed within weeks to months by a variety of other virus-associated proteins.[22,23] However, Western blot analyses do not provide clear delineation of higher molecular weight polypeptides, of which the virus envelope proteins (p120 and p160) are especially important.[23a] To observe these, a radioimmunoprecipate (RIP) blot is done.

The strip preparations themselves will vary in the amount of polypeptide applied and, depending on the culture harvest, even on the relative amount of various polypeptides within the batch. If strips to be used for the Western blot are heavily loaded with protein, the results will enhance sensitivity for specific protein but also bind some antibody nonspecifically, potentially yielding a nonspecific "confirmation." Such reactions are usually weak and have a banding pattern that, while showing reactions, is atypical for the usual profile seen with a seropositive risk group member. Since these tests are intended to provide proof of specificity, it is important to restrict the designation of "positive" to those sera that have a profile essentially equal to that of the known positive control, even while recognizing that sera yielding atypical results could represent either nonspecificity, unusual variants of true positivity, or reactivity to related but different retroviruses.

Several alternative testing approaches may be useful in special circumstances. Among the best is the competitive inhibition system.[24] These tests have been applied most widely in HTLV-I and HTLV-II, but they are also used in HTLV-III. There are methodological questions in the competition inhibition assays that relate to the purity of the reagents used and to the degree of the reduction required to consider a sample as specifically completed. Finally, there are immunofluorescence tests. Performed with an internal control (uninfected cells of the same type on each slide), they can provide impressive evidence of specificity; although in the face of nonspecific immunofluorescence, patterns can be very difficult to interpret.[19]

As is obvious in a rapidly progressing field, more recently developed tests are a large improvement over earlier versions of the same tests. Thus, sera from Africa that proved difficult to analyze because of nonspecificity now can be routinely screened with assurance that the results, while needing confirmation for clinical application, provide a reasonable approximation of the general seroepidemiological profile. Furthermore, advances in technology have enabled many of the polypeptide components of the virus to be isolated with a high degree of purity and even to be molecularly cloned. Availability of these proteins is now enabling the development of new tests based on reactivity to these subcomponents. While these will be of value in helping to verify the specificity of reactivity to those fractions of the virus and in establishing titers, their practical usefulness as screening agents remains to be established since it needs to be shown that any single or subtotal fractional test will detect all of the positives detected by the complete profile, the ultimate function of a screening assay.

HTLV-I

Epidemiology of Clinically Related Conditions

Almost simultaneous with the discovery of HTLV-I, Japanese researchers were describing a new entity, adult T-cell leukemia/lymphoma (ATL).[25] Cases of ATL have now been reported from many areas of the world, but are a substantial fraction of lymphoma cases only in two areas (southern Japan and the nations in or around the Caribbean).[4] Many of the patients with ATL from outside of these areas have been born there. In both areas, patients are generally middle-aged adults (mean 45 years; range 18 to 85 years), with an equal distribution by sex.[4]

The clinical features of typical ATL include leukemia (85% of cases), generalized lymphadenopathy (80%), bone marrow involvement (59%), hepatosplenomegaly (58%), and skin involvement (49%). The skin involvement was the initial manifestation that attracted attention as being unusual, appearing in some cases to resemble a form of mycosis fungoides or cutaneous T-cell lymphoma. In addition, there is evidence for a problem in calcium metabolism, including hypercalcemia (63%) and lytic bone lesions (18%) that are not attributable to the direct effects of malignant involvement. It is speculated that the tumor cells in some cases may be excreting an osteoclast-activating factor.[4]

The histological appearance of the malignant cells is that of a pleomorphic, polylobulated lymphocyte. Although diverse in appearance, the cells can be shown to be clonal in origin.[26] The immunological phenotype is usually T3$^+$, T4$^+$, and T8$^-$.[27] Thus, it is basically of the T-cell helper cell phenotype. Despite the helper phenotype, the great majority of ATL cells act as suppressor cells in vitro, at least in the pokeweed mitogen-induced immunoglobulin test.[27] The significance of this to reports that patients with ATL frequently have opportunistic infections is uncertain. In contrast to other T-cell lymphomas, ATL cells also have receptors for interleukin-2 (originally called T-cell growth factor), and the presence of this receptor is highly correlated with the presence integrated HTLV-I in the genome of the cell.[26]

In addition to the association with ATL, HTLV-I seropositivity has been observed in up to 70% of patients with a rare neurological condition seen in the Caribbean region.[5] This condition, tropical spastic hemiplegia or paraplegia, has no known cause. Since only a subset of patients with this condition are seropositive, HTLV-I is unlikely to be the sole cause. However, assuming the seropositivity is due to specific reactivity, it could play a contributing role or simply reflect common exposures. It is also possible that the reactivity observed is nonspecific, related either to another undiscovered retrovirus or to cross-reactivity to other antigens. In this regard, the correlation between parasitemia and nonspecific reactivity in some of the early ELISA tests should be recalled.

Seroepidemiology

Serological studies of the general populations have shown that those areas with ATL generally also have a high prevalence of HTLV-I, but there are some noteworthy exceptions. Southern Japan and the Caribbean Basin, both areas with a high prevalence of HTLV-I, also have a high frequency of ATL. In contrast, Africa, also with an apparently high incidence of HTLV-I, has a relatively low frequency of ATL.[4] The specificity of the HTLV-I reactivity seen in African sera has recently been challenged,[18-20] which might explain the discrepancy. Alternatively, there may be underdiagnosis of ATL or variation in the natural history of HTLV-I infection in Africa. In a series of lymphoma patients from Africa, there has been no difference in HTLV-I seropositivity between cases and controls (personal data), but it should be noted that ATL is a rapidly fatal malignancy and the case series were prevalence-based rather than incidence-based. Certainly, some of the results reported from seroepidemiological studies in Africa have yielded results no longer considered reliable, but there are still discordant results being reported from various laboratories employing different techniques and it is, therefore, difficult to assess the final profile.

In summary, even in areas with high rates of ATL, the overall HTLV-I seropositivity seems to be no higher than 5 to 10%, with positivity increasing with age and possibly being slightly more common in females. In the low risk areas, such as most of the United States (areas bordering the Caribbean may be slightly higher) and Europe, positivity is less than 1%. Variation between nearby villages in Japan and elsewhere have been interpreted to suggest clustering, such as by person-to-person transmission. In household studies, wives of seropositive husbands are more likely to be positive than either wives of seronegative men or husbands of seropositive women, suggesting that transmission may occur through male/female sexual activity and be more efficient male to female than female to male.[4,26] Recent data also indicate that transmission may occur by male/male sexual activity (W.A. Blattner, personal communication). Transmission may also occur by transfusion and probably by needle-sharing among intravenous drug abusers, who are a subpopulation in the United States with a relatively high prevalence of HTLV-I antibodies.[28]

Children of seropositive women are more likely to be seropositive than those of seronegative women, which suggests that in utero or perinatal transmission may be important modes of spread.[29,30] Postnatal infection of the infant may also be possible since the virus has been isolated from breast milk. So far, however, evidence of infection via this route is lacking in humans. Such transmission has been demonstrated among nonhuman primates.[31]

Conceptually, it remains difficult to completely explain the epidemiology of HTLV-I with the currently available information. If accurate, HTLV-I is relatively difficult to spread, but a few percent of the populations of high prevalence areas will be infected (often without any known exposure source), as will be a fraction of a percent of persons in low risk areas all over the world. Incidence increases with age, yet among Japanese men over 40 years old, prevalence is reported to plateau, whereas among women, it continues to increase. There is a genetically related virus in some primates, STLV-I,[11] but seropositive humans do not appear to have had any contact with such animals in most cases. No insect or animal vectors are known. The mystery of how this virus has spread worldwide and its relationship to diseases may be clarified with the development of more specific and sensitive tests.

HTLV-II

This orphan virus has been hidden from view by the overlapping serological reactivity with the more common HTLV-I antibodies. Serologically, confirmation by competition inhibition or some other assay is required, but the reagents for HTLV-II testing are not widely available. On the basis of isolation attempts, HTLV-II is apparently rare, but this may be because there is no information as to which risk groups/disease types are most likely to be infected. Further screening of hairy cell leukemia patients proved unrewarding, although it should be noted that the original isolate was made from a patient with the very rare T-cell variety (fewer than 20 cases ever reported), whereas those subsequently examined were probably all of the more common B-cell type. The only clearly identified risk group is that of intravenous drug abusers, among whom as many as 10 to 20% in some areas may be seropositive.[28] Indeed, it was among this group that the second isolate was made.[32] Further studies to define specific disease associations and establish the epidemiology have been hampered by the limited availability of specific serological reagents.

HTLV-III and AIDS

Epidemiology of Clinically Related Conditions

In 1981, a number of reports[33-36] first documented the occurrence of unusual diseases related to immunosuppression among young men in the large urban areas, especially New York, San Francisco, and Los Angeles. Most clearly unusual were *Pneumocystis carinii* pneumonia and Kaposi's sarcoma, both illnesses rarely observed among persons in the prime of life without underlying immune disorders. It was striking that the patients were almost all homosexual or bisexual men, with the exception of a few intravenous drug-abusing men.

Following the clinical leads, immunologists soon determined that these patients had a profound abnormality of the immune system, most consistently measurable as a inverted T-lymphocyte helper cell-to-suppressor cell ratio. In the normal individual, helper cells outnumber suppressor cells by a margin of approximately 1.8:1. In these patients, the ratio was usually well below 0.5:1, mainly because of a striking loss of the helper cell component. In addition, functional assays of the immune system were able to show in vitro dysfunction, indicating that the principal defect was an abnormality of the T-helper cell, although there were also abnormalities of other components, not all of which have been fully explained yet. In summary, there was ample evidence both in vivo and in vitro that these patients were severely immunosuppressed.

Thus emerged the epidemic now called AIDS. As greater awareness of the problem spread within the medical community, clinicians were able to extend the range of illnesses recognized among these men to include a wide range of life-threatening infections. These were fungal diseases and virus infections, particularly of the herpesvirus class, already recognized to be problems in immunosuppressed persons, but organisms previously seldom seen to be human pathogens, such as *Mycobacterium avium-intracellulare* and cryptosporidia were also observed.[37,38]

Surveillance and Registry Data

In order to standardize the definition of AIDS for public health purposes, the Centers for Disease Control (CDC) constructed a somewhat restricted surveillance definition of "AIDS," which was limited to life-threatening opportunistic infections and/or Kaposi's sarcoma in persons below the age of 60 years (after which age, Kaposi's sarcoma of a form unrelated to the current epidemic becomes increasingly frequent). (See Appendix: CDC Definition of AIDS.) This public health definition of AIDS, formulated prior to certainty about the etiology, excluded other less severe clinical problems that were being recognized in the same risk groups, principally the appearance of a persistent, generalized lymphadenopathy (PGL),[39,40] also labeled lymphadenopathy syndrome (LAS), and a group of nonlife-threatening illnesses commonly seen in immunosuppressed persons (labeled "lesser AIDS"), which includes herpes zoster, oral thrush, and idiopathic thrombocytopenia.[41] Tuberculosis due to the usual varieties of mycobacteria that cause disease in humans has also been reported.[41,42] In addition, to accommodate observations that non-ill members of the same risk groups had measurable immunological abnormalities, a new definition, AIDS-related complex (ARC), was created, in which the patients were required by definition to have both clinical and immunological abnormalities.[42a] Because of their importance to public health authorities attempting to monitor the epidemic, many of these definitions have persisted. However, now that the cause of AIDS and the related syndromes and immunological abnormalities have been established, these terms may need to be redefined to require evidence of HTLV-III/LAV involvement.

Using the original CDC definition of AIDS, the progression of the epidemic has been dramatic. From retrospective surveys,[43] it appears that the first cases occurred in the United States about 1978/1979 (Fig. 1). Earlier cases may have occurred in Europe, since there are at least two reports of CDC-defined cases among persons previously living in Africa. In general, the incidence of AIDS in Europe appears to be about 10% of that in the United States, and the epidemic curve is following a similar profile but lagging about 2 years behind.[44]

Since 1981, AIDS cases have doubled in number about every 6 months during the first few years, but at a slower rate (every 11 months) by 1985.[46] By the end of 1985, more than 16,000 cases had been reported (Table 1), and, unless there is an unexpected reversal, at least 16,000 more will occur in 1986 alone. Proportionally, *Pneumocystis carinii* pneumonia continues to dominate the list of diagnoses, with more than 60% of cases reporting this illness as the initial life-threatening event. However, the proportional frequency of Kaposi's sarcoma as the initial manifestation has declined steadily over the years.[46] The reasons are not altogether clear. It is now clear that this manifestation is significantly more common (three-fold) among homosexual men than in all other risk groups combined,[47] but the proportion of AIDS cases that are homosexual men has not declined dramatically so far. Thus, it appears that, even among homosexual men, there are proportionally fewer cases of Kaposi's sarcoma than at the onset of the epidemic.

The etiology of Kaposi's sarcoma is not known. Recognized over a century ago to be more common among persons of Jewish and Mediterrean origin,[48] it

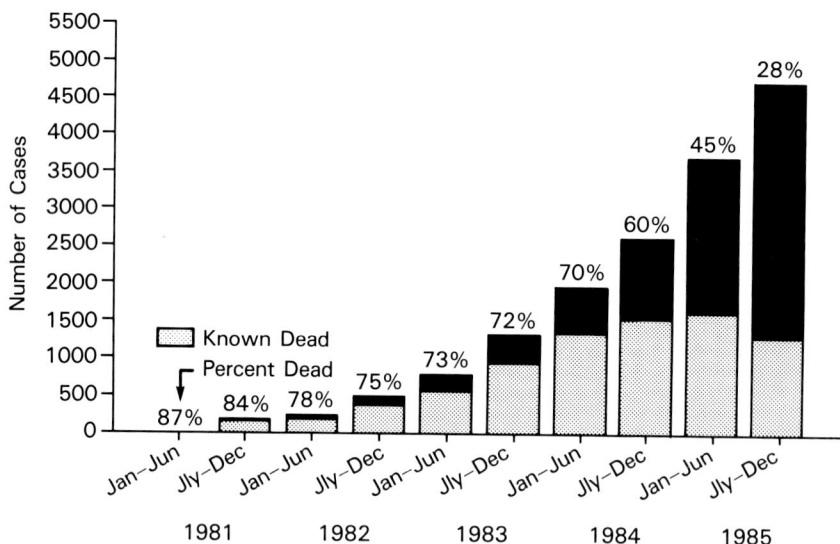

FIGURE 1   AIDS cases by half-year of diagnosis (January 6, 1986; n = 16,138). *Source:* Centers for Disease Control, Atlanta, Georgia (U.S. data).

also has a high prevalence in the population of east/central Africa.[49] Incidence in the pre-AIDS era (0.3 per 100,000 in men; 0.07 per 100,000 in women in the United States) was already three-fold greater in males than females,[50] but in that period, almost all the cases were among the elderly. These "endemic" variety cases appear histologically indistinguishable from the "epidemic" variety seen in AIDS cases, both being characterized by spindle-shaped malignant cells thought to be of endothelial origin and a vascular proliferation.[51]

Clinically, however, the endemic variety is generally nodular, involves the limbs mainly, and progresses only slowly. In contrast, the epidemic variety presents generally as plaques, involves the face and trunk as well as internal organs (particularly the gastrointestinal tract from mouth to rectum) and lymph nodes, and is rapidly progressive. Laboratory studies have shown that the endemic form of Kaposi's sarcoma, whether in non-AIDS risk subjects in the United States, Europe, or Africa, cannot be ascribed to either immunosuppression[52] or HTLV-III/LAV infection.[53] The difference in presentation and prognosis may be related to failure of the compromised immune system in AIDS patients to control a latent disease commonly held in check by the normal immune system. Certainly, even before the epidemic, the AIDS-related form of Kaposi's sarcoma emerged in the early 1980s, Kaposi's was recognized to be a significant complication of immunosuppressive drugs, and in transplant recipients, improvement of the immune system by discontinuation of

TABLE 1   AIDS Cases by Sex and Age at Diagnosis[a]

	Number	Proportion (%)
Sex		
Male	14,880	94
Female	1,029	6
Age (Years)		
<13	229	1
13–19	71	<1
20–29	3,371	21
30–39	7,596	47
40–49	3,355	21
≧50	1,516	9

[a]January 6, 1986; n = 16,138.
Source: Centers for Disease Control, Atlanta, Georgia (U.S. data).

immunosuppressive drugs was associated with improvement or remission of the Kaposi's sarcoma.[48]

In addition to Kaposi's sarcoma, there also may be an association between HTLV-III infection and lymphomas, particularly of B cells with undifferentiated morphology. These tumors are discussed in detail elsewhere in this book. Initially, they were described as Burkitt-like tumors,[54] and an exceptional propensity for developing these tumors in the brain was noted.[55] More recently, the range of histologies described in these lymphomas has broadened to include several varieties of high grade non-Hodgkin's lymphomas (large cell, immunoblastic, lymphoblastic, and Burkitt-like).[56] The CDC now accepts this condition as part of the definition of AIDS when there is evidence of HTLV-III infection as well. It is difficult to assess the strength of this association on the basis of case reports. Analysis of tumor registry data has indicated that in the early years of the AIDS epidemic, there was no significant increase in such tumors (with the exception of the Burkitt-like tumors) in a population clearly at extraordinary risk of getting Kaposi's sarcoma.[57] In 1984, a modest increase was observed in the same group (unpublished data), and it may be that the earlier case reports were harbingers of an association that has a long latent period.

Other tumors have been reported in the risk groups that have AIDS, but their association with HTLV-III or immunodeficiency is unclear. In most instances, they are probably unrelated to the current epidemic since there is no indication in tumor registry data that rates of such tumors are increasing in a manner parallel to the epidemic.[57] Some additional associations are discussed in the chapter by Jaffe et al. Further evaluation of any possible association will require careful epidemiological studies rather than case reports, since it is obvious that with the number of persons now infected with HTLV-III, unrelated cancers will occur frequently.

Risk Groups

In addition to the greater understanding of the clinical dimensions of AIDS, the development of a national surveillance network contributed to the recognition of other groups that were at risk of developing this condition (Table 2). Initially and still today in the United States, homosexual men constitute the greatest percentage of the patients (70 to 75%), but intravenous drug abusers are also involved (15 to 20%). In 1982, the first cases were reported among hemophiliacs, especially those treated for their coagulation disorder with factor VIII concentrate.[58] In addition, Haitian and African patients with diseases that fit the strict CDC AIDS profile began to be observed both in the United States[59] and Europe.[44] Investigations in Haiti[60] and the central African nations of Rwanda[61] and Zaire[62] were able to confirm that cases indigenous to

TABLE 2 Proportion of Adult AIDS Cases by Risk Group[a]

Risk group[b]	Total (%)
Male homosexual	73
IV drug user	17
Transfusion	2
Hemophiliac	1
Heterosexual contact	1
Other/Unknown	6

[a]January 6, 1986; n = 15,909.
[b]Risk group classified according to the most frequently seen risk association; for example, a homosexual drug user with AIDS would be attributed to the homosexual risk group.
Source: Centers for Disease Control, Atlanta, Georgia (U.S. data).

those countries could be found in local hospitals, and that the immune deficiency in those cases resembled closely the profile seen in AIDS cases in the United States. Furthermore, although incidence data were weak, it appeared from the timing of Africans cases referred to Europe that the condition was new to both areas.[63] In addition, it was also soon observed that cases were appearing in subjects who had been transfused with blood or blood products in earlier years.

Beyond these recognized groups, there have always been a number of patients who could not be attributed to a risk group category. Some of these were subjects in whom interview information was considered unreliable because, for example, the patient was critically ill or was diagnosed only at autopsy. Others appeared to have endemic Kaposi's sarcoma unrelated to AIDS, albeit under the age of 60 years. But in approximately half (3% of all AIDS patients), the patient denied any risk group factors. Demographically, these patients resemble drug abusers in that they are concentrated in New York and New Jersey metropolitan areas, tend to be black and Hispanic, and are of lower socioeconomic class. Whether they may represent inaccurate classification or heterosexual transmission from drug-abusing persons remains unclear. These cases provide important indices of the degree to which AIDS might be spreading in the general community and are closely monitored by the CDC. So far there has been a steady increase in the number of such cases, but the proportion relative to all AIDS cases has not increased, probably because the incidence in the risk group members with whom these nonrisk group members are compared has risen so dramatically.

Pathogenesis

It was initially difficult to verify the causal relationship between HTLV-III/LAV and AIDS. While the virus was first isolated from a homosexual man with lymphadenopathy[6] and subsequently from other homosexual men and AIDS patients,[3,7] such subjects were known to harbor many opportunistic virus infections as a consequence of their immunodeficiency. Likewise, cross-sectional studies showing that antibodies against this agent were more likely in AIDS patients than controls could not attribute this to a causal relationship since antibodies to many viruses were higher in titer and more frequent in such patients.[64] Two major observations confirmed the relationship to be a causal one. In a study of transfusion-associated AIDS cases,[65] it was repeatedly possible to find a seropositive donor if sera from all the donors to which the patients had been exposed were available; and in prospective studies of homosexual men,[66,67] only those who had pre-existing exposure, as demonstrated by antibodies, went on to develop the immunodeficiencies and clinical syndromes of AIDS. This convincing evidence of the causal role for HTLV-III in AIDS has enabled a rapid progression of the understanding of the biology of this condition and the risk factors that influence spread of the virus.

HTLV-III can gain access to the cell through the T4 receptor of the helper T cell.[68] Other cells probably also have this receptor. It is clear that some cells in the central nervous system can become infected, but the precise cell type is still unknown.[69-71] In addition, access through other receptors may be possible since some cell lines lacking T4 receptors appear to be capable of being infected in vitro. After infection, the T4 cell population declines gradually.[72,73] There are no clear factors yet shown to influence the rate of decline in vivo, but since this appears to vary from individual to individual, there may be such factors. Among those speculated to influence this are host variations (such as HLA type), frequency of lymphocyte-activating events (such as infections and exposures to foreign antigens), and co-infections with other viruses.

In association with acute infection, symptoms generally similar to mononucleosis but sometimes including encephalopathy may be seen, although probably most infections are asymptomatic. During the period when the immune system is weakened, a number of minor clinical abnormalities, which include the spectrum of diseases seen in lesser AIDS, PGL/LAS, and ARC, may occur. At some point, probably varying with the environmental exposure to infectious agents as well as the residual functional capacity of the remaining cells, the subject will develop a life-threatening opportunistic infection. In this sense, Kaposi's sarcoma should be considered an opportunistic disease to which these persons are susceptible, although no infectious cause is known. From this point onward, the patient is classified as having AIDS. Often more than one infection occurs simultaneously. Even if the clinical problem is controlled through medication, the underlying immune abnormality will not be corrected, and the patient will be subject to repeated problems until one is sufficiently severe or resistant to therapy for death to occur.

Natural History

Animal experiments and prospective epidemiological studies have quantified many aspects of the natural history. The incubation period between exposure and specific antibody production is uncertain. In chimpanzees, animals make antibody within 3 to 12 weeks after parenteral exposure,[74-76] the timing and titer being related to dose of exposure. In humans, antibodies probably appear within the same time, but certainty on this point is confused by occasional reports, still needing confirmation, of virus isolation in an at-risk person months or even more than a year before antibody appears. After parenteral exposure from blood transfusion, antibody appears in 4 to 7 weeks, but there is little known about the appearance of antibodies following sexual exposure.[77]

The frequency of acute illness following HTLV-III infection is unclear, but probably most illnesses are too mild to bring the patient to medical attention. Antibodies against HTLV-III are generally not detectable at the start of illness, appearing from 1 to 3 weeks after illness onset.[78,78a,78b] Symptoms, which generally last about 10 to 14 days, may include fever, fatigue, pharyngitis (sometimes ulcerative), myalgia, arthalgias, rash, and headache.[78,78b,79] Acute encephalopathy, sometimes profound, has also been observed.[78b,80] The importance of central nervous system involvement by HTLV-III is discussed elsewhere in this book. Lymphadenopathy is not uncommon and is variable in extent and timing, being both an early and persistent abnormality in some persons.[77]

The first immunological abnormalities are an elevation in suppressor T cells, to be followed over time by a decline in helper T cells.[23,72,73] Thus, the ratio of helper-to-suppressor cells, being a function of both parameters, is one of the earliest indicators of immunological abnormality. Normally about 1.8:1, less than 5% of HTLV-III-negative healthy subjects will have a ratio of less than 1:1, whereas more than 90% of one group of homosexual men seropositive for more than 3 years had ratios below 1:1.[73] Risk of AIDS development is related to helper cell number rather than suppressor cell number.[68] Among

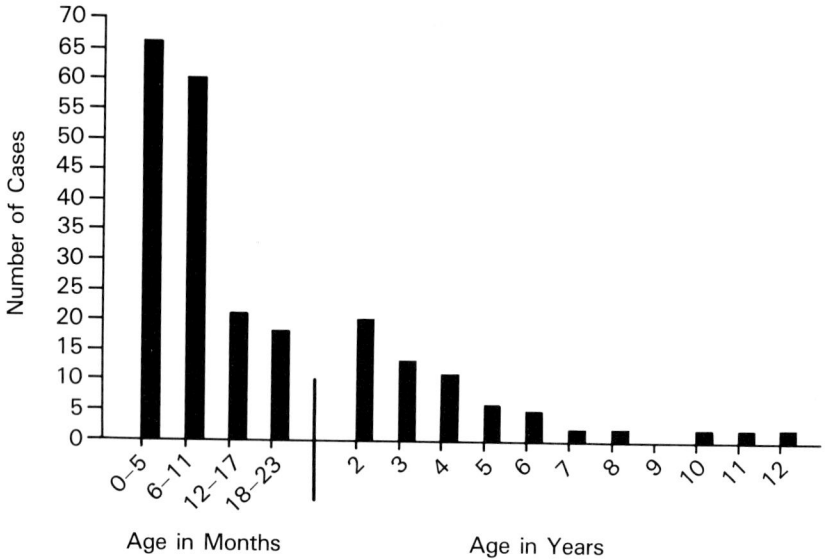

FIGURE 2   Pediatric AIDS cases by age at diagnosis (January 6, 1986; n = 229). *Source:* Centers for Disease Control, Atlanta, Georgia (U.S. data).

seropositive homosexual men with absolute helper cell counts initially below 300/dl, at least 40% were diagnosed with AIDS within 3 years (J.J. Goedert, personal communication).

There are few reports of AIDS in adults known to be infected less than a year, but children appear to run an accelerated course, with the mean age of AIDS development after transfusion exposure as a newborn being 14 months[81] (Fig. 2). Among adults from all AIDS risk groups known to be seropositive for at least 3 years (duration of infection prior to that time unknown), at least 15 to 20% have developed AIDS,[82] and there is no indication that the rate of AIDS development has peaked. Once AIDS has been diagnosed, the average survival is about 1 year, with more than 80% dying within 3 years (Table 3).[46] Most of the long-term survivors have been patients diagnosed only with Kaposi's sarcoma, among whom the immunological abnormality does not appear to be as severe as it is among those developing opportunistic infections.

Seroepidemiology

Risk factors for seroconversion among the various risk groups are fairly well delineated. These will be examined in detail in each risk group, but as a whole, they are directly related to injection of biological products or to homosexual or

TABLE 3 Initial Condition Diagnosed as AIDS Among Adult Cases[a]

Condition	Proportion occurring (%)	Still alive (%)
Both KS and PCP	6	36
KS without PCP	19	62
PCP without KS	57	48
Other conditions	19	45

[a]January 6, 1986; n = 15,909.
Source: Centers for Disease Control, Atlanta, Georgia (U.S. data).
KS = Kaposi's sarcoma; PCP = *Pneumocystis carinii* pneumonia.

heterosexual venereal exposure. There is very little evidence of exposure resulting in infection from any other routes. Although the virus has been isolated from several body fluids such as saliva,[83] tears,[84] and breast milk,[85] there are only rare instances when these fluids are thought to be the route of exposure, and the epidemiological evidence indicates that these are an extremely unlikely vehicle of transmission. It may be that the virus, being quite acid-labile, is destroyed by the normal acidity of the gastric juices. In one instance, breast milk, from which virus can also be cultured, was implicated in transmitting the virus to a nursing infant.[86] Possibly the lack of acidity in the infant stomach and/or the acid-neutralizing capacity of a breast milk diet enabled this infection to occur.

Homosexual men: Among homosexual men, the overwhelming risk factors for being seropositive are the number of partners and frequency of anal-receptive intercourse.[66,67] In areas distant from communities in which HTLV-III infection is frequent, number of partners from the endemic areas supplants total number of partners as being the important risk factor.[66] Other measures that correlate with these factors, such as nitrite inhalant use and fisting (the act of inserting the hand into the anus), will also correlate with seropositivity as they are surrogate measures of anal intercourse. Practices done in preference to anal-receptive intercourse, such as anal-insertive intercourse and oral intercourse, are inversely correlated with seropositivity when that risk is compared with members of the same community who practice anal-receptive intercourse. Even among those denying anal intercourse, there is some risk of seropositivity and AIDS, although the risk appears relatively small and may be because of inaccurate lifestyle information.[87]

The implication of these data is that HTLV-III is spread between homosexual men by exposure to semen, particularly through anal intercourse. This is biologically plausible since the virus has been isolated from semen.[88,89] The degree of risk following oral exposure to HTLV-III-containing semen is difficult to estimate since subjects in most studies performed both oral and anal intercourse.

Following exposure, there are no factors established as influencing progression to immunodeficiency except duration of infection,[68] but the studies examining this question have been based on relatively small numbers of seropositive men. Likewise, factors that influence which clinical manifestation of AIDS will occur first are unknown. Since Kaposi's sarcoma appears to be particularly common as a manifestation of AIDS among seropositive homosexual men,[47] it is tempting to speculate that there may be a necessary co-infection with another agent; so far, however, no such agent has been found. Alternatively, nitrite inhalants have been shown to be mutagenic, and there is some suggestion that homosexual men who develop Kaposi's sarcoma have a history of greater recreational exposure to nitrite inhalants than those who develop opportunistic infections.[90]

Hemophiliacs: The dominant risk factor among hemophiliacs is exposure to commercially produced factor VIII concentrate.[91-93] Cryoprecipitate concentrate is produced by processing the plasma of several thousand donors in batches, and it seems clear that the concentration procedure also efficiently concentrates the virus. Retrospective studies have shown that hemophiliacs began to seroconvert as early as 1979, and that the seroconversion rate increased rapidly in 1981 and 1982,[94,95] to the extent that by 1986 at least 70% of severe hemophiliacs treated during this period with commercial factor VIII concentrate are now seropositive.[91,92] Even among the more mild hemophiliacs, one-third are seropositive. Some countries produce their own factor VIII concentrate, and in one study,[95a] investigators estimated that as few as one or two infectious donors to the entire pool resulted in a batch of factor VIII concentrate that infected half of the recipients. Factor VIII produced commercially in Europe is often made from plasma collected in the United States and, therefore, shared the same infectiousness as factor VIII made in the United States.

Commercially produced factor IX concentrate is also prepared from plasma cryoprecipitates from thousands of donors. Hemophilia B patients treated with this product during the early 1980s have a 20 to 40% prevalence of antibodies against HTLV-III. Whether the lower rate is due to a difference in infectiousness between factor VIII and factor IX or simply to less intensive use of factor IX is unknown. Patients (including those with other bleeding disorders such as von Willebrand's disease) who are treated with either unconcentrated factor products or fresh blood products share the risk of exposure to HTLV-III in proportion to the intensity of exposure.

Initially, it was hoped that the reactivity seen in hemophiliacs might represent immunization with noninfectious parts of the virus, or that lack of co-factors such as venereal and other infections might limit the risk of developing AIDS in this subgroup. However, adjusted for time of exposure, so far, hemophiliacs have followed the same progression to immunodeficiency and AIDS as other risk groups.[82] Prior to the AIDS epidemic, a method of heat-treating the factor products to inactivate the hepatitis virus was developed. This process also appears to be effective in inactivating HTLV-III and has been in standard use since 1985. The currently produced factor concentrates, while more expensive because heat treatment also inactivates some of the coagulation efficiency of the products, are generally considered to be free of infectious HTLV-III,[96-98] although the certainty of this has recently been questioned.[98a]

Contaminated needle contact: Among intravenous drug abusers, use of shared, contaminated needles is presumed to be the major risk factor. The degree of risk with needle-sharing depends on the type of exposure. Hardly any health care workers stuck with needles used on AIDS and HTLV-III-positive subjects have seroconverted.[99] However, drug addicts have vastly greater exposure to shared needles and may further enhance their risk by the practice of "booting," in which blood is drawn back into the syringe to extract any remaining drug in the needle or syringe. The variation in seropositivity between communities of drug addicts in different cities is huge—from none to half of all addicts in treatment programs, with those in New York City and adjacent communities in New Jersey being highest (S.H. Weiss, personal communication). The variation in seroprevalence by community argues that risk is related directly to some aspect of needle-sharing with a drug community with a high HTLV-III prevalence since exposure to other possible risk factors, such as prostitution to support their drug habit, is probably similar in different communities.

Blood product transfusion and transplantation: Transfusion-associated AIDS cases were reported prior to the discovery of the causal role of HTLV-III. Infection required exposure to as little as a single risk group donor. In view of this, blood banks formulated policies to discourage risk group members from blood donation. With the availability of the HTLV-III antibody assay, it has become possible to identify donors who have antibodies (and are, therefore, potential carriers); but the policy requesting risk group members to refrain from donating continues because testing results could be falsely negative and because donors can be infectious prior to the time they develop antibodies.[100,101] Risk to the recipient depends on exposure to a single infectious donor, and the probability of this happening increases with the number of donors to which the recipient has been exposed. Never very high, this risk has dropped to almost zero with the institution of widespread testing.

Exposure to other biological products must be regarded as potential routes of infection. Obviously, organ transplantation involves blood transfusion, for example. Although never shown, exposure to even blood-free transplanted tissues, such as the lens, should be considered potentially hazardous since the virus has been isolated from tear fluid.[84] Exposure to seminal fluid resulted in infection among women artificially inseminated from an HTLV-III-infected donor.[101] Gammaglobulin or other biological products derived from humans have not been definitely associated with HTLV-III transmission, but recent publications suggest the possibility on rare occasions, and this must be carefully monitored in new products. Of initial concern was the hepatitis B vaccine material, but there is no evidence of greater HTLV-III infection in vaccine recipients than controls.[102]

Heterosexual transmission: In the United States and Europe, there is evidence for some degree of heterosexual transmission. The plausibility of such infections has been demonstrated by animal models as well as in women infected by insemination from a seropositive donor.[103] In humans, about 10% of the wives of seropositive hemophiliacs are themselves seropositive,[104,105] presumably as a result of sexual exposure since they are the only family members who are seropositive. Female prostitutes in some cities have an increased prevalence of antibodies,[105a,106] but such women often have other exposures, particularly to intravenous drug abuse, that make interpretation difficult. Still, more than 200 women whose only admitted risk factor was sexual exposure to a man who was a risk group member have developed AIDS.[46] The biological plausibility of female-to-male transmission has recently been enhanced by the demonstration that HTLV-III can be isolated from cervical secretions.[106a,106b] The risk of female-to-male transmission is thought to be low, but there are at least 43 AIDS cases among men whose only admitted exposure was sex acts with a female risk group member (including prostitutes).[46,106]

In central Africa and Haiti, heterosexual transmission appears to be the major route of exposure.[63] Seroprevalence studies have shown that males and females are equally positive, and that seropositivity is restricted to those persons who are in the sexually active ages (unpublished data). Prostitutes in HTLV-III endemic areas of Africa have a high prevalence of antibody,[107,108] and there is some evidence that men who frequent prostitutes and/or have many female sexual partners are more likely to be seropositive.[109] Other routes of exposure, including homosexual sex acts, needle exposure, transfusions and "vectors," do not explain the seroepidemiology now being seen in these regions.[63] However, as HTLV-III infection becomes common, other routes of transmission in Africa, such as exposure through blood transfusion and maternal-infant infection, will increase.

Maternal-infant infection: Infants born to mothers who are seropositive are at increased risk of infection,[81,110,111] as are second children born to mothers who have already had a child with AIDS.[81] The point at which infection occurs is not established, but in the majority it is probably in utero. However, one instance of postnatal infection, probably through breast milk, has been reported.[86]

Nonsexual/nonblood transmission: The risk of becoming infected through casual contact is negligible. A small proportion of AIDS patients, perhaps 3%, deny exposure to known risk factors,[46] but the credibility of these denials may be questionable in some cases. Extensive studies of the families of seropositive hemophiliacs[93,104,112] indicate no risk to household members other than sexual partners. Hospital employees and researchers who have had prolonged and extensive casual physical contact with AIDS patients and AIDS risk group members or who work in a laboratory environment in which exposure to HTLV-III have occurred remain seronegative despite years of exposure.[99,113]

Exceptional cases that indicate nonsexual/nonblood exposure can occur, but the type of exposure is not casual. Examples of such cases include the infant who apparently seroconverted after exposure to breast milk from a seropositive mother,[101] a mother who provided (without any precautions) colostomy and wound dressing care for a seropositive retarded child with multiple birth defects,[114] a nurse who provided home nursing care involving extensive contact with body fluids from a terminally ill African patient with AIDS,[115] and the spouse of an elderly seropositive hemophiliac who denied any sexual contact with her husband for many years. As the number of cases increases, examples of nonsexual/nonblood product transmission will no doubt increase, perhaps to sufficient levels that new routes of transmission may be deduced. Nevertheless, from the few examples of such transmission described, it can be seen that this type of transmission involves unusual, high-intensity exposures unlike anything that the average citizen would experience, and even with these unusual exposures, transmission is rare. These examples further support the concept that this virus is not transmitted by casual contact.

Projecting the Future

The profile of the AIDS epidemic to date can be well understood by the current understanding of HTLV-III transmission. The origin of the HTLV-III virus is not known, but it probably arose as a mutant of another as yet unknown human or animal retrovirus.[63] The widespread distribution in central Africa has promoted the idea that it arose there, but there is no proof of this; indeed, available evidence supports the idea that it is new in Africa as well, appearing about the same time as in the United States and Europe.[63]

Following the adaption of this new agent to the human host, the virus was transmitted readily through sexual activity and exposure to blood and other biological products. The route by which the virus spread through various communities depended on the frequency of opportunities to spread. Thus, subgroups of the community who were first recognized as at increased risk of developing AIDS were those who engaged in sexual activity with greater numbers of partners than did the usual community members.

Blood products also served to spread the agent both nationally and internationally. Individuals only now known to be at risk of carrying HTLV-III frequently served as blood donors before the recognition of an infectious agent in this epidemic. Their donations would have been added to the plasma pools used to make factor VIII, and since this process efficiently concentrates the virus, it resulted in extensive infection of the commercial factor VIII concentrate-using hemophiliac population throughout the world.[116] Simple blood transfusion also contributed, especially to women and children. Among men, where other risk factors, such as homosexuality, drug abuse, and hemophilia, dominated exposure risk, the proportion attributed to blood donations was small. But for women and infants, transmission via transfusion was considerable. Women were also exposed in the United States and Europe through sexual intercourse with seropositive hemophiliacs, drug abusers, and bisexual men. Because of the exceptional increases in the other groups, the proportion of AIDS cases who were female (7%) remained low despite gradually increasing numbers. From these women, infants were born who developed AIDS. It is also probable that these women sometimes transmitted HTLV-III to their male sexual partners. Data from Africa indicate that heterosexual transmission may occur efficiently enough to sustain the epidemic spread of HTLV-III in the general population. Whether there are particular factors in Africa, such as number of partners or concomitant venereal disease, that enhance the probability of transmission is unknown.

Within the United States, estimates of the number of seropositive persons vary from 500,000 to 2 million persons. Extrapolating from the number of AIDS cases, between 50,000 and 200,000 persons in Europe may be positive. In Africa, there are no reliable data. However, if 5 to 10% of urban populations in central Africa are seropositive, this adds several hundred thousand seropositive persons. From natural history studies in the United States, at least 20% of seropositive persons (and probably more) will develop AIDS.[82] Thus, within the next few years, there may be as many as several hundred thousand AIDS cases worldwide, most of whom will progress to death within 1 to 2 years. (See also the chapter by Hardy and Curran.) In addition, there may be diseases other than AIDS that are related to HTLV-III itself or to the immunosuppression associated with it, such as malignancies or neurological disorders, that will appear in the coming years. These sobering figures indicate the need for intervention strategies that will interrupt the dissemination of the virus and treat those already seropositive. Such strategies are discussed in other chapters of this book.

Acknowledgments

I am grateful for the comments on the manuscript by Drs. William A. Blattner, James J. Goedert, and Mads Melbye from the Environmental Epidemiology Branch, National Cancer Institute, Bethesda, Maryland.

Appendix: CDC Definition of AIDS

1. Presence of reliably diagnosed diseases at least moderately indicative of cellular immunodeficiency.
2. Absence of known causes of underlying reduced resistence to those diseases, other than that due to HTLV-III/LAV infection.

Diseases Considered at Least Moderately Indicative of Underlying Immunodeficiency

---

Protozoan infection
Pneumocystis carinii pneumonitis
Toxoplasma gondii encephalitis or disseminated infection (excluding congenital infection)
Chronic *Cryptosporidium* enteritis (>1 month)

Fungal diseases
Candida esophagitis
Candida bronchial infection (with positive HTLV-III test)
Cryptococcal meningitis or disseminated infection
Disseminated histoplasmosis (with positive HTLV-III test)
Chronic enteric Isosporiasis (with positive HTLV-III test)

Bacterial infection
Disseminated *Mycobacterium avium* complex or *M. Kansasii*

Noncongenital virus infections
Chronic mucocutaneous herpes simplex (>1 month)
Cytomegalovirus infection of an organ other than liver or lymph node
Progressive multifocal leukoencephalopathy

Cancers
Kaposi's sarcoma (positive test for HTLV-III required if age $\geqq 60$ years)
Primary brain lymphoma (limited to the brain)
Helminthic infections
Strongyloidiasis (disseminated beyond the gastrointestinal tract)
Other
Diffuse interstitial lymphoid pneumonitis (unless HTLV-III test is negative)

Source: Centers for Disease Control, Atlanta, Georgia, January 1986.

References

1. Poiesz BJ, Ruscetti FW, Gazdar AF, et al. Detection and isolation of type-C retrovirus particles from fresh and cultured lymphocytes of a patient with cutaneous T cell lymphoma. Proc Natl Acad Sci USA 1980; 77:7415–7419.
2. Kalyanaraman VS, Sarngadharan MG, Robert-Guroff M, et al. A new subtype of human T cell leukemia virus (HTLV-II) associated with a T cell variant of hairy cell leukemia. Science 1982; 218:571–573.
3. Popovic M, Sarngadharan MG, Read E, Gallo RC. Detection, isolation, and continuous production of cytopathic retrovirus (HTLV-III) from patients with AIDS and pre-AIDS. Science 1984; 244:497–500.
4. Blattner WA, Clark JW, Gibbs WN, et al. HTLV: epidemiology and relationship to human malignancy. In: Gallo RC, Essex M, Gross L, eds. Cancer cells, volume 3: human T cell leukemia viruses. New York: Cold Spring Harbor Press, 1984.
5. Gessain A, Barin F, Vernant JC, et al. Antibodies to human T-lymphotropic virus type-I in patients with tropical spastic paraparesis. Lancet 1985; ii:407–409.
6. Barré-Sinoussi F, Chermann JC, Rey F, et al. Isolation of a T-lymphotropic retrovirus from a patient at risk for acquired immune deficiency syndrome (AIDS). Science 1983; 220:868–870.
7. Gallo RC, Salahuddin SZ, Popovic M, et al. Frequent detection and isolation of cytopathic retroviruses (HTLV-III) from patients with AIDS and at risk for AIDS. Science 1984; 224:500–503.
8. Schupbach J, Popovic M, Gilden RV, Gonda MA, Sarngadharan MG, Gallo RC. Serological analysis of a subgroup of human T-lymphotropic retroviruses (HTLV-III) associated with AIDS. Science 1984; 224:503–505.
9. Levy JA, Hoffman AD, Kramer SM, et al. Isolation of lymphadenopathic retroviruses from San Francisco patients with AIDS. Science 1984; 225:840–842.
10. Chiu IM, Yaniv A, Dahlberg JE, et al. Nucleotide sequence evidence for relationship of AIDS retrovirus and lentiviruses. Nature 1985; 317:366–368.
11. Komuro A, Watanabe T, Miyoshi I, et al. Detection and characterization of simian retroviruses homologous to human T-cell leukemia virus type I. Virology 1984; 138:373–378.
12. Daniel MD, Letvin NL, King NW, et al. Isolation of T-cell tropic HTLV-III-like retrovirus from macaques. Science 1985; 228:1201–1204.

13. Kanki PJ, McLane MF, King NW Jr, Letvin NL, Hunt RD, Sehgal P, Daniel MD, Desrosiers RC, Essex M. Serologic identification and characterization of a macaque T-lymphotropic retrovirus closely related to HTLV-III. Science 1985; 228:1999–1201.

14. Kanki PJ, Kurth R, Becker W, Dreesman G, McLane MF, Essex M. Antibodies to simian T-lymphotropic retrovirus type III in African green monkeys and recognition of STLV-III viral proteins by AIDS and related sera. Lancet 1985; i:1330–1332.

15. Letvin NL, Daniel MD, Sehgal PK, et al. Induction of AIDS-like disease in macaque monkeys with T-cell tropic retrovirus STLV-III. Science 1985; 230:71–73.

16. Centers for Disease Control. Provisional public health service inter-agency recommendations for screening donated blood and plasma for antibody to the virus causing acquired immunodeficiency syndrome. MMWR 1985; 34:1–5.

17. Weiss SH, Goedert JJ, Sarngadharan MG, et al. Screening test for HTLV-III (AIDS-agent) antibodies: specificity, sensitivity, and applications. JAMA 1985; 253:221–225.

18. Biggar RJ, Gigase PL, Melbye M, Kestens L, Sarin P, Bodner AJ, Demedts P, Stevens WJ, Paluku L, Delacollette C, Blattner WA. ELISA HTLV retrovirus antibody reactivity associated with malaria and immune complexes in healthy Africans. Lancet 1985; ii:520–523.

19. Karpas A, Maayan S, Raz R. Lack of antibodies to adult T-cell leukaemia virus and to AIDS virus in Israeli Falashas. Nature 1986; 319:794.

20. Weiss RA, Cheingsong-Popov R, Clayden S, et al. Lack of HTLV-I antibodies in Africans. Nature 1986; 319:794–795.

21. Towbin H, Staehelin T, Gordon J. Electrophoretic transfer of proteins from polyacrylamide gels to nitrocellulose sheets: procedures and some applications. Proc Natl Acad Sci USA 1979; 76:4350–4354.

22. Sarngadharan MG, Popovic M, Bruch L, et al. Antibodies reactive with human T-lymphotropic retrovirus (HTLV-III) in the serum of patients with AIDS. Science 1984; 224:506–508.

23. Biggar RJ, Melbye M, Ebbesen P, Alexander S, Nielsen JO, Sarin P, Faber V. Variation in antibodies to human T cell lymphotropic virus III (HTLV-III) in homosexual men: decline prior to the onset of acquired immunodeficiency disease syndrome (AIDS). Br Med J 1985; 91:997–998.

23a. Barin F, McLane MF, Allan JS, Lee TH, Groopman JE, Essex M. Virus envelope protein of HTLV-III represents major target antigen for antibodies in AIDS patients. Science 1985; 228:1094–1096.

24. Serwadda D, Mugerwa RD, Sewankambo NK, et al. Slim disease: a new disease in Uganda and its association with HTLV-III infection. Lancet 1985; ii:849–852.

25. Takatsuki K, et al. Adult T-cell leukemia proposal as a new disease and cytogenetic, phenotypic, and functional studies of leukemic cells. Gann Monogr Cancer Res 1982; 28:13.

26. Blattner WA. Human retroviruses. In: Feigin RD, Cherry DS, eds. Textbook of pediatric infectious diseases. Philadelphia: W. B. Saunders, 1986.

27. Yamada Y. Phenotypic and functional analysis of leukemic cells from 16 patients with adult T cell leukemia/lymphoma. Blood 1983; 61:192.
28. Robert-Guroff M, Weiss SH, Giron JA, et al. Prevalence of antibodies to HTLV-I, -II, and -III in intravenous drug abusers from an AIDS endemic region. JAMA (in press).
29. Robert-Guroff M, Kalyanaraman VS, Blattner WA, et al. Evidence for HTLV-infections of family members of HTLV positive T cell leukemia-lymphoma patients. J Exp Med 1983; 157:248–258.
30. Hino S, Yamaguchi K, Katamine S, et al. Mother-to-child transmission of human T-cell leukemia virus type-I. Jpn J Cancer Res (Gann) 1985; 76:474–480.
31. Yamanouchi K, Kinoshita K, Moriuchi R, et al. Oral transmission of human T-cell leukemia virus type-I into a common marmoset (Callithrix jacchus) as an experimental model for milk-borne transmission. Jpn J Cancer Res (Gann) 1985; 76:481–487.
32. Hahn BJ, Popovic M, Kalyanaraman VS, et al. Detection and characterization of an HTLV-II provirus in a patient with AIDS. In: Gottlieb MS, Groopman JE, eds. Acquired immune deficiency syndrome. UCLA symposium on molecular and cellular biology, new series, volume 15. New York: Alan R. Liss, 1984:73–81.
33. Gottlieb MS, Schroff R, Schanker HM, et al. Pneumocystis carinii pneumonia and mucosal candidiasis in previously healthy homosexual men: evidence of a new acquired cellular immunodeficiency. N Engl J Med 1981; 305:1425–1431.
34. Masur H, Michelis MA, Greene JB, et al. An outbreak of community-acquired Pneumocystis carinii pneumonia: initial manifestation of cellular immune dysfunction. N Engl J Med 1981; 305:1431–1438.
35. Hymes KB, Cheung T, Greene JB, et al. Kaposi's sarcoma in homosexual men: a report of eight cases. Lancet 1981; ii:598–600.
36. Gottlieb GJ, Rayaz A, Vogel JV, et al. A preliminary communication on extensive disseminated Kaposi's sarcoma in young homosexual men. Am J Dermatopathol 1981; 3:111–114.
37. Masur H. Mycobacterium avium-intracellulare: another scourge for individuals with the acquired immunodeficiency syndrome. JAMA 1982; 248:3018.
38. Zakowski P, Fligiel S, Berlin OG, Johnson BL. Disemminated Mycobacterium avium-intracellulare in homosexual men dying of acquired immunodeficiency. JAMA 1982; 248:2980–2982.
39. Centers for Disease Control. Persistent, generalized lymphadenopathy among homosexual males. MMWR 1982; 31:249–251.
40. Metroka CE, Cunningham-Rundles S, Pollack MS, et al. Generalized lymphoadenopathy in homosexual men. Ann Intern Med 1983; 99:585–591.
41. Goedert JJ, Weiss SH, Biggar RJ, Landesman SH, Weber J, Grossman RJ, Robert Guroff M. Lesser AIDS and tuberculosis. Lancet 1985; ii:52.
42. Pitchenik AE, Cole C, Russell BW, Fischl MA, Spira TJ, Snider DE. Tuberculosis, atypical mycobacterium, and the acquired immunodeficiency syndrome among Haitian and non-Haitian patients in south Florida. Ann Intern Med 1985; 101:641–645.
42a. Quinn T. Early symptoms and signs of AIDS and the AIDS-related complex. In:

Ebbesen P, Biggar RJ, Melbye M, eds. AIDS. A basic guide for clinicians. Copenhagen/Philadelphia: Munksgaard/WB Saunders, 1985:69–83.

43. Allen JR. AIDS epidemiology, United States. In: Ebbesen P, Biggar RJ, Melbye M, eds. AIDS. A basic guide for clinicians. Copenhagen/Philadelphia: Munksgaard/WB Saunders, 1985:15–28.

44. Melbye M, Biggar RJ, Ebbesen P. Epidemiology—Europe and Africa. In: Ebbesen P, Biggar RJ, Melbye M, eds. AIDS. A basic guide to clinicians. Copenhagen/Philadelphia: Munksgaard/WB Saunders, 1985:29–41.

45. Centers for Disease Control. Update: acquired immunodeficiency syndrome—Europe. MMWR 1986; 35:35–46.

46. Centers for Disease Control. Update: acquired immunodeficiency syndrome—United States. MMWR 1986; 35:17–21.

47. Haverkos H, Drotman DP, Morgan M. Prevalence of Kaposi's sarcoma among patients with AIDS. N Engl J Med 1985; 312:1518.

48. Safai B, Good RA. Kaposi's sarcoma: a review and recent developments. Clin Bull 1980; 10:62–69.

49. Hutt MS. The epidemiology of Kaposi's sarcoma. Antibiot Chemother 1981; 29:3–8.

50. Biggar RJ, Horm J, Fraumeni JF Jr, Greene MH, Goedert JJ. Incidence of Kaposi's sarcoma and mycosis fungoides in the United States including Puerto Rico, 1973–81. J Natl Cancer Inst 1984; 73:89–94.

51. Safai B, Parris A, Urmacher C. Histopathology of Kaposi's sarcoma and other neoplasms. In: Ebbesen P, Biggar RJ, Melbye M, eds. AIDS. A basic guide for clinicians. Copenhagen/Philadelphia: Munksgaard/WB Saunders, 1985:123–131.

52. Kestens L, Melbye M, Biggar RJ, Stevens WJ, Piot P, de Muynck A, Taelman H, de Feyter M, Paluku L, Gigase PL. Endemic African Kaposi's sarcoma is not associated with immunodeficiency. Int J Cancer 1985; 36:49–55.

53. Biggar RJ, Melbye M, Kestens L, Sarngadharan MG, de Feyter M, Blattner WA, Gallo TC, Gigase P. Kaposi's sarcoma in Zaire is not associated with HTLV-III infection. N Engl J Med 1984; 311:1051–1052.

54. Ziegler JL, Drew WL, Miner RC, Mintz L, Rosenbaum E, Gershow J, Lennette ET, Greenspan J, Shillitoe E, Beckstead J, Casavant C, Yamamoto K. Outbreak of Burkitt's-like lymphoma in homosexual men. Lancet 1982; ii:631–633.

55. Ziegler JL, Beckstead JA, Volberding PA, et al. Non-Hodgkin's lymphoma in 90 homosexual men. Relation to generalized lymphadenopathy and the acquired immunodeficiency syndrome. N Engl J Med 1984; 311:565–570.

56. Boring CC, Brynes RK, Chan WC, et al. Increase in high-grade lymphomas in young men. Lancet 1985; i:857–859.

57. Biggar RJ, Horm J, Lubin JH, Goedert JJ, Greene MH, Fraumeni JF. Cancer trends in a population at risk of AIDS. J Natl Cancer Inst 1985; 74:793–797.

58. Centers for Disease Control. Pneumocystis carinii pneumonia among persons with hemophilia A. MMWR 1982; 31:365–367.

59. Viera J, Frank E, Spira TJ, Landesman SH. Acquired immunodeficiency in Haitians: opportunistic infections in previously healthy immigrants. N Engl J Med 1983; 308:125–128.

60. Pape JW, Liaulaud B, Thomas F, et al. Characteristics of the acquired immune deficiency syndrome in Haitians. N Engl J Med 1983; 309:945–950.
61. Perre P, Rouvroy D, Lepage P, Bogaerts J, Kestelyn P, Kayihigi J, Hekker AC, Butzler JP, Clumeck N. Acquired immunodeficiency syndrome in Rwanda. Lancet 1984; ii:62–65.
62. Piot P, Quinn TC, Taelman H, et al. Acquired immunodeficiency syndrome in a heterosexual population in Zaire. Lancet 1984; ii:65–69.
63. Biggar RJ. The AIDS problem in Africa. Lancet 1986; i:79–83.
64. Melbye M, Biggar RJ, Ebbesen P, Andersen HK, Vestergaard BF. Lifestyle and antiviral antibody studies among homosexual men in Denmark. Acta Pathol Microbiol Immunol Scand [Sect B] 1983; 91:357–364.
65. Jaffe HW, Sarngadharan MG, DeVico AL, et al. Infection with HTLV-III/LAV and transfusion associated acquired immunodeficiency syndrome. JAMA 1985; 254:770–773.
66. Melbye M, Biggar RJ, Ebbesen P, et al. Seroepidemiology of HTLV-III in Danish homosexual men: prevalence, transmission and disease outcome. Br Med J 1984; 289:573–575.
67. Goedert JJ, Sarngadharan MG, Biggar RJ, et al. Determinants of retrovirus (HTLV-III) antibody and immunodeficiency conditions in homosexual men. Lancet 1984; ii:711–716.
68. Kalish RS, Schlossman SF. The T4 lymphocyte in AIDS. N Engl J Med 1985; 313:112–113.
70. Ho DD, Rota TR, Schooley RT, Kaplan JC, Allan JD, Groopman JE, Resnick L, Felsenstein D, Andrews CA, Hirsch MS. Isolation of HTLV-III from cerebrospinal fluid and neural tissues of patients with neurologic syndromes related to the acquired immunodeficiency syndrome. N Engl J Med 1985; 313:1493–1497.
71. Carne CA, Tedder RS, Smith A, Sutherland S, Elkington SG, Daly HM, Preston FE, Craske J. Acute encephalopathy coincident with seroconversion for anti-HTLV-III. Lancet 1985; ii:1206–1208.
72. Schwartz K, Visscher BR, Dtel R, Taylor J, Nishauian P, Fahey JL. Immunological changes in lymphadenopathy virus positive and negative symptomless male homosexuals: two years of observation. Lancet 1985; ii:831–832.
73. Melbye M, Biggar RJ, Ebbesen P, et al. Long term HTLV-III seropositive homosexual men without AIDS develop measurable immunologic and clinical abnormalities. A longitudinal study. Ann Intern Med 1986; 104:496–500.
74. Alter HJ, Eichberg JW, Masur H, et al. Transmission of HTLV-III infection from human plasma to chimpanzees: an animal model for AIDS. Science 1984; 226:549–552.
75. Francis DP, Feorino PM, Broderson JR, et al. Infection of chimpanzees with lymphadenopathy-associated virus. Lancet 1984; ii:1276–1277.
76. Gajdusek DC, Amyx HL, Gibbs CJ, et al. Infection of chimpanzees by human T-lymphotropic retrovirus in brain and other tissue from AIDS patients. Lancet 1985; i:55–56.
77. Melbye M. The natural history of human T lymphotropic virus-III infection: the cause of AIDS. Br Med J 1986; 292:5–12.

78. Cooper DA, Gold J, Maclean P, Donovan B, Finlayson R, Barnes TG, Michelmore HM, Brooke P, Penny R. Acute AIDS retrovirus infection: definition of a clinical illness associated with seroconversion. Lancet 1985; i:537–540.

78a. Ho DD, Sarngadharan MG, Resnick L, et al. Primary human T-lymphotropic virus type III infection. Ann Intern Med 1985; 103:880–883.

78b. Biggar RJ, Johnson BK, Musoke SS, et al. Severe illness associated with HTLV-III seroconversion in an African. Br Med J 1986 (in press).

79. Tucker J, Ludlum CA, Craig A, Philp I, Steel CM, Tedder RS, Cheingsong-Popov R, Macnicol MF, McClelland DBL, Boulton FE. HTLV-III infection associated with glandular-fever-like illness in a haemophiliac. Lancet 1985; i:585.

80. Carne CA, Tedder RS, Smith A, Sutherland S, Elkington SG, Daly HM, Preston FE, Craske J. Acute encephalopathy coincident with seroconversion for anti-HTLV-III. Lancet 1985; ii:1206–1208.

81. Scott GB, Fischl MA, Klimas N, et al. Mothers of infants with the acquired immunodeficiency syndrome. Evidence for both symptomatic and asymptomatic carriers. JAMA 1985; 253:363–366.

82. Goedert JJ, Biggar RJ, Weiss SH, et al. Three-year incidence of AIDS in five cohorts of HTLV-III-infected risk group members. Science 1986; 231:992–995.

83. Groopman JE, Salahuddin SZ, Sarngadharan MG, Gonda M, Sliski A, Gallo RC. HTLV-III in saliva of people with AIDS-related complex and healthy homosexual men at risk for AIDS. Science 1984; 226:447–449.

84. Fujikawa LS, Salahuddin SZ, Palestine AG, Masur H, Nussenblatt RB, Gallo RC. Isolation of human T-lymphotropic virus type III from the tears of a patient with the acquired immunodeficiency syndrome. Lancet 1985; ii:529–530.

85. Thiry L, Sprecher-Goldberger S, Jonckheer T, et al. Isolation of AIDS virus from cell-free breast milk of three health virus carriers. Lancet 1985; ii:891–892.

86. Ziegler JB, Cooper DA, Johnson RO, Gold J. Postnatal transmission of AIDS-associated retrovirus from mother to infant. Lancet 1985; i:896–898.

87. Schekter MT, Boyko NJ, Douglas B, et al. Can HTLV-III be transmitted orally? Lancet 1986; i:379.

88. Zagury D, Bernard J, Leibowitch J, et al. HTLV-III in cells cultured from semen of two patients with AIDS. Science 1984; 226:449–451.

89. Ho DD, Schooley RT, Rota TR, et al. HTLV-III in the semen and blood of a healthy homosexual man. Science 1984; 226:451–453.

90. Haverkos HW, Pinsky PF, Drotman DP, Bregman DJ. Disease manifestation among homosexual men with acquired immunodeficiency syndrome (AIDS): a possible role of nitrites in Kaposi's sarcoma. Sex Transm Dis 1985; 12:203–208.

91. Melbye M, Froebel KS, Madhok R, et al. HTLV-III seropositivity in European haemophiliacs exposed to factor VIII concentrate imported from the USA. Lancet 1984; ii:1444–1446.

92. Goedert JJ, Sarngadharan MG, Eyster ME, et al. Antibodies reactive with human T-cell leukemia viruses (HTLV-III) in the sera of hemophiliacs receiving factor VIII concentrate. Blood 1985; 65:492–495.

93. Jason J, McDougal S, Holman RC, et al. Human T-lymphotropic retrovirus type

III/lymphadenopathy-associated virus antibody. Association with hemophiliacs immune status and blood component usage. JAMA 1985; 253:3409–3415.

94. Madhok R, Melbye M, Lowe GDO, et al. HTLV-III antibody in sequential plasma samples: from haemophiliacs 1974–84. Lancet 1985; i:524–525.

95. Eyster ME, Goedert JJ, Sarngadharan MG, et al. Development and early history of HTLV-III antibodies in persons with hemophilia. JAMA 1985; 253:2219–2223.

95a. Ludlum CA, Tucker J, Steel CM, et al. Human T-lymphotropic virus (HTLV-III) infection in seronegative haemophiliacs after transfusion of factor VIII. Lancet 1985; ii:233–236.

96. Rouzioux C, Charmaret S, Montagnier L, et al. Absence of antibodies to AIDS virus in haemophiliacs treated with heat-treated factor VIII concentrate. Lancet 1985; ii:271–272.

97. Moseler J, Schimpf K, Auerswald G, et al. Inability of pasteurised factor VIII preparations to induce antibodies to HTLV-III after long-term treatment. Lancet 1985; i:1111.

98. Felding P, Nelsson IM, Hansson BG, Biberfeld G. Absence of antibodies to LAV/HTLV-III in haemophiliacs treated with heat-treated factor VIII concentrate of American origin. Lancet 1985; ii:832–833.

98a. White GC, Matthews TJ, Weinhold KJ, et al. HTLV-III seroconversion associated with heat-treated factor VIII concentrate. Lancet 1986; i:611–612.

99. Weiss ST, Saxinger WC, Rechtman MH, et al. HTLV-III infection among health care workers: association with needle-stick injuries. JAMA 1985; 254:2089–2093.

100. Dodd RY, Sandler G. Transfusion-associated AIDS. In: Ebbesen P, Biggar RJ, Melbye M, eds. AIDS. A basic guide for clinicians. Copenhagen/Philadelphia: Munksgaard/WB Saunders, 1985:123–131.

101. Centers for Disease Control. Provisional public health service inter-agency recommendations for screening donated blood and plasma for antibody to the virus causing acquired immunodeficiency syndrome. MMWR 1985; 34:1–5.

102. Poiesz B, Tomar R, Lehr B, Moore J. Hepatitis B vaccine: evidence confirming lack of AIDS transmission. MMWR 1984; 33:685–687.

103. Stewart GT, Tyler JPP, Cunningham AL, et al. Transmission of human T-cell lymphotropic virus type III (HTLV-III) by artificial insemination by donor. Lancet 1985; ii:581–584.

104. Melbye M, Ingerslev J, Biggar RJ, et al. Anal intercourse as a possible factor in heterosexual transmission of HTLV-III to spouses of hemophiliacs. N Engl J Med 1985; 312:857.

105. Kreiss JK, Kitchen LW, Prince HE, et al. Antibody to human T-lymphotropic virus type III in wives of haemophiliacs. Ann Intern Med 1985; 102:623–626.

105a. Centers for Disease Control. Heterosexual transmission of human T-lymphotropic virus type III/lymphadenopathy-associated virus. Morbid Mortal Wk Rep 1985; 34:561–563.

106. Redfield RR, Markham PD, Salahuddin SZ, Wright DC, Sarngadharan MG, Gallo RC. Heterosexually acquired HTLV-III/LAV disease (AIDS-related complex and AIDS). JAMA 1985; 254:2094–2096.

106a. Vogt MW, Witt DJ, Craven DE, et al. Isolation of HTLV-III/LAV from cervical secretions of women at risk for AIDS. Lancet 1986; i:525–527.

106b. Wofsy CB, Cohen JB, Hauer LB, et al. Isolation of AIDS-associated retrovirus from genital secretions of women with antibodies to the virus. Lancet 1986; i:527–529.

107. Van de Perre P, Clumeck N, Carael M, et al. Female prostitutes: a risk group for infection with human T-cell lymphotropic virus type III. Lancet 1985; ii:524–526.

108. Kreiss JK, Koech D, Plummer FA, et al. AIDS virus infection in Nairobi prostitutes: spread of the epidemic in East Africa. N Engl J Med 1986; 314:414–418.

109. Clumeck N, Van de Perre P, Carael M, Rouvroy D, Nzaramba D, Heterosexual promiscuity among African patients with AIDS. N Engl J Med 1985; 313:182.

110. Cowan MJ, Hellman D, Chudwin D, et al. Maternal transmission of acquired immune deficiency syndrome. Pediatrics 1984; 73:382–386.

111. Centers for Disease Control. Recommendations for assisting in the prevention of perinatal transmission of human T-lymphotropic virus type III/lymphadenopathy associated virus and acquired immunodeficiency syndrome. MMWR 1985; 34:721–732.

112. Kaplan JE, Oleske J, Getshell JP, et al. Evidence against transmission of human T-lymphotropic virus/lymphadenopathy-associated virus (HTLV-III/LAV) in families with the acquired immunodeficiency syndrome. Pediatr Infect Dis 1985; 4:468–469.

113. Hirsh MS, Wormser GP, Schooley RT, et al. Risk of nosocomial infection with human T-cell lymphotropic virus III (HTLV-III). N Engl J Med 1985; 312:1–4.

114. Centers for Disease Control. Apparent transmission of human T-lymphotropic virus type-III/lymphadenopathy-associated virus from a child to a mother providing health care. MMWR 1986; 35:76–79.

115. Editorial: Needlestick transmission of HTLV-III from a patient infected in Africa. Lancet 1984; ii:1376–1377.

116. Tsuchie H, Kurimura T, Hinuma Y. Survey of the prevalence of AIDS-associated virus (LAV) infection in Japan. J Infect 1985; 10:272–276.

8

Psychiatric and Psychosocial Aspects of AIDS

David R. Rubinow
Biological Psychiatry Branch
National Institute of Mental Health
National Institutes of Health
Bethesda, Maryland

Russell T. Joffe
St. Michael's Hospital
and University of Toronto
Toronto, Ontario, Canada

The impact of acquired immunodeficiency syndrome (AIDS) on social consciousness is epitomized by its recent horror movie-like billing in *Life Magazine* (July 1985), "Now no one is safe from AIDS!" The terror and revulsion that AIDS seems capable of evoking are the product of reactions to all that AIDS has come to represent: the plague, infection, death, venereal disease, homosexuality, drug abuse, contamination, uncertainty. These associative aspects of AIDS are so pervasive that they have lead to the suggestion that AIDS is a psychological crisis as well as a medical crisis.[1] Many of the concerns expressed in the lay media have no basis in fact (see chapters by Hardy and Curran and by Biggar elsewhere in this book).

Precise description of the extent and nature of the impact of AIDS on behavior and psychological well-being clearly requires identification of the social groups under consideration. In this chapter, we will describe the impact of AIDS on several groups of people—AIDS patients, members of the high risk groups, the "public," and health care workers. We also will briefly review the AIDS-associated organic brain syndromes and their management, and discuss strategies that health care workers may employ when working with AIDS or AIDS-related complex (ARC) patients. Finally, particular aspects of the relationship between AIDS and alterations of cognition or behavior that require further research will be discussed.

AIDS Patients

The impact of AIDS on patients can be characterized as a pervasive and catastrophic loss of health, job, financial autonomy, normal life style, friends, and social supports. Peace of mind may be shattered by unresolved feelings about sexual preference, by guilt over exposing others to a devastating illness, or by the self-accusation experienced by many people with a serious illness. All of these factors can be amplified by the cruelty of others. Patients experience the loss of physical strength, mental acuity, control of life's activities, self-esteem, and, ultimately, life. Sexual activity, if not lost, is corrupted as it becomes identified as the mode of transmission of the illness. The specter of death for AIDS patients can create hopelessness; moreover, the ability of patients to negotiate the stages of dying and to deal with their illness and their anticipated death may be made more difficult by their frequent abandonment by family and friends. The despair, anger, anxiety, and loneliness experienced by AIDS patients do not pose surprises. It is also no surprise that AIDS patients vary greatly in their response to the illness, largely as a product of pre-illness personality, coping skills, the personal meaning of their illness, past experience with stress and illness, and availability of social support.

When the mood disturbances that have been reported in patients with AIDS[2-6] are evaluated, it is important to distinguish those emotional symptoms that are understandable and expectable from specific clinical psychiatric syndromes that may require different therapeutic interventions. For example, a major depression or anxiety disorder that may be amenable to treatment with conventional psychopharmacological agents should not be mistaken for the sadness and fear that occur in reaction to AIDS and its consequences. In this context, one must also constantly bear in mind that HTLV-III, the etiological agent, can infect the brain and cause organic disease. (See the chapter by Berger and Resnick.)

Alterations in mood and behavior have been reported to occur with increasing frequency in AIDS patients with central nervous system (CNS) complications. It has been suggested by some[7-9] that 70 to 80% of AIDS patients have CNS involvement and that one-third to two-thirds of these patients manifest clinical symptoms of this CNS involvement. The likelihood of CNS complications increases with time, although CNS symptoms may be the presenting manifestation of AIDS, and may antedate a proven immunodeficiency syndrome. Further, behavioral disturbances may be the first or most dramatic symptom of AIDS-related CNS involvement. These mood and behavioral disturbances include agitation, depression, apathy, socially inappropriate behavior, hallucinations, delusions, anxiety, and memory impairment. As has been reviewed elsewhere,[10] a variety of organic mental syndromes is seen in AIDS patients, including dementia, delirium, and organic personality syndrome. One of the most common of these syndromes is an indolent, progressive HTLV-III-induced CNS dysfunction called subacute encephalitis.[11] Subacute encephalitis may present as a delirium, or patients may appear to suffer from a mood disorder as their apathy, anergy, and withdrawal are mistaken for depression.[12] The syndrome progresses over time to a severe chronic encephalopathy characterized by dementia, seizures, and, finally, death.[11] These observations underscore once again how important it is that antiviral approaches to the therapy of AIDS include strategies for controlling the virus in the brain.

Obviously, management of AIDS-related mood and behavioral disturbances requires immediate identification of the major determinants of these disturbances, that is, "illness behavior" (reactions to having the illness), recurrence of premorbid psychopathology (e.g., substance abuse disorder), or an AIDS-related organic mental syndrome.

The distress accompanying the diagnosis of AIDS is most effectively managed by education, symptom relief, psychological support, and social assistance. Provision of pharmacological and behavioral strategies for management of pain and opportunistic infection-related somatic symptoms (e.g., gastrointestinal) may not only enhance the patient's physical comfort, but also may create a welcomed area of control in an otherwise uncontrollable illness and, therefore, may greatly diminish anxiety. The patient should be educated with respect to the following: the potential course and complications of his illness; options for therapeutic trials; permitted and proscribed practices to reduce the likelihood of viral transmission and ensure "safe sex;" and resources available for psychological support and social assistance. In general, psychological support may best be provided by asking and listening; one should actively inquire about the patient's problems, concerns, fears, and fantasies, and create an environment in which the patient feels comfortable expressing his/her myriad reactions and concerns. Many patients will, in addition, require formal psychological support in the form of support groups or individual psychotherapy. The profound stress that AIDS creates may precipitate interpersonal maladjustment, intensify pre-illness psychopathology, or reactivate earlier areas of personal conflict or distress. Thus, the patient with AIDS may receive less rather than more support from his/her significant others, may re-initiate or intensify substance abuse, may re-experience anxiety and guilt around areas of unresolved conflict (e.g., homosexuality, particularly if this is viewed as the behavior responsible for the acquisition of AIDS), or may express previously controlled rage through self-destructive acts (e.g., suicide) or acts injurious to others (e.g., increased promiscuity). Patients with AIDS, then, often require assistance negotiating help with family, friends, and society. Education and support must be supplemented with active efforts to identify problems and facilitate successful referral to ancillary treatment and social assistance agencies.

The importance of serving as a patient advocate in his social network is underscored by several recent studies demonstrating evidence of neuropsychological deficits in patients with AIDS, but without overt evidence of CNS involvement. In our study at the National Institute of Mental Health,[13] we performed standardized psychiatric interviews and neuropsychological evaluations on 13 AIDS patients and 13 medically well homosexual controls matched for age, sex, and level of education. At the time of testing, AIDS patients were relatively well and showed no clinical evidence of systemic infection or neurological complications. Several AIDS patients fulfilled diagnostic criteria for adjustment disorder with depressed mood at the time of evaluation, consistent with the high incidence of adjustment disorders reported in terminally ill cancer patients.[14] AIDS patients, compared with controls, had significantly lower full-scale IQ and verbal IQ scores on the Wechsler Adult Intelligence Scale—Revised (WAIS-R), a standard IQ test.[15] Furthermore, AIDS patients scored significantly lower on the vocabulary and the digit symbol subtests of the WAIS-R. In addition, AIDS patients, compared with controls, had significantly lower scores on tests of attention, concentration, and visual motor and visual-spatial performance. These neuropsychological data suggest that AIDS patients, relative to a group of age- and education-matched controls, show signs of generalized cerebral dysfunction and possibly localized cerebral dysfunction as evidenced by the reduced vocabulary subtest scores. Similar findings were reported by Tross et al.,[16] who observed impairment of motor and language skills, memory loss, and other forms of neuropsychological compromise in patients with AIDS, but without overt evidence of neurological complications. The full clinical significance of these preliminary findings is presently unclear. Nonetheless, the isolation of the HTLV-III virus from the brains and CSF[17,18] of patients with AIDS, as well as the recent description of an HTLV-III receptor in brain,[19] suggest that the neuropsychological dysfunction evident in the studies by Joffe et al.[13] and Tross et al.[16] may represent a clinical expression of HTLV-III infection of the CNS. This possibility is supported by several reports of HTLV-III viral syndromes involving the CNS in the absence of other clinical or laboratory evidence of AIDS.[20,21]

The general management recommendations for the AIDS patient (outlined previously) require modification when there is evidence of an organic brain syndrome. Treatment under these conditions is directed toward identifying the causes of the delirium or dementia and improving or eliminating them to the greatest extent possible. Management consists of several elements. First, the patient must be protected from self-harm by providing a safe, closely monitored, physical environment in the case of the hospitalized patient, or by arranging support services to assist the outpatient with routine tasks of daily living, such as shopping or taking medications. Second, pharmacotherapy may be required to mitigate suffering or control dangerous behavior. Psychotropic agents should be prescribed with appropriate caution and with recognition that the CNS side effects of these agents are far more common in the brain-damaged and the elderly.[22,23] Acute symptoms of psychosis and/or agitation may be effectively controlled in hospitalized patients by titrating low doses of a neuroleptic such as haloperidol (0.5 to 1.0 mg every 30 minutes to 1 hour).[24] One-half to two-thirds of the dose required during the first 24 hours may be sufficient thereafter to manage these symptoms. For patients with dementia or organic personality syndrome, a low dose of neuroleptic (e.g., 1 or 2 mg of haloperidol) administered at bedtime may improve sleep and reduce behavioral lability and anxiety. Minor tranquilizers should, in general, be avoided in patients with organic mental syndrome because these medications may paradoxically disinhibit the patient and/or exacerbate cognitive or behavioral symptoms of the organic mental syndrome. Finally, a structured environmental program should be developed to assist the organically impaired AIDS patient in his or her adaptation to their impairment. In the hospital, such a program consists largely of frequent explanation and reorientation. Information should be presented clearly and repeatedly to the patient, with the expectation that much may quickly be forgotten. Patients should be frequently reoriented to time and place, and should be provided with orienting objects (e.g., calendar or familiar items from home). Familiar faces (friends, family, or staff with whom the patient feels comfortable) may reduce anxiety and can, with the other orientation measures mentioned, dramatically reduce the amount of psychotropic medication required.[25] At home, the family and friends can perform a similar reorientation process and assist the organically impaired patient with tasks of daily living. Family and friends, therefore, must be carefully educated about the problems that the AIDS patient with CNS dysfunction may manifest, such as impaired memory, reduced concentration, labile mood, irritability, and inability to perform or sustain a variety of activities. It is important to acknowledge to these significant others that caring for a patient with dementia may be both demanding and frustrating. The reorientation and support that can be provided by community and social service groups should not be underestimated.

High Risk Groups

AIDS-Related Complex (ARC)

ARC patients, as described elsewhere in this volume, are those who are symptomatic, but do not meet full criteria for the AIDS syndrome. Many of the psychosocial issues described in relation to the AIDS patient are relevant to the ARC patient. Although they do not necessarily have to face the more devastating consequences of fulminant AIDS, ARC patients, nonetheless, are continually confronted with the prospect of developing an illness that is uniformly fatal. In many respects, the anxiety experienced by these patients in anticipation of possibly developing AIDS is perhaps more stressful in certain settings than the knowledge that one, indeed, has AIDS. Anxiety may precipitously increase with the development of any new, even minor, symptom that may signify to patients that their worst fear has been realized. Preoccupation with fears about developing AIDS may become pervasive and profoundly disabling. Like patients with AIDS, ARC patients may experience social isolation and cruel discrimination that exacerbate feelings of anxiety, depression, and anger. Drastic changes in lifestyle may occur, including loss of job, income, housing, and customary social contacts. ARC patients suffer the stigma of AIDS patients or of those social groups that are at highest risk for developing AIDS (homosexuals and intravenous drug abusers). In addition, the somatic symptoms experienced by ARC patients may compound their social problems and interfere with their ability to work and participate in usual activities. Thus, while the major theme for AIDS patients may be seen as "loss," ARC patients also experience considerable loss, but in the context of even more overwhelming uncertainty. In the treatment of the ARC patient, emphasis should be placed on acknowledgment of their dilemma, elucidation of their concerns, education about the course and prognosis of their illness, and recognition that ARC patients may not have access to some of the financial and support systems available to patients with AIDS.

HTLV-III Antibody-Positive Individuals

Members of this group, like the ARC patients, are estimated to have a 10 to 20% chance of developing AIDS in some studies. However, unlike the ARC patients, they are frequently asymptomatic when they learn that they carry the antibody to the AIDS virus. Apart from the sword of Damocles that is suddenly poised above their heads, members of this group are faced with an extremely difficult set of problems. The presence of the HTLV-III antibody that may have resulted from a clandestine bisexual or past homosexual affair may be painfully difficult to explain to a spouse, children, other family members, or friends. Overwhelming guilt may accompany the realization that a spouse or even, indirectly, a child has inadvertently been exposed to the HTLV-III virus and, therefore, is at risk for developing a fatal disease.

The widespread ramifications of the availability of HTLV-III antibody testing are becoming gradually apparent. The decision by the U.S. Defense Department to screen all recruits (August 1985) as well as all active personnel (October 1985) has already resulted in considerable complexities involving areas that overlap disciplines of medicine and bioethics. Recruits who have been denied admission to the Navy on the basis of their HTLV-III antibody have described their fear, resentment, anger, and helplessness in response to a testing process that may provide only limited counselling and education about AIDS or the significance of an HTLV-III titer, legal advice regarding their right of appeal, or confidentiality.[26] Some would-be recruits have described ostracism by other personnel, as well as concerns that their relationships with their families have been irreparably damaged. " 'Everybody is rude. People are afraid to touch us. They are afraid of being with us. They're afraid of getting AIDS. And we aren't even diagnosed as having it.' "[26] The range and severity of reactions to learning that one is HTLV-III antibody-positive have yet to be determined. However, it is clear that the knowledge that one is HTLV-III antibody-positive produces considerable interpersonal disruption and psychological distress and, therefore, such information must be conveyed with the same sensitivity, compassion, education, and support as that required by patients with AIDS.

Worried Well

For the worried well, members of those groups at high risk for acquiring AIDS, two major concerns have emerged. First and most obvious is the concern about possible contraction of AIDS as a result of past or future exposure. In addition to a preoccupation with health—the sense that the next sore throat or skin blemish may be the first sign of impending death—fears about AIDS have contributed to lifestyle changes as evidenced by marked reductions in multiple partner exposures reported in the gay community. However, for the gay community in particular, AIDS has raised a second major concern—the threat to homosexual civil rights posed by the public reaction to AIDS. Several states have already passed antisodomy and other legal measures in response to AIDS.[27] A Houston mayoral candidate recently "joked" that one way to control AIDS was to "shoot the queers."[28] A proposed congressional resolution would cut off federal funds to local governments that allow gay bathhouses to operate.[29] The availability of HTLV-III antibody testing has intensified concerns about loss of civil liberties as the majority of people who are HTLV-III antibody-positive are homosexual or will be labeled as such. Critics of the U.S. Defense Department's screening policy have suggested that the HTLV-III antibody test will be used to identify and discriminate against homosexuals. Furthermore, the problem of confidentiality and regulation of access to information about HTLV-III antibody test results is far from resolved. For example, are insurance companies or employers entitled to know the results of HTLV-III testing, and, if so, how will the lives of those with positive screening tests be affected? Thus, despite its obvious importance in protecting against transfusion-related AIDS, HTLV-III antibody testing may be associated with psychosocial consequences in the worried well as a product of the societal response to AIDS and the groups at risk. This is an area that merits a great deal of attention.

The Public

AIDS has certainly captured the public attention and imagination. Initially, there was an observer horror—a visceral response to the brutal destructive power of AIDS, tempered by a relative sense of security and, in some cases, moral satisfaction as evidenced by those who viewed AIDS as the wages of sin or God's punishment of societal deviants. As the numbers of AIDS patients increased at an alarming rate, the public demanded information that would allow them to assess and assure their safety. Could AIDS be transmitted by a mosquito bite, a vaccination, a sauna, or food handled by an HTLV-III-infected person? What precautions, if any, should the average person take to avoid exposure to the AIDS virus? If the AIDS virus has been found in tears and saliva, how can one be sure that AIDS may not be acquired by contact with these "bodily fluids"? These and many similar questions are expressed in the increasing number of legal and ethical dilemmas that surround the AIDS patient. Should children with AIDS be permitted to attend public school, or should they be quarantined? Should such a question be decided purely on public health grounds, or are there legal and ethical considerations? Should the siblings of children with AIDS be barred from public school attendance? Should AIDS patients who continue to engage in sexual activity be quarantined as proposed in Virginia[30] or subject to felony charges as in San Antonio?[31] Should all people participating in blood-sampling procedures be screened for HTLV-III? If an AIDS patient requests that his family not be notified of his illness and/or impending death, can his request be honored? If an HTLV-III antibody positive person does not wish to tell his/her spouse, does the health care worker have an obligation to notify the spouse or attempt to obtain the names of other sexual partners? These problems defy easy solution and suggest, along with estimates that up to a million people or more have been infected with the HTLV-III virus, that the involvement of the public in AIDS-related issues will expand rather than decrease in the near future.

Health Care Workers

AIDS poses several major problems for health care workers. First, there exists the fear, despite evidence to the contrary, that one will contract AIDS and/or inadvertently transmit it to a family member. This fear is fueled by several features of AIDS: (1) it is transmitted by bodily fluids that are frequently handled by health care workers; (2) it evokes anxiety and dread, and is viewed as a malignant process destroying the body in a way different from other fatal degenerative diseases; (3) it has a relatively long latency of onset, which allows for greater uncertainty and more time to vigilantly respond to any somatic symptom as possible evidence of the disease; and (4) it is uniformly fatal.

Concerns about acquiring AIDS are enhanced by recent reports[32] suggesting that, "in rare instances the AIDS virus may also be spread to hospital workers who, in turn, may infect their sexual partners." In addition to illness-related factors, there are care-related and patient-related factors that may profoundly affect health care workers. AIDS victims are usually young, male and female patients who experience a rapid, fulminating, destructive illness culminating in their death. The relentless suffering and loss of young patients despite the best efforts of health care workers constitute a frustrating and demoralizing process. The infectious disease precautions that are required considerably increase the work load of the health care staff, and the psychological needs as well as the cognitive and behavioral deterioration of patients create intense and, for some, unfamiliar demands that may overwhelm staff members. Ambiguous policies regarding participants in the informed consent process, confidentiality, and the rights of lovers may further enhance staff anxiety. The social characteristics of many AIDS patients may contribute to the burden of care. Homosexuality is capable of evoking intense, disparate, and potentially upsetting responses in many people. If a health care worker reacts with discomfort to an affectionate exchange between a patient and his or her lover, it is unclear how that reaction influences the staff member's behavior. It is also uncertain how staff behavior is influenced by the fear of contagion, by a sense of being overburdened by the special needs of AIDS patients, and by feelings of demoralization or hopelessness in response to the inevitability of their patients' death. The ability of the health care worker to deal with AIDS patients is determined by individual coping strategies, meaning of death, personal support, tolerance of anxiety, and a host of individual-specific factors. Health care workers experience varied and often conflicting feelings, which may be difficult to tolerate when working with suffering young patients who are struggling to live.

The cumulative effect of the multiple stresses that confront the health care worker results in a short-circuiting of one's customary adaptive strategies; a belief that one's stated concerns are not being heard; an inability to hear didactic information about AIDS in a convincing way; and, in time, "burn-out."[33] This process can be most effectively prevented or reversed by helping staff members to recognize and articulate their varied responses to working with patients with AIDS. The ability to express and compare concerns with others can reduce anxiety and allow staff members to accept their responses and recognize that certain aspects of their predicament are unavoidable. Only then can health care workers believe that they are being heard, a prerequisite for a meaningful and salutary dialogue among staff and between staff and patients. Patients with AIDS require assistance in their attempts to improve the quality of life that remains for them. Health care workers can provide that assistance only when they come to recognize, without judgment, the difficulty of their task.

Conclusion

The psychosocial aspects of AIDS have become more prominent as the extent of the illness and its potential threat to the general population become more apparent. Given the nature of AIDS and all that it represents, the fear that it has generated in the general population as well as in specific groups, directly or indirectly involved with the disease, is understandable. Additionally, the predilection of AIDS for certain high risk groups has created new and height-ened existing social tensions. In the future, closer clinical and research atten-tion should be directed to the psychological problems that have arisen in people who are affected by the illness, both patients and health care workers. Research should include systematic evaluation of the psychiatric and neuro-psychological morbidity of patients with HTLV-III-related illnesses and should assess the clinical and prognostic implications of these findings. Should suc-cessful treatment of AIDS eventually be accomplished (see the chapter by Yarchoan and Broder in this book), the neuropsychological impairment ob-served early in the course of AIDS may represent a potential source of residual morbidity. At present, those most closely affected by AIDS are, in most cases, best treated with the opportunity to express their concerns, education, and support.

References

1. Morrin SF, Batchelor WF. Responding to the psychological crisis of AIDS. Public Health Rep 1984; 99:4–9.
2. Ochitill HN, Perl M, Dilley J, Volberd P. Case reports of psychiatric disturbance in patients with acquired immune deficiency syndrome. Intl J Psychiatry Med 1984; 14:259–263.

3. Loewenstein RJ, Sharfstein SS. Neuropsychiatric aspects of acquired immune deficiency syndrome. Intl J Psychiatry Med 1983/1984; 13:255–260.
4. Kermani E, Drob S, Alpert M. Organic brain syndrome in three cases of acquired immune deficiency syndrome. Comp Psychiatry 1984; 25:294–297.
5. Nurnberg G, Prudic J, Fiori M. Psychopathologic complications of acquired immune deficiency syndrome (AIDS). Am J Psychiatry 1984; 141:95–96.
6. Kermani EJ, Borod JC, Brown PH, Tunnel G. New psychopathologic findings in AIDS: case report. J Clin Psychiatry 1985; 46:240–241.
7. Levy RM, Bredesen DE, Rosenblum ML. Neurological manifestation of the acquired immune deficiency syndrome (AIDS): experience at UCSF and review of the literature. J Neurosurg 1985; 62:475–495.
8. Reichert CM, O'Leary TM, Levens DL, Simrell CR, Macher AM. Autopsy pathology in the acquired immune deficiency syndrome. Am J Pathol 1983; 112:357–382.
9. Welch K, Finkbeiner W, Alpers CE, Blumenfeld W, Davis RL, Smuckler EA, Beckstead JH. Autopsy findings in the acquired immune deficiency syndrome. JAMA 1984; 252:1152–1159.
10. Loewenstein RJ, Rubinow DR. Psychiatric aspects of AIDS: the organic mental syndromes. In: Kurstak E, Lipowski ZJ, Morozov PV, eds. Viruses, immunity, and mental illness. New York: Plenum (in press).
11. Snider WD, Simpson DM, Nielsen S, Gold JWM, Metroka CE, Posner JB. Neurological complications of acquired immune deficiency syndrome: analysis of 50 patients. Ann Neurol 1983; 14:403–418.
12. Loewenstein RJ, Sharfstein SS. Neuropsychiatric aspects of acquired immune deficiency syndrome. Intl J Psychiatr Med 1983/1984; 13(40):255–260.
13. Joffe RT, Rubinow DR, Squillace K, Lane CH, Duncan CC, Fauci AS, Mirsky AF. Neuropsychiatric manifestations of acquired immune deficiency syndrome. Presented at the Annual Meeting of the American College of Neuropsychopharmacology, Maui, Hawaii, December 9–13, 1985, p. 29.
14. Derogatis LR, Morrow GR, Fetting J, Penman D, Piasetsky S, Schmale AM, Henrichs M, Carnicke SLM, Jr. The prevalence of psychiatric disorders among cancer patients. JAMA 1983; 249:751–757.
15. Weschsler D. Wechsler adult intelligence scale-revised. New York: The Psychological Corporation, 1981.
16. Tross S, Price R, Sidtis J, Holland J, Wolf L, Navia B. Neuropsychological complications of AIDS. Presented at the Annual Meeting of the American College of Neuropsychopharmacology, Maui, Hawaii, December 9–13, 1985, p. 28.
17. Shaw GM, Harper ME, Han BH, Epstein LG, Gajdusek DC, Price RW, Navia BA, Petito CK, O'Hara CJ, Groopman JE, Cho ES, Oleske JM, Wong-Staal F, Gallo RC. HTLV-III infections in brains of children and adults with AIDS encephalopathy. Science 1985; 227:177–182.
18. Levy JA, Shimabururo J, Hollander H, Mills J, Kaminsky L. Isolation of AIDS-associated retroviruses from cerebrospinal fluid and brain of patients with neurological symptoms. Lancet 1985; i:586–588.
19. Pert CB, Hill JM, Farrar WL, Ruscetti FW. Autoradiographical distribution of the AIDS virus receptor (entry protein) in primate brain. Presented at the Annual Meeting of the American College of Neuropsychopharmacology, Maui, Hawaii, December 9–13, 1985, p. 30.

20. Cooper DA, Maclean P, Finlayson R, Michelmore HM, Gold J, Donovan B, Barnes TG, Penhy R. Acute AIDS retrovirus infection. Lancet 1985; i:537–540.

21. Goldwater PN, Synek BJL, Koelmeyer TD, Scott PJ. Structures resembling scrapie-associated fibrils in AIDS encephalopathy. Lancet 1985; ii:447–448.

22. Thompson TL, Moran MG, Nies AS. Psychotrophic drug use in the elderly (first of two parts). N Engl J Med 1983a; 308:134–138.

23. Thompson TL, Moran MG, Nies AS. Psychotropic drug use in the elderly (second of two parts). N Engl J Med 1983b; 308:194–199.

24. Steinhart MJ. The use of haloperidol in geriatric patients with organic mental disorder. Curr Ther Res 1983; 33(1):132–143.

25. Loewenstein RJ. Evaluation and management of the neuropsychiatric complications of acquired immune deficiency syndrome. Medicine et Science (Switzerland) (in press).

26. Washington Post, p. A8, November 23, 1985.

27. Appleson G. Litigation imminent on AIDS issues. Natl Law J 1983; 25:3.

28. Washington Post, p. A4, October 26, 1985.

29. American Bar Assoc J 1985; 71:22.

30. Washington Post, p. D3, November 9, 1985.

31. Washington Post, p. A18, October 18, 1985.

32. Washington Post, p. A1, October 18, 1985.

33. Gardner ER, Hall RC. The professional stress syndrome. Psychosom 1981; 22:672–680.

9

Spectrum of HTLV-III Infection

Jerome E. Groopman
New England Deaconess Hospital
and Harvard Medical School
Boston, Massachusetts

Introduction

The acquired immunodeficiency syndrome (AIDS) serves as an important example in which clinical observation moves rapidly into basic biological studies in the laboratory in order to provide insights into the pathophysiological mechanisms of clinical phenomena. It is likely that the etiological agent of AIDS [a newly described human retrovirus termed human T-lymphotropic virus type III (HTLV-III),[1] lymphadenopathy/AIDS virus (LAV),[2] and AIDS-related virus (ARV)[3]] results in clinical syndromes far beyond that of full-blown AIDS. AIDS was described for purposes of epidemiological surveillance by the Centers for Disease Control[4] as a reliably diagnosed disease such as Kaposi's sarcoma, or opportunistic infections, such as *Pneumocystis carinii* pneumonia, occurring in the setting of cellular immune deficiency with no clear cause such cellular immune dysfunction. Knowing now that AIDS is caused by HTLV-III/LAV, and being able to accurately diagnose infection with this human retrovirus on the basis of antibodies that develop against HTLV-III/LAV antigens (as well as by recovery of virus from culture), we are able to more accurately define the spectrum of disease consequent to retroviral infection. AIDS is, indeed, only the "tip of the iceberg" and may represent only 5 to 10% of persons who have been infected with HTLV-III/LAV.[5] Several recent reviews on the clinical manifestations of AIDS provide a knowledge base for the clinician in diagnosis and management of Kaposi's sarcoma and the opportunistic infections that develop in these patients.[6,7] The discussion here will focus on HTLV-III/LAV-related diseases other than full-blown AIDS.

AIDS-Related Complex (ARC)

The AIDS-related complex (ARC) is a collection of clinical signs and laboratory abnormalities that has not yet been identified in a uniformly accepted fashion. Nonetheless, working definitions have been developed both by the National Institutes of Health and the Centers for Disease Control.[8] Detailed epidemiological surveillance data have not yet been obtained on ARC, so the numbers of cases in the United States and elsewhere are not known. Although it is widely recognized that there is considerable morbidity and ultimate mortality in nearly all cases of AIDS, it has been far less appreciated both by physicians and the general public that ARC is a serious medical condition in many of the cases and may lead to death.

The cardinal clinical finding in ARC is that of generalized lymphadenopathy.[9] Lymphadenopathy should be present for at least 3 months duration, not be explicable by any clear infectious or neoplastic cause, and have nodes measuring at least 1.5 cm in two distinct extrainguinal areas. The histopathology of these lymph nodes generally shows follicular hyperplasia, with an abundance of B-lymphocytes. This probably represents the B-cell immune response to HTLV-III infection in T-lymphocytes, as well as possible reactivation of latent Epstein-Barr virus infection. The lymph nodes may wax and wane in size, may occasionally cause discomfort to the patient, but are rarely so large as to result in obstructing symptoms. The need for lymph node biopsy to document follicular hyperplasia is still somewhat controversial in these patients. We studied 35 consecutive asymptomatic homosexual men with generalized lymphadenopathy at the New England Deaconess Hospital and performed lymph node biopsy. In no case was the diagnosis changed to AIDS on the basis of biopsy. For that reason, unless there is a change in the clinical status (such as fever, weight loss, or rapid change in the size of the lymph nodes), there is little justification for routine lymph node biopsy.

Two "minor" opportunistic infections, herpes zoster and oral candidiasis, are frequently seen in patients with ARC.[10] These infections are thought to be too common in the general population to include them under the criteria for full-blown AIDS. Nonetheless, these pathogens are clearly handled by the cellular immune system, and the development of either oral candidiasis or herpes zoster is often an ominous sign in an ARC patient. In some series, a significant proportion of patients with ARC who manifested oral candidiasis and/or herpes zoster progressed to AIDS.[9] It is clear that one should suspect HTLV-III infection in any person with oral candidiasis or herpes zoster who is epidemiologically at risk for this retrovirus. Particular concern should occur among patients who are immunocompromised for other reasons, such as patients with lymphoma or leukemia, who have been transfused and develop herpes zoster.[11] Previously, the clinician might ascribe this to the underlying immune deficiency that occurs with certain neoplasms. Because HTLV-III might have been acquired by transfusion, it is clinically valuable to test such patients for evidence of infection with this retrovirus if minor opportunistic infections occur.

Diarrhea, either persistent or intermittent, is also frequently seen in ARC. There appears to be a nonspecific enteropathy associated with HTLV-III infection.[6] The pathophysiological basis for this enteropathy has not yet been established, but it appears to be a secretory diarrhea in most cases. Extensive evaluation should be performed by the clinician for evidence of an opportunistic bowel pathogen such as *Cryptosporidium* or *Mycobacterium avium*. In the absence of finding such pathogens, the diarrhea can be ascribed to HTLV-III infection. The management of such patients can be quite difficult. Generally, palliative therapy with opiates as well as avoiding excessive ingestion of milk products may have some success.

The hematological manifestations of HTLV-III infection are part of the laboratory abnormalities seen in ARC.[9] Patients may present with an isolated cytopenia, such as leukopenia (nearly always lymphopenia and often granulocytopenia), thrombocytopenia, and anemia. The bone marrow often shows a mildly dysplastic picture in patients with ARC and cytopenias. The pathogenesis of these abnormalities has not yet been fully determined. It has been demonstrated that there are circulating immune complexes in patients with HTLV-III infection, which coat the surface of their platelets.[12] Such nonspecific coating of the platelet surface by antibody-antigen complexes, with premature destruction by the macrophages of the spleen, may result in thrombocytopenia. Other data indicate that there may be an autoantibody directed against a platelet surface antigen in patients with ARC and thrombocytopenia.[13] Antibodies to white cell antigens have not yet been demonstrated in patients with leukopenia and ARC. Similarly, the pathogenesis of the anemia (which is usually normochromic normocytic) is not known. It is possible that destruction of the T4$^+$-lymphocyte population with subsequent failure to generate growth factors for hematopoietic cells normally produced by this lymphocyte class results in cytopenias. Similarly, it is possible that HTLV-III might directly infect bone marrow stem cells, leading to ineffective hematopoiesis.

Nervous System Disease Associated with HTLV-III

The neurotropic properties of HTLV-III have been recently recognized,[14-16] and are discussed elsewhere in this book by Berger and Resnick. Shaw and co-workers[14] elegantly demonstrated by in situ hybridization techniques infection of brain in patients with AIDS who had central nervous system dysfunction. It has become abundantly clear that HTLV-III has a wide spectrum of neurological abnormalities consequent to its infecting a host. We have seen many patients who presented initially with dementia before developing opportunistic infections and/or Kaposi's sarcoma. Cognitive dysfunction can be quite subtle in these patients early in the disease and only demonstrated by formal neuropsychiatric testing. Such patients usually have a progressively downhill course over 6 months to 1 year. The virus appears to be distributed throughout the neuraxis and does not appear to infect any particular area of brain.

We have also seen patients who presented with neurological disorders other than dementia, which now can be attributed to HTLV-III infection. Such patients were initially diagnosed as having multiple sclerosis, amyotrophic lateral sclerosis, mononeuritis multiplex, and Guillain-Barré syndromes. A vacuolar myelopathy has been described in many of these patients with progressive deterioration of spinal cord and peripheral nerves. Studies by Ho and co-workers[15] have demonstrated recovery of HTLV-III in cell-free spinal fluid from many patients with this syndrome. Similarly, Resnick and co-workers[16] found in such patients a disproportionate level of spinal fluid immunoglobulin specifically directed against HTLV-III compared with serum levels of such antibodies. The spinal fluid generally shows a mild to moderate mononuclear cell pleocytosis, a normal glucose, and a normal or mildly elevated protein. This formula (and, most importantly, the exclusion of other infectious and neoplastic processes as accounting for the neurological syndromes) should assist the clinician in making the diagnosis of HTLV-III-related central nervous system disease.

In addition to focal neurological abnormalities associated with HTLV-III infection, it has been the clinical impression of this author and others that there may be psychiatric disorders due to HTLV-III infection. This is clearly quite difficult to document, but certain psychiatric abnormalities including paranoia, hallucinations, night terrors, and severe depression have occurred in some patients with HTLV-III infection preceding clinical dementia. Such psychiatric syndromes probably reflect early central nervous system dysfunction due to infection with the retrovirus.

Acute HTLV-III Infection

It has been extraordinarily difficult to ascertain the symtomatic host response after initial exposure to HTLV-III. Nonetheless, certain serendipitous cases have been evaluated and appear to represent acute HTLV-III illness. The clinical presentation is that of fever, headache, myalgias, lymphadenopathy, photophobia, headache, meningismus, and occasionally a transient erythematous rash. Such symptoms are of course highly nonspecific and can be seen in a variety of common virual illnesses such as Coxsackie and Epstein-Barr virus infections. These cases were diagnosed as HTLV-III illness on the basis of recovery of the retrovirus from peripheral blood lymphocytes and/or spinal fluid in the absence of detectable antibody to HTLV-III. There was later seroconversion, with appearance of anti-HTLV-III antibodies and resolution of the acute illness. No other infectious pathogen could be identified in these cases. Interestingly, many patients with established AIDS or ARC report a similar episode or illness like this 1 to 3 years before the diagnosis of AIDS or ARC. Similarly, primates that are experimentally exposed to HTLV-III may demonstrate an acute illness of this type with seroconversion after 12 to 16 weeks. Thus, in the spectrum of HTLV-III infection, one must consider an acute and highly nonspecific viral-like illness, which may be diagnosed only with viral cultures or retrospectively by seroconversion.

Neoplasms Associated with HTLV-III Infection

Kaposi's sarcoma and central nervous system lymphoma were included as two neoplasms that formed the original criteria for the diagnosis of AIDS prior to the recognition of HTLV-III as the etiological agent of the syndrome. These neoplasms frequently arise in persons with cellular immune deficiency, either on an acquired or congenital basis. It has become abundantly clear that extra-CNS non-Hodgkin's lymphoma of the B-cell type, particularly with an unfavorable histology, is occurring at an increasing rate in homosexual men at risk for AIDS.[17] This led to the revision of the surveillance definition by the Centers for Disease Control to include persons with such B-cell lymphomas and a positive HTLV-III status. Our studies have suggested that the pathogenesis of such B-cell lymphomas in the setting of HTLV-III infection might be related to Epstein-Barr virus infection;[18] that is, a detailed molecular biological study of one such patient demonstrated that the malignant B cells contained Epstein-Barr virus genome, had a rearrangement of the c-myc oncogene, and did not contain the HTLV-III-related sequences. This molecular phenotype of the AIDS-related B-cell lymphoma is quite similar to that of patients with Burkitt's lymphoma unrelated to AIDS. Other investigators[19] have described an 8;14 translocation as well as an 8;22 translocation in the B-cell tumors in patients with AIDS. Such translocations are also seen in Burkitt's lymphomas related to HTLV-III infection.

Preliminary reports[20] have focused on the occurrence of Hodgkin's disease among homosexual men at risk for HTLV-III infection. We and others have noted an apparently disproportionate number of cases of Hodgkin's disease occurring among HTLV-III-infected persons at an age where Hodgkin's disease is unusual and in a clinical fashion atypical for Hodgkin's. We have seen six patients with Hodgkin's disease over the last year at the New England Deaconess Hospital who had HTLV-III infection. Two of these patients subsequently developed AIDS as defined by the Centers for Disease Control. In two patients, ARC had been present for 6 months to 2 years prior to the development of Hodgkin's disease. All patients presented with "B" symptoms of fever, weight loss, and night sweats, and all had palpable lymphadenopathy. What was most interesting is that the two patients with ARC had had lymphadenopathy, which had been biopsied in the past and demonstrated reactive follicular hyperplasia, the histopathological picture seen in ARC. Rebiopsy of the lymph nodes demonstrated mixed cellularity Hodgkin's disease in both cases. Some patients have presented with extensive cervical and axillary nodal disease and involved bone marrow without mediastinal disease. Other patients have had skin involvement that demonstrated Reed-Sternberg cells.

There has been considerable speculation that Hodgkin's disease was related to a transmissable agent due to its occasional occurrence in geographic clusters. Most persons with immune deficiency diseases not caused by HTLV-III, such as congenital immune deficiencies or iatrogenic immune deficiency with corticosteroid or chemotherapy treatment, do not have an increased incidence of Hodgkin's disease. Therefore, the occurrence of Hodgkin's disease in the setting of HTLV-III infection is quite unusual and may provide an important opportunity to study Hodgkin's disease as to its pathophysiological basis. Preliminary studies conducted in collaboration with Dr. Mary Harper at the National Cancer Institute on the spleen of a patient with HTLV-III and Hodgkin's disease demonstrated, using in situ hybridization, HTLV-III infection in the lymphocytes in the spleen, but not in the Reed-Sternberg cells. It is possible that a second virus or other transmissable agent is being passed among populations also at risk for HTLV-III. Attempts are underway to culture Reed-Sternberg cells and probe the cells for HTLV-III or other retroviruses.

The clinical management of both B-cell lymphomas and Hodgkin's disease in the setting of HTLV-III infection is quite complex.[21] Since these patients have a high propensity to opportunistic infections, aggressive combination chemotherapy with cytotoxic agents and corticosteroids (the mainstay of current approaches to lymphoma) may actually exacerbate the risk for opportunistic infection. Most centers that treat these patients have found that survival is quite short in HTLV-III-infected persons with lymphoma, and that these patients generally succumb to opportunistic infections. Nonetheless, since the neoplasms are quite aggressive, it is justified to treat them in the hope of obtaining a remission. We have generally employed regimens such as CHOP (cyclophosphamide, adriamycin, vincristine, and prednisone) for B-cell lymphomas, and ABVD (adriamycin, bleomycin, vinblastine, and DTIC) for Hodgkin's disease. We chose ABVD because it lacks the corticosteroid that might be the most important drug in potentiating the development of *Pneumocystis carinii* pneumonia.

Anecdotal cases have also been noted of unexpected neoplasms in HTLV-III-infected persons. We have seen three HTLV-III-infected patients with squamous carcinoma of the head and neck, who had no clear risk factor for such neoplasm (no alcohol or tobacco ingestion). One patient developed full-blown AIDS with Kaposi's sarcoma of the head and neck after the diagnosis of squamous carcinoma of the tongue. We have also seen two patients with aggressive adenocarcinoma of unknown origin. Anecdotal reports include adenocarcinoma of the pancreas, small cell carcinoma of the pancreas, and aggressive seminoma in persons epidemiologically at risk for HTLV-III infection. It is, of course, unclear whether these represent "background" cases or are actually neoplasms that develop in the setting of cellular immune deficiency due to retroviral infection. One might speculate that other viruses that have been implicated in the pathogenesis of neoplasms, such as papilloma viruses in squamous carcinoma, could be more oncogenic in the setting of HTLV-III infection. We and others have also speculated that the coincidence of infection with HTLV-III and hepatitis B virus in populations at risk for AIDS (homosexual men, intravenous drug abusers, and hemophiliacs) might lead to the development of hepatoma in the ensuing decades.

Conclusion

It is clear that the clinical spectrum of HTLV-III infection goes well beyond that of AIDS as defined by the Centers for Disease Control for purposes of epidemiological surveillance. Physicians and basic scientists are confronted with a wide array of disorders that appear to be the result of infection with this new retrovirus. It is also clear that this retrovirus is not only lymphotropic, but also neurotropic. One of the most prominent of its clinical manifestations is central and peripheral nervous system dysfunction. It is also apparent that we are afforded a unique opportunity to study the pathogenesis of a number of neoplasms beyond Kaposi's sarcoma and central nervous system lymphoma that arise consequent to HTLV-III infection in the host. The clinical dimensions of this epidemic have not yet been fully defined. Registries should be established to accurately define and delineate the spectrum of HTLV-III-related disorders.

References

1. Gallo RC, Salahuddin SZ, Popovic M, et al. Science 1984; 224:500.
2. Barré-Sinoussi F, Chermann JC, Rey R, et al. Science 1983; 220:868.
3. Levy JA, Hoffman AD, Kramer SM, Landis JA, Shimabukuro JM, Oshiro LS. Science 1984; 225:840.
4. Centers for Disease Control. MMWR 1981; 25:305.
5. Francis DP, Jaffe HW, Fultz PN, Getchell JP, McDougal JS, Feorino PM. Ann Intern Med 1985; 103:719.
6. Armstrong DA, Gold JWM, Dryjanski J, Whimbey E, Polsky B, Hawkins C, Brown AE, Bernard E, Kiehn TE. Ann Intern Med 1985; 103:738.
7. Safai B, Johnson KG, Myskowski PL, Koziner B, Yang SY, Cunningham-Rundles S, Godbold JH, Dupont B. Ann Intern Med 1985; 103:744.
8. Fauci AS, Macher AM, Longo DL, et al. Ann Intern Med 1984; 100:92.
9. Jaffe HW, Darrow WW, Echenberg DF, et al. Ann Intern Med. 1985;103:210.
10. Goedert JJ, Sarngadharan MG, Biggar RJ, et al. Lancet 1984; ii:711.
11. Groopman JE, Allan JD, Sallan SE, Hammer SM. J Clin Oncol (in press).
12. Morris L, Distenfeld A, Amorosi E, Karpatlan S. Ann Intern Med 1982; 96:714.
13. Stricker RB, Abrams BI, Corash L, Schuman MA. N Engl J Med (in press).
14. Shaw GM, Harper ME, Hahn BH, et al. Science 1985; 227:177.
15. Ho DD, Rota TR, Schooley RT, Kaplan JC, Allan JD, Groopman JE, Resnick L, Felsenstein D, Andrews CA, Hirsch MS. N Engl J Med 1985; 313:493.
16. Resnick L, DiMarzo-Veronese F, Schupbach J, Tourtellotte WW, Ho DD, Muller F, Shapshak P, Vogt M, Groopman JE, Markham PD, Gallo RC. N Engl J Med 1985; 313:1498.
17. Ziegler JL, Miner RC, Rosenbaum E, et al. Lancet 1982; ii:631.
18. Groopman JE, Sullivan JL, Mulder C, et al. Blood (in press).
19. Chaganti RS, Jhanwar SC, Koziner B, et al. Blood 1983; 61:1265.
20. Schoeppel SL, Hoppe RT, Dorfman RD, Horning SJ, Collier AC, Chew TG, Weiss LM. Ann Intern Med 1985; 102:68.
21. Kelter SP, Riggs SA, Cabanilas F, et al. Blood 1985; 66:665.

10

Pathology of AIDS

Elaine S. Jaffe
Laboratory of Pathology
National Cancer Institute
National Institutes of Health
Bethesda, Maryland

David A. Katz
National Institute of Neurological
and Communicative Diseases and Stroke
and Laboratory of Pathology
National Cancer Institute
National Institutes of Health
Bethesda, Maryland

Abe M. Macher
Registry of AIDS Pathology
Armed Forces Institute of Pathology
Washington, D.C.

Introduction

The pathology of the acquired immunodeficiency syndrome (AIDS) and HTLV-III is primarily the pathology of the infectious, proliferative, and neoplastic conditions that ensue as the disease progresses.[1-6] The changes that are most closely attributable to the etiological agent itself are those of profound lymphoid depletion secondary to the lympholytic effects of the virus. In addition, evidence is now emerging that HTLV-III may have a primary effect on the central nervous system. However, most of the clinical and pathological features of AIDS are secondary.

The destruction of T-lymphocytes throughout the lymphoid system disrupts the essential balance of the immune system. There is a failure in B-cell regulation, which leads to multiple autoimmune phenomena, polyclonal and oligoclonal B-cell proliferation, and B-cell lymphomas. The severe immune

143

defect leads to disseminated opportunistic infections. Several malignancies, most importantly Kaposi's sarcomas (KS), also occur with an increased frequency, suggesting that they too may have an infectious basis. Nevertheless, despite the widespread and devastating clinical consequence of AIDS, it is perhaps surprising the degree to which there has emerged a common clinico-pathological picture. The outpouring of medical literature generated by this worldwide epidemic has indicated a striking repetition from center to center and city to city in the clinicopathological features encountered.

Lymphoid and Hematological Lesions Associated with AIDS

Lymph Nodes

Lymph node biopsies exhibit a spectrum of characteristic, though not specific, histopathological changes that roughly correlate with the time course of disease progression.[7-13]

1. Reactive follicular hyperplasia, observed in patients with the AIDS-related complex (ARC) and perhaps early AIDS
2. Selective paracortical lymphoid depletion, often heralding the appearance of serious opportunistic infections
3. Severe lymphoid depletion and eventual "burn-out," an ominous prognostic indicator frequently seen at autopsy

The enlarged lymph nodes biopsied from patients with ARC exhibit florid follicular hyperplasia and plasmacytosis, with mild or minimal paracortical hyperplasia. The markedly hyperplastic germinal centers frequently exhibit attenuated lymphoid cuffs and may appear naked. However, they are well demarcated and readily distinguished from follicular lymphoma. Focally, the germinal centers may contain collections of small lymphocytes, and may appear fragmented and disrupted. The interfollicular zone is minimally affected at this stage. However, the medulla of the lymph node shows an intense plasmacytosis.

These histological features are seen in patients with persistent generalized lymphadenopathy (PGL) who are seropositive for HTLV-III. These changes may persist for many months without progression to overt AIDS. However, the natural history of patients with ARC or PGL is not yet established, and it is not yet determined what percentage of patients in this group will ultimately develop AIDS. These histological features may also persist for an interval after a diagnosis of AIDS has been established.

Correlating with the histological findings of follicular hyperplasia and plasmacytosis is in vivo and in vitro evidence of polyclonal B-cell activation in AIDS. Clinically, patients manifest polyclonal hypergammaglobulinemia and autoimmune hemolytic anemia, thrombocytopenia, Sjögren's syndrome, and related phenomena. Spontaneous polyclonal B-cell activation can be demonstrated in vitro.[14,15] The relationship of HTLV-III to these changes in unclear. A direct effect of HTLV-III on B-cell function has not been shown. The B-cell hyperactivity could be secondary to the presence of Epstein-Barr virus (EBV), a polyclonal B-cell activator, or an absence of normal suppressor T-cell function.

Stage II, or lymphoid depletion, is progressive and appears to parallel the degree of lymphopenia within the peripheral blood. At first, there is a decrease of lymphocytes within the paracortical (T-cell) zones, accompanied by an attenuation of the follicular mantles, plasmacytosis, and variable hyalinization of the germinal centers.[7,8] Biberfeld et al.[16] have described progressive changes in the lymphoid follicle, consisting of follicular fragmentation and follicular atrophy. The germinal center borders become serrated, and lymphocytic infiltration into the germinal center becomes more pronounced. Immunohistochemical studies of frozen sections of lymph nodes reveal a selective loss of helper T-lymphocytes, as well as increased numbers of suppressor/cytotoxic lymphocytes within germinal centers, where normally they are not found.[16-20] Correlating with alterations in the germinal centers, destruction of dendritic reticulum cells has been described.[16]

Other changes in nonlymphoid elements include an increase in angiogenesis, within both the germinal center and the paracortex. Atrophic germinal centers may contain prominent vascularity, especially in patients with lymphadenopathic KS. In the paracortex, postcapillary venules are prominent and may exhibit endothelial proliferation.

With disease progression, there is loss of both T- and B-lymphocytes. This phase has been termed stage III by Ewing et al.,[12] and is only seen in patients with fully developed AIDS. Erythrophagocytosis, as well as phagocytosis of other cellular elements, may be prominent in these lymph nodes. It is likely that the pathogenesis is similar to that seen in the infection-associated hemophagocytic syndromes and may be the result of excessive lymphokine production. These "burned-out" lymph nodes, most often seen at autopsy, may harbor surprising numbers of opportunistic pathogens. Because of the profound degree of immunosuppression at this stage, there is usually little evidence of a host response (i.e., granuloma or microabscess formation). At this late stage, it would appear that therapeutic regimens aimed only at immune modulation and enhancement are doomed to failure.

Lymphadenopathic KS may be the initial manifestation of AIDS. Early lymph node involvement by KS is characteristically subcapsular, with subsequent invasion of the lymph node by involvement of cortical and medullary sinuses. Peripheral "hemorrage" on gross inspection is usually evident, and small foci of KS may be missed without careful gross examination. The follicles in KS nodes may resemble the follicles of Castleman's disease or angiomatous lymphoid hamartoma,[21-23] but in all other respects, the lesions differ clinically and pathologically from the true isolated Castleman's lesion, which resembles a hamartomatous mass.[24]

Bone Marrow and Peripheral Blood

The bone marrow in AIDS is usually normocellular or hypercellular.[25] However, more than half the patients will exhibit either neutropenia or thrombocytopenia, and greater than 80% of patients will be anemic.[25,26] These cytopenias are present with apparently normal numbers of erythroid, myeloid, and megakaryocytic precursors; thus, peripheral destruction of hematopoietic elements is likely.[27-32]

The mechanism of anemia and thrombocytopenia in many patients appears autoimmune.[27-32] Plasmacytosis in the bone marrow is seen in most patients, correlating with the plasmacytosis found in peripheal lymphoid organs[25] Serum immunoglobulins show a polyclonal elevation of all immunoglobulin classes. However, high-resolution zone electrophoresis is capable of demonstrating small monoclonal and oligoclonal bands in the majority of patients.[15] The presence of monoclonal bands is independent of whether or not the patients have experienced opportunistic infection. It is felt that this limited clonal expansion of B cells is an important step in B-cell lymphoma genesis in these patients. On occasion, the bone marrow may be the site of lymphoma diagnosis.

The bone marrow biopsy frequently contains either focal lymphoplasmacytic aggregates or poorly formed granulomas. These cellular infiltrates are usually associated with a focal increase in reticulin fibers. *Mycobacterium avium-intracellulare* is the organism most frequently associated with granulomas. However, in a signficant number of cases, mycobacteria may be obtained by culture in marrows lacking demonstrable granulomas. Special stains may also commonly identify the organism in scattered histiocytes.

Lymphopenia is a constant finding in AIDS, with inversion of the T4:T8 ratio and severe reduction in the absolute numbers of helper T cells. The early search for a viral agent in AIDS led to the demonstration of tubuloreticular inclusions in circulating lymphocytes by transmission electron microscopy.[33,34] Elevation of serum interferon was found in all individuals demonstrating such inclusions, and in the past, interferon has been linked to their production. Most patients having inclusions also exhibited active infection by DNA viruses. Using monoclonal antibodies, the inclusions were localized to the cytotoxic/suppressor (T8-CD8-positive) T-lymphocytes.[34]

Lymphoid Lesions in Other Organs

The polyclonal B-cell activation seen in lymph nodes and bone marrow can also lead to lymphoid proliferation in other organs. Lung biopsies in patients with interstitial pulmonary infiltrates may show lymphoid interstitial pneumonitis. We have seen three cases of Sjögren's syndrome in males with the AIDS-related complex and polyclonal hypergammaglobulinemia, who clinically manifested the sicca syndrome.[35] Biopsy of salivary gland lesions demonstrated marked lymphoid infiltration with florid follicular hyperplasia. There was atrophy of acinar tissue and destruction of ducts with conspicuous myoepithelial islands. Cervical lymphadenopathy was also present, and lymph node biopsy demonstrated a florid follicular hyperplasia. One other similar case has also been demonstrated.[36]

Opportunistic Infections in Patients with AIDS

AIDS is characterized by an acquired, irreversible, profound immunosuppression that predisposes the patient to multiple opportunistic infections and malignancies. Thus, patients with AIDS are particularly susceptible to a variety of protozoal, viral, fungal, and bacterial infections. In patients with AIDS, such opportunistic infections are often severe, persistent, and/or relapsing despite appropriate therapy. Furthermore, numerous simultaneous opportunistic infections frequently occur. The etiological agents of opportunistic infections in patients with AIDS are given in Table 1.

The pathology of AIDS is divided into three general categories; (1) morphological manifestations of severe lymphoid depletion; (2) unusual neoplasms, most frequently KS or high-grade lymphomas; and (3) opportunistic infections. Because of the multiplicity of infections encountered in patients with AIDS, and because of the potential hazards of the various therapeutic agents involved, specific pathological diagnoses are essential for a rational approach to therapy.

Protozoa

Pneumocystis carinii: P. *carinii* was originally described in 1907 in experimental animals infected with *Trypanosoma* parasites. By 1909, the organism was recognized as distinct from trypanosomes and was given its present name. P. *carinii* is a protozoan parasite of the Sporozoa family. The mature P. *carinii* cyst contains up to eight miniature nucleated structures called sporozoites. After excystation, these sporozoites mature into trophozoites. The trophozoites are unicellular organisms that ultimately attach to host cells (i.e., alveolar-

TABLE 1 Etiological Agents of
Opportunistic Infections in
Patients with AIDS

Protozoa
> *Pneumocystis carinii*
> *Cryptosporidium*
> *Isospora belli*
> *Toxoplasma gondii*

Viruses
> Cytomegalovirus
> Herpes simplex
> Herpes zoster
> Polyomavirus

Fungi
> *Candida* sp.
> *Cryptococcus neoformans*
> *Histoplasma capsulatum*
> *Histoplasma duboisii*
> *Coccidioides immitis*

Bacteria
> *Mycobacterium avium-intracellulare*
> *Mycobacterium tuberculosis*
> *Legionella* sp.
> *Nocardia* sp.
> *Salmonella* sp.
> *Shigella* sp.
> *Listeria monocytogenes*

lining cells in the lung) and develop a true cyst wall. They then undergo internal nuclear division, resulting in the formation of eight new sporozoites.

P. carinii causes pulmonary infections in a variety of domestic and wild animals. The first human isolations were from malnourished and premature European infants suffering from interstitial plasma cell pneumonia; subsequently, it has been reported in all parts of the world. It has come into prominence in recent years as a recent cause of pneumonia in patients with congenital and acquired immunological disorders, as well as in the increasing group subjected to immunosuppressive therapy for indications ranging from neoplasia or collagen diseases to organ transplantation.

Approximately 60% of patients with AIDS develop *P. carinii* pneumonia (PCP); this is frequently their first diagnosed opportunistic infection.[37-39] AIDS patients with PCP present with fever, a cough, dyspnea, and/or shortness of breath. The condition is usually subacute, but it may be fulminant with severe hypoxemia and rapid progression. Ultimately, AIDS patients with untreated PCP will develop life-threatening pulmonary insufficiency as a result of extensive pulmonary consolidation.

The physician must maintain a high index of suspicion of PCP in patients with AIDS. The respiratory symptoms are often mild, with a persistent nonproductive cough being the only symptom for weeks or months. Roentgenograms of the chest may reveal unilateral or bilateral interstitial and/or alveolar infiltrates; however, initial radiographs may be normal in association with only borderline abnormal or normal arterial blood gas studies. Gallium scanning may show diffuse pulmonary uptake or may be unremarkable.

A noninvasive bronchoscopy with bronchial lavage and/or washings often demonstrates *P. carinii*. In patients without coagulopathies, a simultaneous transbronchial biopsy should be performed. The diagnosis of PCP is based on the demonstration of *P. carinii* in bronchial secretions or in sections of lung. Bronchial secretions and touch imprints of unfixed lung tissues may be stained with toluidine blue,[40] Gram-Weiger, or methenamine silver techniques to demonstrate the cyst forms. Sometimes confused for fungal yeast, these nonbudding cysts of *P. carinii* are oval, round, or collapsed, measure 3 to 7 μm, and frequently exhibit a crescent-shaped thickening of the wall.[41] Gram's,[42] Wright's,[43] and methylene blue staining techniques will demonstrate up to eight internal sporozoites per cyst; although the cyst walls are transparent, the cysts are indirectly outlined by thin, clear, nonstaining halos. Toluidine blue or methenamine silver staining of frozen sections or formalin-fixed, paraffin-embedded transbronchial and open lung biopsy tissues will demonstrate the cyst forms within alveoli. Unlike fungi, the cyst walls of *P. carinii* do not stain well with periodic acid-Schiff (PAS).

Grossly, lung tissues are heavy and consolidated and cut with increasing resistance. Early involvement is characteristically patchy, but postmortem examination frequently reveals an almost homogeneous gray-white consolidation of the lungs bilaterally; despite this generalized distribution, pleural effusion is rarely present. Histopathologically, there are thickened alveolar septae associated with an interstitial infiltrate composed of a mixture of lymphocytes, plasma cells, and histiocytes. The clue to diagnosis, however, is the characteristic intraalveolar, eosinophilic, foamy, and honeycombed exudates that contain the characteristic clustered cysts of *P. carinii*.

Unfortunately, *P. carinii* cannot be routinely cultured, and serological tests for pneumocystis antigen or antipneumocystis antibody have no proven diagnostic value. Therapeutically, PCP in the patient with AIDS may respond to trimethoprim-sulfamethoxazole and/or pentamidine isethionate. Nevertheless, overall survival from PCP is approximately 50 to 60% per episode.

Because PCP may present with other concomitant opportunistic pulmonary infections, bacterial, mycobacterial, fungal, and viral pathogens should also be searched for. Tissue specimens should, therefore, always be stained with acid-fast, Gram's, Giemsa, PAS, methenamine silver, and toluidine blue techniques; tissues should also be cultured for bacterial (i.e., *Legionella* and *Nocardia* spp.), mycobacterial, and fungal pathogens.

Although human infection by *P. carinii* has been typically associated with pneumonitis, extrapulmonary infections may be seen in patients with AIDS. We recently autopsied a male homosexual patient with AIDS and discovered a widely disseminated *P. carinii* infection involving lymph nodes, liver, spleen, kidneys, heart, thyroid, adrenals, etc.

Cryptosporidium: Cryptosporidium is a protozoa coccidian originally reported as a parasite of the intestinal tracts of many different vertebrates, including reptiles, birds, and mammals; these infected animals may be asymptomatic or may suffer from chronic enteritis, poor growth, and loss of vigor. As a zoonosis, calves and other animals may serve as sources of human infection.[44] Human infection with *Cryptosporidium* was first reported in 1976. One patient was a 3-year-old child, previously in good health and with no evidence of altered immune status, in whom this organism produced a severe but self-limited enterocolitis. The other infection affected a 39-year-old man with bullous pemphigoid who, in the course of treatment for that disease with corticosteroids and cyclophosphamide, developed a severe diarrhea with malabsorption, which cleared 2 weeks after discontinuation of the latter drug.[45] It has since become apparent that this enteric parasite may cause a self-limited diarrheal illness of 1 to 2 weeks duration in individuals with intact immunity (i.e., traveler's diarrhea). However, in immunocompromised hosts, the disease may be fulminant and intractable.

Persistent or recurrent diarrhea is a frequent problem among patients with AIDS. Although some patients have several loose stools per day, others may have copious volumes of watery diarrhea that can reach 15 liters/day. Homosexuals with AIDS may have a range of bowel problems due to the enteric organisms that cause symptomatic disease in the general homosexual population, including *Entamoeba histolytica, Giardia lamblia, Salmonella* sp., and *Campylobacter* sp. Appropriate antimicrobial treatment that eliminates these pathogens often fails to eliminate the copious water diarrhea. Some patients with persistent watery stools have cryptosporidiosis.

As an enteric protozoan, *Cryptosporidium* attaches to the epithelial surface of the small and large intestine and causes chronic, profuse, watery diarrhea in patients with AIDS.[46] The 2 to 6 μm oocyst form of the protozoan is demonstrated in stool specimens using a modified Sheather's sucrose flotation technique. In brief, after centrifugation of 0.5 gram of stool specimen in a sucrose solution, the oocysts accumulate on the surface; the oocysts are then transferred to a microscopic slide with a wire loop and observed by phase-contrast microscopy.[44] The Cryptosporidium oocysts are differentiated from yeast cells by their bright refractile quality. Because the oocysts are acid-fast, the diagnosis may also be established by a modified Ziehl-Neelsen technique[47,48] or by a fluorescent auramine stain of either fecal smear or formalin-ether and formalin concentrates of stool.[49]

Histopathologically, hematoxylin- and eosin-stained sections of small bowel biopsies demonstrate cryptosporidia arranged in rows along the mucosal brush borders of intestinal villi, which may appear blunted[50] or normal.[51] Cryptosporidia may also be observed lying free within the crypts. The organisms are not seen in the lamina propria. The parasites may also be attached to the mucosal epithelial surface of the rectum or gallbladder. Rarely, the organism may infect the respiratory tract.[52,53] With a Masson stain, a small red nucleus and blue cytoplasm may be distinguished in many of the cryptosporidia. Transmission electron microscopy has demonstrated several different stages of development of the parasite, including trophozoite, schizont, oocyst, macrogametocyte, and merozoite forms.[54] The mechanism of the diarrhea is unknown. The absence of significant light microscopic alterations suggests the possibility of toxin elaboration.

Isopora belli: I. *belli* is a protozoal coccidian that causes enteritis in man. It is a parasite of the epithelial cells of the intestine, in which it may undergo repeated asexual development with consequent destruction of considerable portions of the surface layer of the intestine. The parasites may be found by small bowel biopsy. In addition to asexual stages, which serve to spread the infection within the bowel wall, sexual stages occur, and these culminate in oocysts passed in the feces. Immature oocysts are ellipsoid or spindle (banana)-shaped with blunt ends. They average 30×12 μm. Contained within the immature oocyst is a spherical mass of protoplasm, which divides to form two sporoblasts. These sporoblasts, still within the oocyst, develop thick cyst walls and are known as sporocysts. With each sporocyst, four curved sausage-shaped sporozoites develop. All stages, from immature oocysts containing nothing but an undivided mass of protoplasm to those containing fully developed sporocysts and sporozoites, may be seen in the feces.

In immunocompetent hosts, I. *belli* causes self-limited infections associated with symptoms ranging from mild gastrointestinal distress to severe dysentery.[55] In patients with AIDS, however, enteric infections are protracted due to the underlying immunodeficiency.

I. *belli* oocysts may be seen on direct examination of the stool or may be detected in concentrates. They concentrate well with the zinc sulfate technique, but are so light that they float even in the customary zinc-sulfate-iodine mixture, and will only be seen if the area directly beneath the coverslip is carefully examined with reduced illumination. Unless iodine-stained, the oocysts and contained material (sporocysts and sporozoites) are quite transparent and very difficult to recognize.

Although iosoporiasis has been reported in intracellular parasites restricted to the columnar cells of the intestinal mucosa both in humans and animals, *extraintestinal*-disseminated infections may be seen in patients with AIDS. We studied a male homosexual patient with AIDS who had a history of *I. belli* infestation treated with trimethoprim-sulfamethoxazole. Postmortem examination demonstrated intracellular and extracellular *I. belli* oocysts within the lamina propria of small and large intestine, as well as in mesenteric and tracheobronchial lymph nodes where an associated granulomatous reaction was also present. The oocysts in tissue stain with hemtoxylin and eosin and PAS techniques.

Toxoplasma gondii: T. gondii is an intracellular protozoal coccidian. Its name derives partly from the comma shape of the characteristic $2 \times 6 \mu$ trophozoite stage (i.e., toxon is Greek for arc). The species name derives from the gondi, the rodent in which *T. gondii* was first described in 1908. The cat is the definitive host harboring the sexual stage of reproduction (the oocyst). Man and many other mammalian species are intermediate hosts who harbor the other two stages of the organism, the proliferating trophozoite and the dormant tissue cyst. The most common modes of acquisition of *T. gondii* infection include: (1) ingestion of oocysts through contact with cats, (2) ingestion of tissue cysts in poorly cooked beef or pork, and (3) transplacental infection of the fetus during primary maternal infection.

T. gondii is the most common cause of parasitic infestation in the United States. Despite the high frequency of the infection, clinical illness of any kind due to *T. gondii* is rare. A small percentage of primarily infected adults will develop a mononucleosis-like illness. After primary infection, *T. gondii* becomes latent within host tissues (i.e., brain). Reactivation of acquired latent infection with the production of clinically significant disease probably occurs exclusively in the immunosuppressed host. Toxoplasmic encephalitis with or without hematogeneous dissemination to other organs may then occur.

In patients with AIDS, toxoplasmosis presents as a severe acute, subacute, or chronic necrotizing encephalitis with fevers and focal neurological signs and/or chorioretinitis.[56,57] Characteristically, single or multiple contrast-enhancing intracerebral defects appear on computed tomographic (CT) scans;[58-60] nevertheless, intracerebral abscesses due to *Cryptococcus neoformans*, mycobacteria, cytomegalovirus, *Nocardia,* and lymphoma should also be considered in the differential diagnosis.[61,62] Despite active disease, IgM toxoplasma titers are frequently negative and IgG titers are frequently elevated, reflecting past exposure.[58] These serological findings suggest that in AIDS patients, central nervous system toxoplasmosis results from reactivation rather than from primary infection.[56]

Definitive diagnosis requires demonstration of the characteristic tachyzoites and cysts within hematoxylin and eosin- or Giemsa-stained biopsy specimens or Wright-Giemsa-stained smears. During acute infection, the 2 × 6 μm tachyzoites multiply asexually within engorged human host cells; host cells eventually rupture, releasing freed tachyzoites that infect additional cells. Progressive destruction of parasitized cells results in foci of suppurative, necrotizing, intracerebral lesions that may be detected grossly or microscopically. There appears to be a predilection for involvement of deep gray matter.[57,62,66] Histopathologically, intracerebral lesions are characterized by foci of suppurative necrosis; encysted forms are most often seen at the periphery of the necrotic lesions. Free tachyzoites are usually most easily detected at the interface between viable and necrotic tissues. The clue to diagnosis is an accompanying prominent arteritis with concentric fibrosis of vessel media and adventitia.[65] In addition to the brain, toxoplasma lesions appear in the heart and lungs of patients with AIDS.[67]

When numbers of tachyzoites are too few for direct visualization, the organisms may be detected by the inoculation of suspected material into uninfected mice or through the use of specific immunoperoxidase staining of tissues.[64,68] Prolonged institution of pyramethamine and sulfadiazine therapy is essential to reverse neurological defects.

Viruses

Cytomegalovirus: Cytomegalovirus (CMV) may be isolated from several sites, including throat washings, urine, or blood from nearly all patients with AIDS. Clinically significant infections with CMV occur in the majority of these patients.[49] Serological testing for CMV infections is unreliable; high levels of IgG antibodies to CMV are frequently seen in healthy male homosexuals, and AIDS patients with tissue-destructive CMV lesions commonly fail to produce specific IgM antibody during reactivated infections.[69]

Although pneumonia caused by *P. carinii* is the most common life-threatening opportunistic infection in patients with AIDS, it can often be successfully treated and retreated. Nevertheless, despite apparently appropriate antipneumocystis therapy, the patient's profound immunodeficient state persists and the clinical course may ultimately be complicated by other opportunistic life-threatening pulmonary infections, including those caused by viral, fungal, and/or other unusual pathogens. After pneumonia caused by *P. carinii,* CMV infection is the next most common cause of life-threatening pneumonitis in patients with AIDS. Typically, CMV pneumonia appears late in the clinical course of patients with AIDS and signals a poor prognosis. These patients are often viremic, and postmortem histopathology frequently reveals that the interstitial pneumonitis is but part of a disseminated CMV infection.

The diagnosis of pneumonia caused by CMV may be established by detection of the characteristic viral inclusions. The virus exhibits a predilection for growth in endothelial and epithelial cells. A member of the herpes group of DNA viruses, CMV induces cellular gigantism (cytomegaly) with characteristic intranuclear and intracytoplasmic inclusions. The enlarged nucleus of an infected cell possesses a ground-glass eosinophilic inclusion with a peripheral halo (seen with hematoxylin and eosin staining). Numerous coarse intracytoplasmic viral inclusions are also evident.

Disseminated infections with CMV may involve a wide variety of organs in patients with AIDS and cause devastating sequelae. Infection of the lungs results in focal or severe diffuse interstitial and hemorrhagic pneumonitis that is frequently fatal. In the lungs, CMV may be the sole pathogen, or it may coexist with *P. carinii,* other infections, KS, or lymphoma.[70] CMV infection of the adrenal glands may cause bilateral hemorrhagic necrosis, with preferential involvement of the medullae.[71] Infection of the gastrointestinal tract by CMV is characterized by ulceration anywhere for the esophagus to the rectum.[72] There is a reported predilection of CMV ulcers for involvement of the cecum.[73] CMV intestinal ulcers may provide a portal of entry into the bloodstream and lymphatics for a variety of enteric organisms (i.e., *Salmonella* and *Shigella* spp., *Streptococcus bovis, I. belli,* etc.). Retinitis caused by CMV is the major cause of progressive loss of vision in patients with AIDS. Affected retinas show varying degrees of perivascular exudative hemorrhagic lesions, and histological sections reveal foci of necrosis and characteristic viral inclusions within retinal, choroidal, and optic nerve tissues.[74,75] In the central nervous system, CMV may cause subacute encephalitis, peripheral neuropathies, and Guillain-Barré syndromes.[76,77] In AIDS patients with encephalitis, microglial nodules are frequently seen in the gray matter;[62] CMV inclusion cells may be seen centrally within such microglial nodules, which may represent a host response to CMV infection of the central nervous system. CMV infections may result in foci of necrotic intracerebral lesions that may be detected grossly and microscopically.

Until recently, there had been no effective therapy for CMV infections, but a new antiviral drug, dihydroxy propoxymethyl guanine (DHPG), shows promise. Initial studies suggest that DHPG suppresses the spread of CMV infections.

Herpes simplex and herpes zoster: Chronic mucocutaneous herpes as well as herpetic esophagitis are opportunistic infections in patients with AIDS. The painful, vesicular, erythematous lesions of herpes simplex typically appear in oral, anal, and genital areas; lesions may also involve the esophageal and tracheobronchial mucosa. Herpes infections may result in extensive areas of chronic ulceration in patients with AIDS.[78] Herpes zoster infections may present within single or multiple dermatomes in patients with AIDS.

Histopathologically, the characteristic mucocutaneous herpetic lesion consists of an intraepidermal vesicle produced by marked acantholysis and ballooning degeneration of epithelial cells. Eosinophilic viral inclusion bodies may be detected in the center of the enlarged nuclei of balloon cells. Infected cells may coalesce to form syncytial multinucleated giant cells.[79] Herpetic infections may be successfully managed with acyclovir therapy.

Polyomavirus: Progressive multifocal leukoencephalopathy is a central nervous system demyelinating disorder caused by polyomaviruses of the papova family.[80] Infections develop in adults who are immunologically suppressed, and cases have been described in patients with AIDS.[81,82] Neurological signs and symptoms, which indicate a diffuse but asymmetrical disease, include slowly progressive dementia. CT scans of the brain may show focal hypodense white-matter lesions without contrast enhancement or mass effect.[62]

Gross pathological examination reveals a granular yellow softening of white matter. Confluent lesions may attain several centimeters in size. Histopathologically, there are patchy areas of demyelination, necrosis, and gliosis. The plaques of demyelination are especially well seen by myelin stains. Within these areas are scattered oligodendroglia, whose nuclei are filled with eosinophilic to amphophilic viral inclusions, gigantic bizarre astrocytes, and numerous foamy macrophages. Polyomavirus inclusions can be demonstrated by immunohistochemical staining, employing a polyclonal antibody with reactivity among JC, SV40, and BK types of polyomaviruses.

Fungi

Candida species: Oral candidiasis (thrush) frequently occurs in patients with AIDS. The diagnosis is established by the presence of characteristic white intraoral mucosal lesions; examination of gram-stained or wet-mounted mucosal scrapings reveals budding yeast cells and pseudohyphae. Candidial esophagitis is also a frequent opportunistic infection in patients with AIDS. Patients with esophageal lesions complain of dysphagia and odynophagia; mucosal ulcerations may be demonstrated by esophagoscopy or barium swallow esophagrams. Hematoxylin and eosin staining of esophageal biopsies demonstrates hematoxylinophilic, $3 \times 4 \mu$ budding yeast, and pseudohyphae invading ulcerated epithelium.[83] *Candida albicans* is the most common species identified, but other species may also cause disease. In its most recent revision of the case definition of AIDS, the Centers for Disease Control have added bronchial or pulmonary candidiasis as a disease indicative of AIDS if the patient has a positive serological test for HTLV-III/LAV.[84] Although candidiasis is often a serious disseminated disease in debilitated or immunosuppressed non-AIDS patients, widespread visceral dissemination is infrequent in patients with AIDS.

Cryptococcus neoformans: Relapsing *C. neoformans meningoencephalitis* as a manifestation of disseminated cryptococcus is yet another complication of the profound T-helper lymphocyte depletion found in patients with AIDS. Any AIDS patient complaining of persistent headache should undergo a spinal tap. Cerebrospinal fluid must be examined for presence of encapsulated budding yeast (using an India ink wet-mount method)[40] and cryptococcal antigen; a portion should be submitted for fungal cultures (blood and urine fungal cultures are also frequently positive). At autopsy, we have demonstrated disseminated *C. neoformans* infections in the lungs, central nervous system, lymph nodes, adrenal glands, liver, spleen, and bone marrow. Hematoxylin- and eosin-stained tissue sections reveal pale hematoxylinophilic cell walls of narrow pore budding yeast 4 to 7 μ across. Positive mucicarmine stains distinguish cryptococcal yeast cells from those of *Blastomyces* or *Histoplasma*; unlike the other opportunistic yeasts, *C. neoformans* is surrounded by a characteristic carminophilic pink capsule.[85] In patients with AIDS, there is minimal to absent inflammation accompanying the organisms, which may be intracellular within macrophages or extracellular. Despite aggressive therapy with antifungal agents, relapses are common.

Histoplasma capsulatum/Histoplasma duboisii: Histoplasmosis is acquired by inhalation of *H. capsulatum* microcinidia (spores) from soil contaminated by the feces of bats and others. Lymphohematogeneous dissemination from the lungs may result in lesions at distant sites, including the liver, spleen, lymph nodes, meninges, adrenals, and bone marrow. AIDS patients with dissemi- nated histoplasmosis variously present with fevers of unknown origin, unex- plained hepatosplenomegaly, abnormal liver function tests, lymphadenopathy, pancytopenia, chorioretinitis, and meningitis.[86] We studied the case of a male homosexual with AIDS in whom budding *H. capsulatum* yeast cells were noted within leukocytes on a Wright-Giemsa-stained peripheral blood smear; cul- tures of blood grew *H. capsulatum,* and postmortem examination demon- strated a disseminated histoplasma infection and bilateral *H. capsulatum* cho- rioretinitis.

Histopathologically, characteristic 2 × 4 μ budding yeast are typically found clustered into and expanding the cytoplasm of histiocytes or hematox- ylin- and eosin-stained tissues; the yeast are best demonstrated using PAS and methenamine silver stains. We have not seen caseating granulomas in the setting of AIDS.

As a saprophytic fungus endemic in and peculiar to Central and West Africa, *Histoplasma duboisii* characteristically causes chronic necrotizing le- sions of skin and bone in patients without AIDS. We studied a heterosexual male from Zaire with aggressive visceral (intestinal) KS and disseminated anergic *H. duboisii* infection involving lungs, lymph nodes, liver, spleen, pancreas, kidneys, and adrenals. The yeast had no capsule, did not stain with mucicarmine, and were up to 8 μm across. They were clustered into and expanded both histiocytes and giant cells. Disseminated infection by *H. du-*

boisii should be added to the list of opportunistic infections associated with AIDS in Africans.

Coccidioides immitis: C. *immitis* is a dimorphic fungus that is endemic in the southwestern United States. Following inhalation of airborne arthrospores, a primary pulmonary infection ensues; thereafter, the organisms may hematogeneously disseminate to extrapulmonary sites. Biopsied tissues demonstrate thick-walled, 30 to 60 μm spherules containing numerous endospores. Disseminated coccidioidomycosis occurs in patients with AIDS.[87,88]

Bacteria

Mycobacterium avium-intracellulare/M. tuberculosis: Before AIDS, this ubiquitous, atypical acid-fast bacillus was an uncommon human pathogen; M. *avium-intracellulare* was an infrequent cause of disseminated infections in patients with impaired immune defenses. Disseminated M. *avium-intracellulare* is a uniquely common infection in patients with AIDS;[89] these patients are often mycobacteremic,[90] and M. *avium-intracellulare* may be cultured from lymph nodes, bone marrow, liver, lung, gastrointestinal tract, and other sites.

In contrast to the caseating granulomas that are classically observed in mycobacterial infections, histological sections of infected AIDS tissues commonly show sheets of foamy histiocytes, with otherwise minimal inflammation and poorly formed or absent granulomas. For this reason, M. *avium-intracellulare* infections may go undetected unless special stains are performed. Acid-fast stains of affected tissues will reveal surprisingly large numbers of mycobacteria within the cytoplasm of distended histiocytes, reminiscent of the "globi" seen in patients with lepromatous leprosy. Involvement of the small bowel may mimic Whipple's disease.[91] M. *avium-intracellulare* infections are persistent in patients with AIDS as the organism is most resistant to conventional antituberculous therapy.

There is a high prevalence of M. *tuberculosis* among patients with AIDS. Histopathologically, this acid-fast bacillus is indistinguishable from M. *avium-intracellulare.*

Other Bacteria: Opportunistic bacterial agents causing infections in patients with AIDS include species of *Legionella* (pneumonitis),[70] *Nocardia* (pneumonitis/disseminated infections), *Salmonella* or *Shigella* (enteritis/bacteremias), and *Listeria monocytogenes* (bacteremia).

Malignancies and AIDS

Kaposi's Sarcoma

The most common neoplasm in patients with AIDS is KS.[92-98] The most common sites of involvement are the skin, lymph nodes, and spleen. Lymph node involvement is more frequent in AIDS than in endemic KS in African and Mediterranean populations. For example, in Africa, the lymphadenopathic form of KS occurs primarily in children.[99] Other common sites of involvement include the upper and lower gastrointestinal tracts and the respiratory system. Virtually any mucosal surface can be involved. Due to the concomitant presence of opportunistic infections in sites such as the gastroinestinal tract and lungs, it is often difficult to assess the clinical significance of the lesions. However, significant hemorrhage has occasionally been observed in the lung and small intestine.

The Kaposi's lesions consist of collections of spindle cells in predominantly parallel arrays. Extravasated red cells are numerous and suggest the presence of poorly formed vascular spaces. With time, there is an accumulation of hemosiderin pigment. Cytologic atypia is usually inconspicuous in the proliferating spindle cells, a feature that may distinguish KS in AIDS from KS in some African patients. Hyaline eosinophilic PAS-positive globules are usually identified, often appearing within cellular elements. These globules do not stain for factor VIII, and their exact pathogenesis is unclear.

Although it has long been suggested that KS is a tumor of endothelial cells, proof of an endothelial cell origin is uncertain. While some studies[100,101] have reported the presence of factor VIII in the proliferating cells by immunoperoxidase stains, others have interpreted the positive-staining cells as residual normal endothelial cells[102] and have provided evidence for a lymphatic origin.[99,103]

The lesions in lymph nodes appear to arise in the capsule adjacent to the subcapsular sinus and spread along lymphatic channels or sinuses. In many organs, the lesions appear to follow large vessels, such as along coronary arteries in the heart.[104] This distribution would also be in keeping with a lympatic origin of the process.

The bland nature of the proliferating cells and the multicentric origin of the process have led to speculation that KS is not truly a neoplasm, but a reversible transformation of endothelium, possibly secondary to a viral agent.[105] KS occurs frequently in immunosuppressed individuals and in transplant recipients for whom immunosuppression can be withdrawn.[106-112] Spontaneous regression of the lesions may occur after restoration of immune function. A clonal origin for KS has not been demonstrated.

The lymph nodes bearing KS frequently show a hyalinization and vascularity of the germinal centers resembling that seen in Castleman's disease.[22,23] Plasmacytosis is also usually marked, a feature which is also seen in Castleman's disease. However, Castleman's disease, as it was originally described, is a localized hamartomatous mass. Symptoms, if present, usually regress following surgical removal, and immunodeficiency is not reported. Thus, it is likely that the follicular changes are not related or identical to those of Castleman's or angiofollicular lymphoid hamartoma.

Non-Hodgkin's Lymphoma

The most common neoplasm in the AIDS population, other than KS, is non-Hodgkin's lymphoma.[3,4,113-118] These lymphomas are typically the high-grade, diffuse B-cell neoplasms of the undifferentiated small noncleaved cell (Burkitt's and non-Burkitt's) or large noncleaved cell types.[4,115] They frequently present in extranodal locations, a feature also seen in Burkitt's lymphomas and lymphomas in immunosuppressed (post-transplant) individuals. Notably, like Burkitt's lymphoma in Africa but unlike the nonendemic form, these neoplasms are frequently EBNA-positive.[119,120]

It is likely that the pathogenesis of these lymphomas is related to the polyclonal B-cell proliferation which is a constant feature of early AIDS and the persistent lymphadenopathy syndrome associated with HTLV-III. EBV, a polyclonal B-cell activator, may be an important component in B-cell proliferation, which may be further promoted by the absence of effective T-cell regulation. In this setting of rapid B-cell proliferation, a spontaneous cytogenetic translocation would not be unexpected.

Notably, the cytogenetic translocations noted in the AIDS lymphomas are similar to those of Burkitt's lymphomas and involve the c-*myc* oncogene and the immunoglobulin gene loci.[121-123] Croce et al.[124] have noted the parallels between the AIDS lymphomas and classical African Burkitt's lymphoma. In Africa, chronic malaria infection plus a high incidence of EBV may contribute to both T-cell suppression and polyclonal B-cell activation.

An excess incidence of low-grade B- or T-cell lymphomas has not been noted in the HTLV-III-positive population.[118] However, one case of multiple myeloma has been reported,[125] as well as an instance of plasmacytoma.[126]

Hodgkin's Disease

A relationship of AIDS with Hodgkin's disease is more difficult to establish. Homosexual men with Hodgkin's disease and clinical stigmata of AIDS have been identified.[13,118,127-131] However, since Hodgkin's disease itself is associated with defective T-cell function, in the absence of HTLV-III it is difficult to conclude that these individuals also have AIDS. Moreover, because Hodgkin's disease is a neoplasm that occurs with some frequency in the young adult male population, a statistically increased incidence of Hodgkin's disease must be shown in the HTLV-III-positive population before an association is drawn.

In three cases of Hodgkin's disease diagnosed in HTLV-III-positive homosexual men, we noted a prevalence of advanced stage (IIIB or IVB) and high-grade (mixed cellularity or lymphocyte-depleted) disease.[13] Other unusual or aggressive features, such as cutaneous and rectal involvement (sites of involvement extremely unusual for conventional Hodgkin's disease), have also been reported in HTLV-III-positive individuals with Hodgkin's disease.[127,131]

Regarding the aggressive nature of Hodgkin's disease seen in the AIDS population, it is likely that the ability of the host to mount an effective immune response alters the clinical behavior of the underlying disease. It is accepted that lymphocyte-predominant Hodgkin's disease is associated with low-stage disease and an excellent prognosis, whereas lymphocyte-depleted Hodgkin's disease is associated with advanced stage disease and a more aggressive course. Because of the lymphoctyopenia of AIDS, Hodgkin's disease in this population is invariably lymphocyte-depleted.

If there is an increased incidence of Hodgkin's disease in AIDS patients, there would still be several possible explanations. For one, it is possible that the immunodeficiency of Hodgkin's disease leads to an increased susceptibility to HTLV-III infection. Alternatively, the immunodeficiency of AIDS could lead to an increased susceptibility to the putative "Hodgkin's disease agent." Such cases might provide an excellent opportunity to search for the etiological agent of Hodgkin's disease.

Small Cell Carcinomas

Several cases of small cell undifferentiated carcinoma or "oat" cell carcinoma have been reported in individuals with AIDS.[132-134] Small cell carcinomas are primitive neuroendocrine tumors that are most common in the lung, but can occur in many sites including the gastrointestinal tract and pancreas. Sites of origin in the AIDS patient have included the rectosigmoid, pancreas, and lung.

It is of interest that malignant small cell tumors of neuroendocrine origin have been induced in the pancreas of hamsters inoculated with human BK papova virus.[135] BK virus is often found in patients with immunodeficiency disorders, and has been isolated from the urine of patients with Wiskott-Aldrich syndrome.[136] Thus, small cell carcinoma might be another virally induced neoplasm occurring with increasing frequency in the AIDS population. BK virus has also been recovered from a brain tumor in a patient with Wiskott-Aldrich syndrome, and has been shown to cause ependymomas in hamsters.

These observations are provocative and warrant further investigation. It would be desirable to investigate further cases for BK-associated antigens or BK sequences in the DNA of malignant cells.

Other Malignancies

Other malignant tumors have been reported sporadically in the AIDS population. Homosexual men practicing anal intercourse have an increased incidence of anal and venereal warts (condylomata acuminata).[137] These lesions have been associated with members of the papilloma virus family. Some of these lesions have shown evidence of in situ carcinoma or intraepithelial malignant change, and both oral and anal squamous cell carcinomas have been reported.[137-142] Papilloma viruses have been linked to squamous cell carcinomas of the cervix in women, and it has been postulated that members of the papilloma virus family are also linked to these epithelial and possibly sexually transmitted malignancies in homosexual men.[137,143,144]

Other tumors reported sporadically in patients with AIDS include malignant melanoma[128] and embryonal cell carcinoma.[145] It is notable that melanomas, like small cell carcinomas, are of neuroendocrine origin. However, the occurrence of embryonal cell carcinoma would appear to be coincidental in this young male patient population.

Neuropathology of AIDS

Introduction

Neurological disease complicates the clinical course of over one-third of patients with AIDS;[146] at autopsy, over 80% of cases may show neuropathological involvement.[147,148] In this section, selected neuropathological features of AIDS are discussed and illustrated. Because a complete discussion of this subject is beyond the scope of this chapter, the reader is referred to any of the numerous recent reviews for details.[3-5,62,68,146,147,149-152] Of particular interest are those of Snider,[62] Levy,[146] and their co-workers; these include algorithmic approaches to diagnosis, which should prove equally useful to the pathologist and clinician.

Microglial Nodules

Microglial nodules (MN) are microscopic inflammatory foci found within the central nervous system parenchyma, in either gray or white matter (Fig. 1). Contrary to their name, the cells forming these lesions are not of glial origin, but are derived from cells of the monocyte-macrophage series and are hematogenous in origin (Fig. 2). They are nonspecific in that they may be seen in a number of central nervous system parenchymal infections, which may be variously of viral, rickettsial, fungal, or protozoan etiology.[153]

MN are, overall, the single most common histopathological finding in the brains of AIDS patients.[62,147] If one eliminates those associated with "specific" identifiable agents (fungi, *Toxoplasma*), there remain many cases with variable numbers of MN as the sole neuropathological finding; the MN in the white matter may be associated with focal demyelination (Fig. 3).[62,147,154,155] However, a small number (i.e., less than 10%)[151,155,156] of MN in this setting may contain, at their center, a large cell with an intranuclear (and sometimes

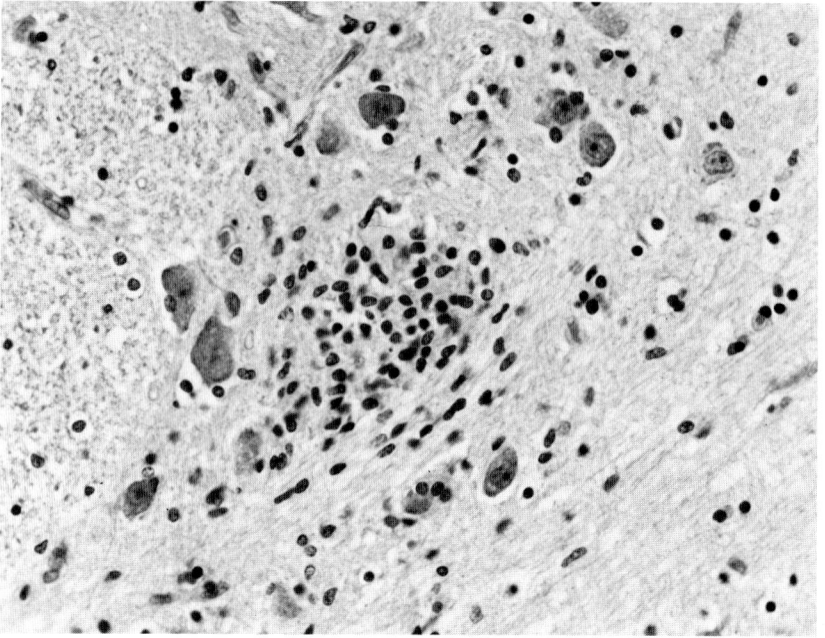

FIGURE 1 Microglial nodule in gray matter. (Hematoxylin and eosin, 330×.)

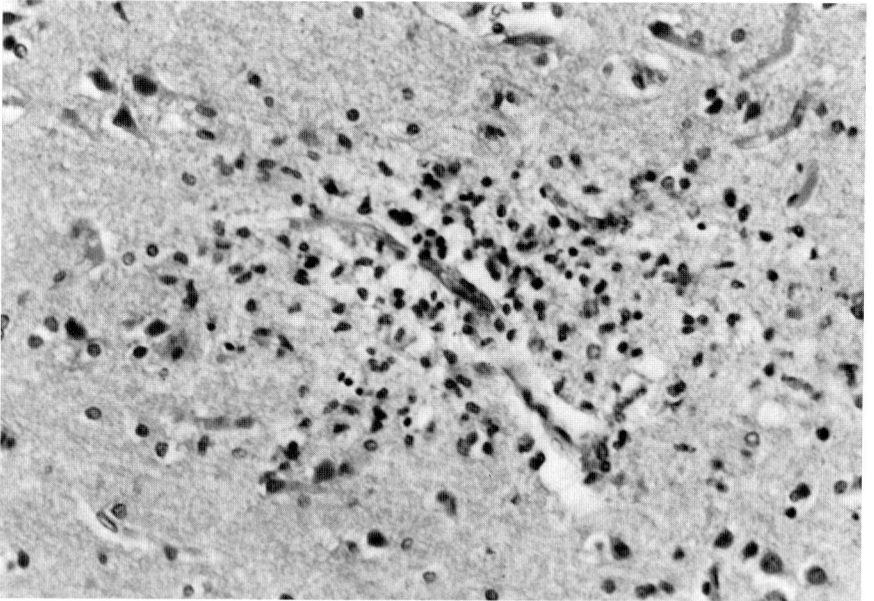

FIGURE 2 Hematogenous mononuclear cells exiting cerebral capillary to form a microglial nodule. (Hematoxylin and eosin, 300×.)

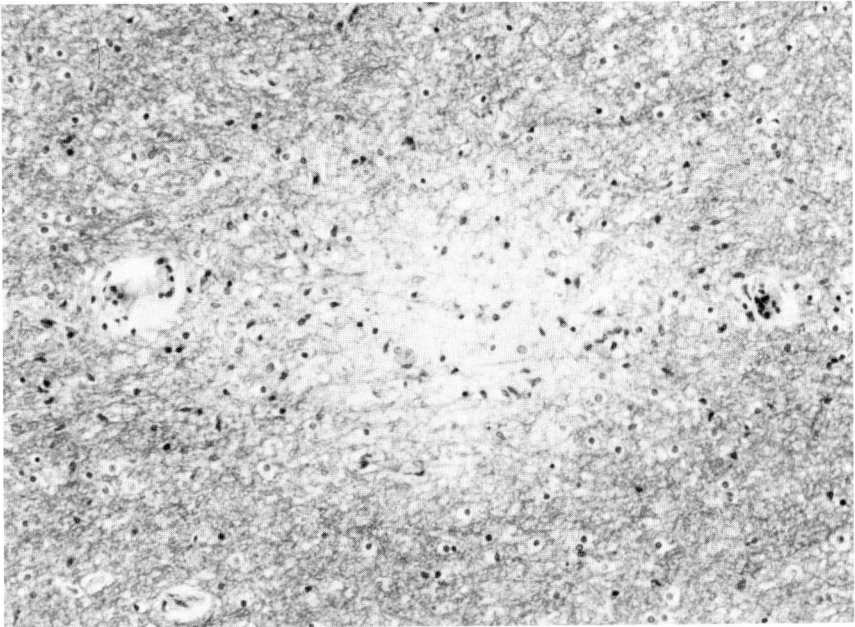

FIGURE 3 Focal zone of myelin loss in cerebral white matter. (Luxol fast blue-PAS, 200×.)

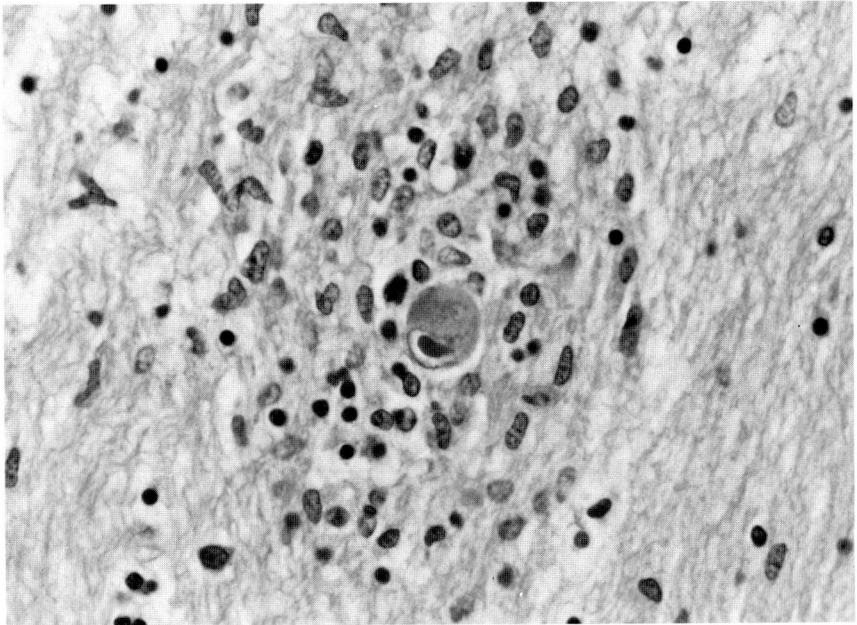

FIGURE 4 Microglial nodule with cytomegalic cell (intranuclear inclusion, ballooned cell body with granular cytoplasm) in center. (Hematoxylin and eosin, 400×.)

intracytoplasmic) inclusion, typical of cytomegalovirus (CMV) infection, and permitting a diagnosis of CMV encephalitis (Fig. 4).

Study of these inclusion-bearing cells has confirmed the presence of CMV by electron microscopy[157] and immunocytochemistry.[151] In addition, in situ hybridization has shown infection of histologically normal cells.[158] Infection of endothelial cells[156] and ependymal cells[158] may be of pathogenetic importance in this context.

Subacute Encephalitis

The above considerations concerning MN and CMV are central to current investigations of the progressive encephalopathy with dementia often seen in

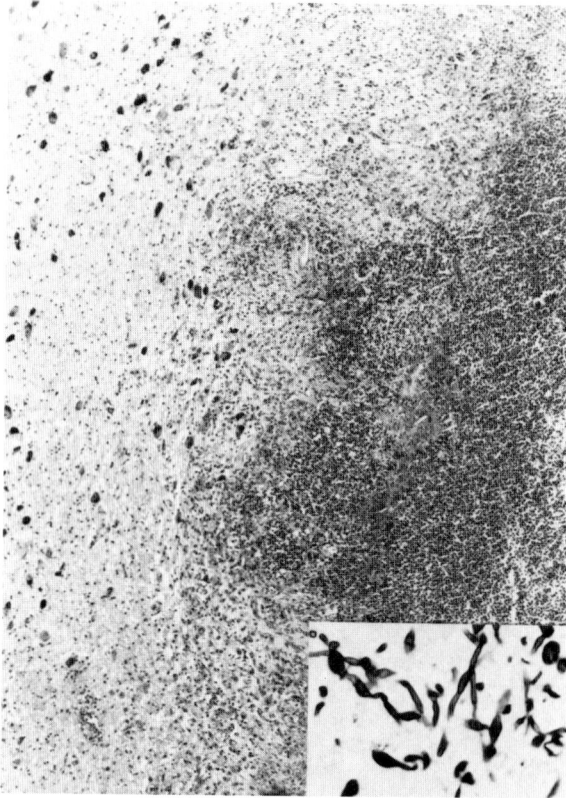

FIGURE 5 Abscess formation in the midbrain due to *Candida*. On the right, there is extensive necrosis with suppurative inflammation. (Hematoxylin and eosin, 54×.) The inset shows fungal elements consistent with *Candida*. (Methenamine silver, 430×.)

AIDS patients. In these patients, in whom no other "specific" (identifiable) clinical or neuropathological substrate for dementia is present, one most often finds neuropathological findings referred to as "subacute encephalitis" (SE)[146-148,151,155] consisting of MN (predominantly in gray matter) with or without foci of demyelination in white matter. Other evidence of inflammation is absent. It should be noted that the extent and severity of these findings are extremely variable from case to case and that precise correlation with the clinical history of encephalopathy is not always possible.

The demonstration of CMV by various methods in some of these cases, as just noted, has raised the possibility that *all* cases of SE might be due to CMV;

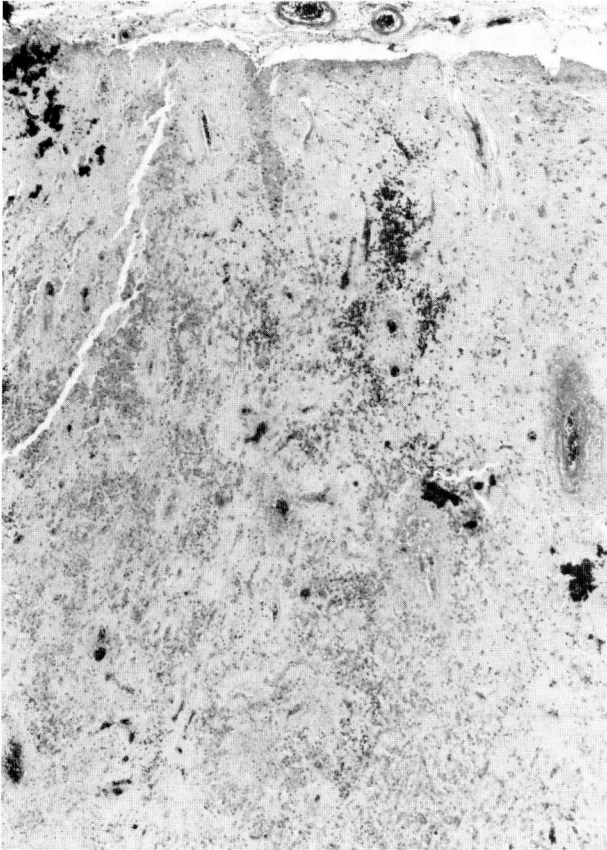

FIGURE 6   Necrotizing encephalitis due to toxoplasmosis. The cerebral cortex, particularly on the left, shows extensive vasculocentric necrosis and inflammation. (Hematoxylin and eosin, 54×.)

it is clear that some are—at least in part. However, the recent demonstration of HTLV-III infection in the brains of AIDS patients makes it possible that AIDS encephalopathy is, in fact, due to HTLV-III, with or without a "secondary" complicating entity such as CMV encephalitis. Evidence for CNS infection by HTLV-III in AIDS encephalopathy includes the presence of viral-specific RNA as shown by Southern analysis and in situ hybridization[159] and isolation of HTLV-III from cerebrospinal fluid (CSF) and brain of affected patients.[160] In addition, synthesis within the blood-brain barrier of HTLV-III-specific IgG has been shown in neurologically symtomatic AIDS patients.[161] Furthermore, it appears that some of the previously unexplained neurological manifestations of AIDS, such as aseptic meningitis, vacuolar myelopathy, and peripheral neuropathy, may also be due to infection by HTLV-III.[160-164]

Specific Secondary Infections

Under this heading, which encompasses much of the neurology of AIDS, are included a very wide range of clinically and pathologically identifiable infec-

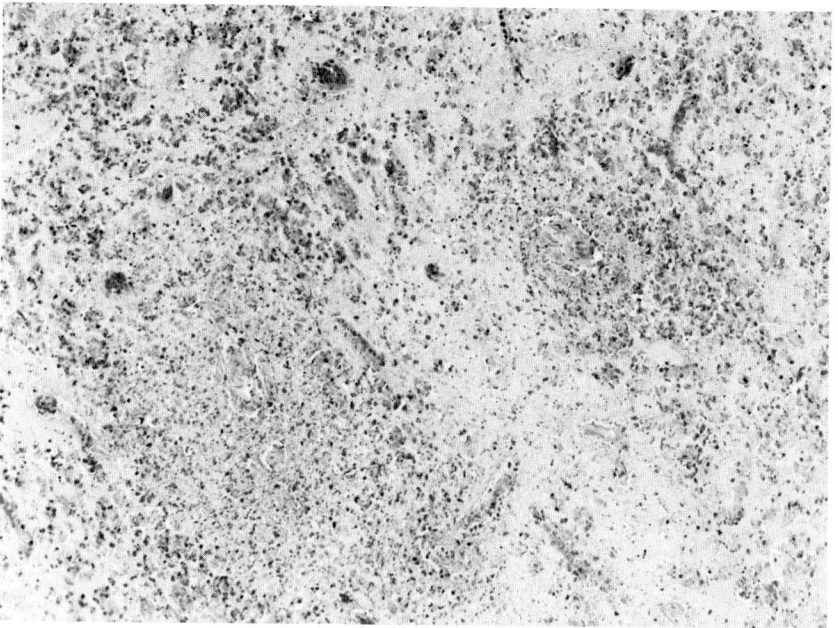

FIGURE 7　Area near edge of affected area in *Toxoplasma* encephalitis. It is within such microscopic fields that organisms are most easily found. (Hematoxylin and eosin, 130×.)

tions due to bacteria, fungi, protozoa, and viruses. Because of the nature of the underlying disease, these are often part of a disseminated systemic infection, as described earlier.

Bacterial infections, both systemic and CNS, have been notably unusual in AIDS. However, *Mycobacterium avium-intracellulare,* a frequent systemic infection in these patients, occasionally involves the CNS.[146]

Fungal infection of the CNS is more frequent, most commonly *Cryptococcus neoformans* and *Candida albicans,* resulting in meningitis and/or encephalitis and sometimes (*Candida*) abscess formation.[62,146,150] This is illus-

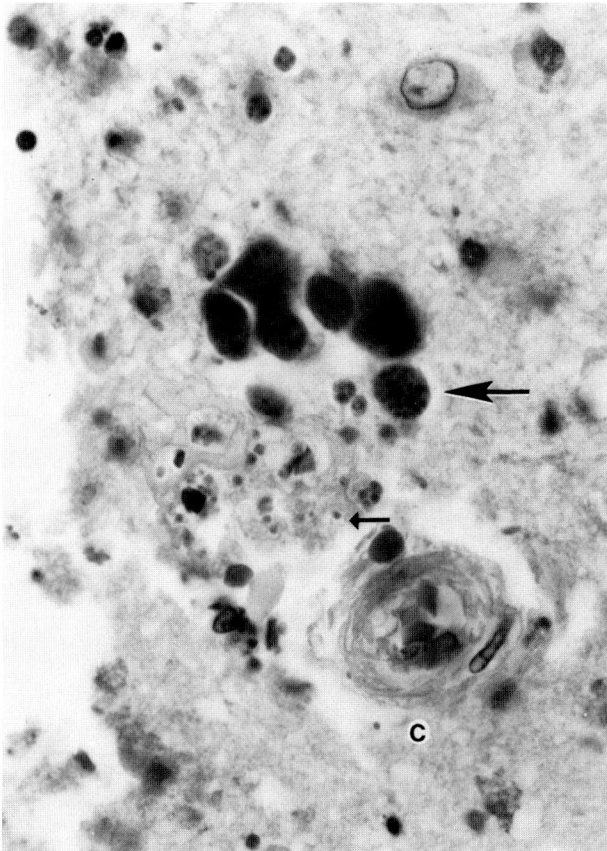

FIGURE 8   High power examination reveals both encysted (large arrow) and free organisms (small arrow) adjacent to a capillary (c). (Hematoxylin and eosin, oil, 860×.)

trated in Figure 5, which shows a focal area of suppurative inflammation containing fungal elements.

Toxoplasma gondii, a protozoan, is the most common organism infecting the CNS of AIDS patients.[62,68,146,147,151,152] Infection with this organism is described in detail elsewhere in this chapter. Pathologically, *Toxoplasma* causes a necrotizing encephalitis that often leads to abscess formation, illustrated in Figures 6, 7, and 8.

Viral infections within the CNS may cause meningitis, encephalitis, or myelitis. The majority of CNS viral illness in AIDS is due to infection by CMV and/or HTLV-III (as discussed). In addition to its possible role in SE, CMV may

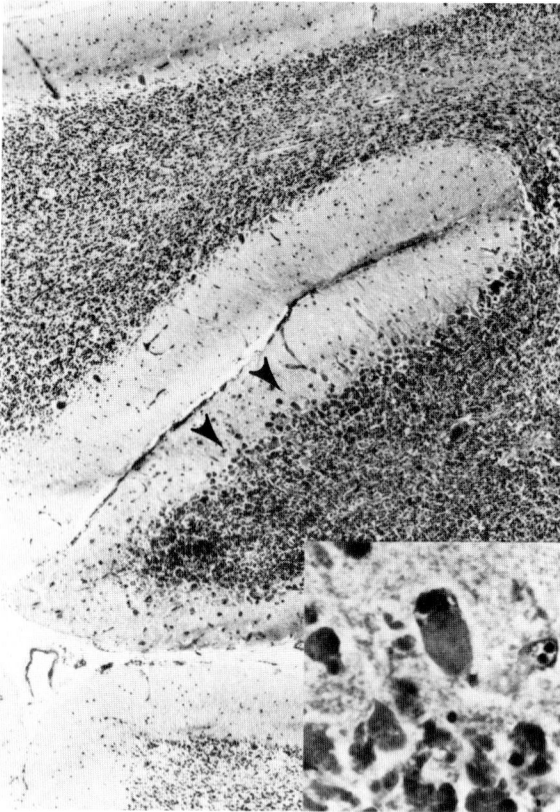

FIGURE 9   Focal encephalitis due to CMV in the cerebellar cortex, predominantly in the Purkinje cell layer (arrows). (Hematoxylin and eosin, 54×.) The inset reveals a typical cytomegalic cell. (Hematoxylin and eosin, 430×.)

cause a focal encephalitis (Fig. 9), which can be clinically silent, and meningoencephalitis, in which virus may be isolated from inflammatory cells in the CSF.[165] Other viruses that may cause these types of illnesses in AIDS include herpes simplex virus I and II and varicella zoster (encephalitis).[146,166,167]

Another somewhat different but important viral infection is progressive multifocal leukoencephalopathy (PML).[62,146,147,151,168-170] This subacute, almost always fatal, disease is due to infection of oligodendrocytes (Fig. 10) by a human papovavirus in compromised hosts. Virus can be demonstrated in these cells by electron microscopy, immunocytochemistry, and in situ hybridization.[168] Infection of these cells, which are responsible for myelination of CNS axons, results in progressive multifocal demyelination, as illustrated in Figures 11 and 12, with resulting neurological deterioration.

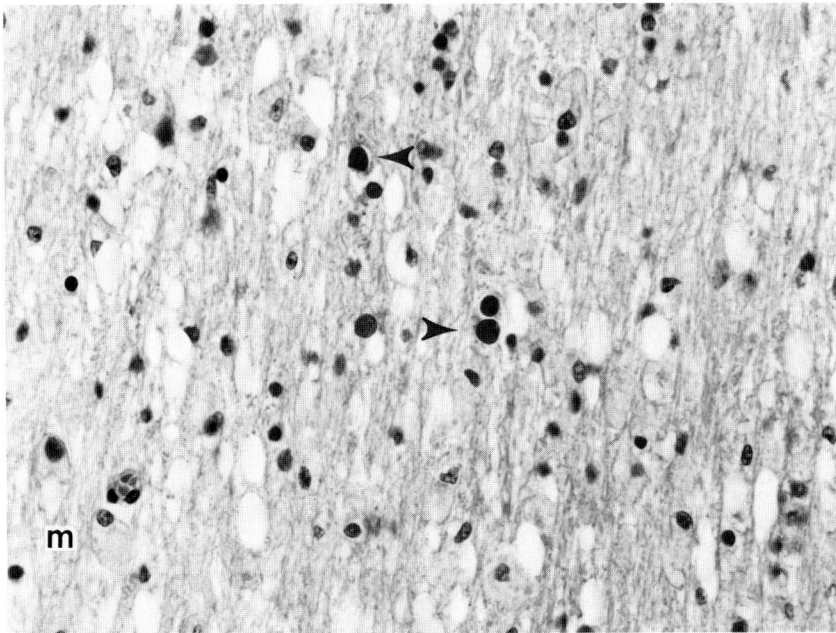

FIGURE 10   Margin of lesion in progressive multifocal leukoencephalopathy (PML). Several darkly staining, enlarged oligodendrocytes are seen (arrows); these are infected with papovavirus. The white matter is vacuolated, and scattered macrophages (m) are seen. (Hematoxylin and eosin, 330×.)

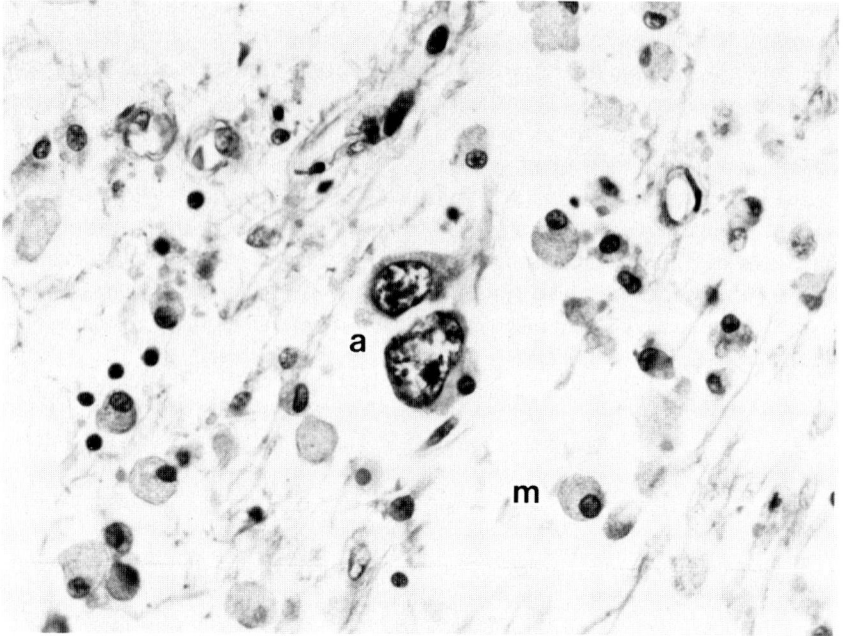

FIGURE 11   Area of severely affected white matter in progressive multifocal leukoen-cephalopathy (PML). There are numerous macrophages (m) and two enlarged bizarre astroctyes (a). The relationship of these latter to the papovavirus infection is unclear. (Hematoxylin and eosin, 500×.)

Cerebral Mass Lesions

Cerebral mass lesions are not uncommon in AIDS patients. Study of these cases has revealed a number of etiologies, including abscesses (particularly those due to *Toxoplasma* or fungus) and lymphoma.[61] Cerebral abscesses result from progression (liquefaction, encapsulation) of the encephalitic stage of infection ("cerebritis"), as described for *Candida* and *Toxoplasma*.

The intracranial lymphomas are histologically comparable with those seen in other immunosuppressed states, and may occur as primary nervous system tumors or in conjunction with systemic lymphoma. It should be noted that CNS lymphomas, especially when secondary to systemic lymphomas, can be diffusely infiltrative and often spread through the CSF pathways; thus, they may present as a diffuse encephalopathy rather than as an intracranial mass lesion (Figs. 13, 14, and 15).[62,146,147,150,151]

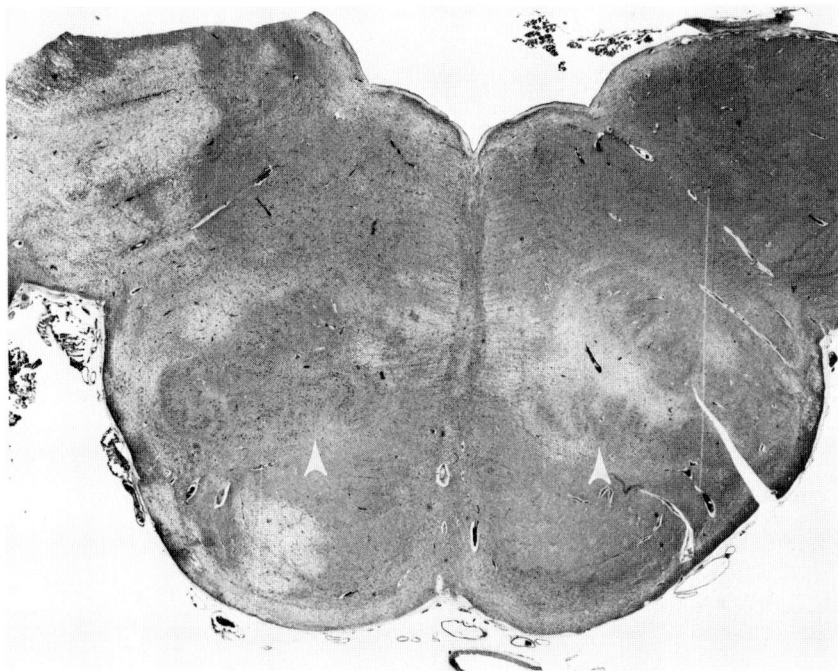

FIGURE 12   Macroscopic findings in progressive multifocal leukoencephalopathy (PML). The multiple pale foci in the white matter of the medulla are areas of demyelination. Note clearcut sparing of gray matter, such as the inferior olives (arrows). (Hematoxylin and eosin, 6×.)

Although Kaposi's sarcoma (KS) is a major systemic feature of AIDS,[150] involvement of the CNS by KS is extremely rare. Only seven cases have been reported.[61,171]

Peripheral Nerve Involvement

Disease of the peripheral nervous system (PNS) is diagnosed relatively infrequently in AIDS patients, perhaps partly because the severity of the systemic and CNS illnesses found in these patients renders diagnosis of PNS disease difficult. A variety of cranial and peripheral nerve syndromes have been described in AIDS patients, many of which do not appear at present to have a known specific etiology except, for example, cases of herpes zoster radiculitis.[146] These are discussed elsewhere in this book. An "inflammatory"

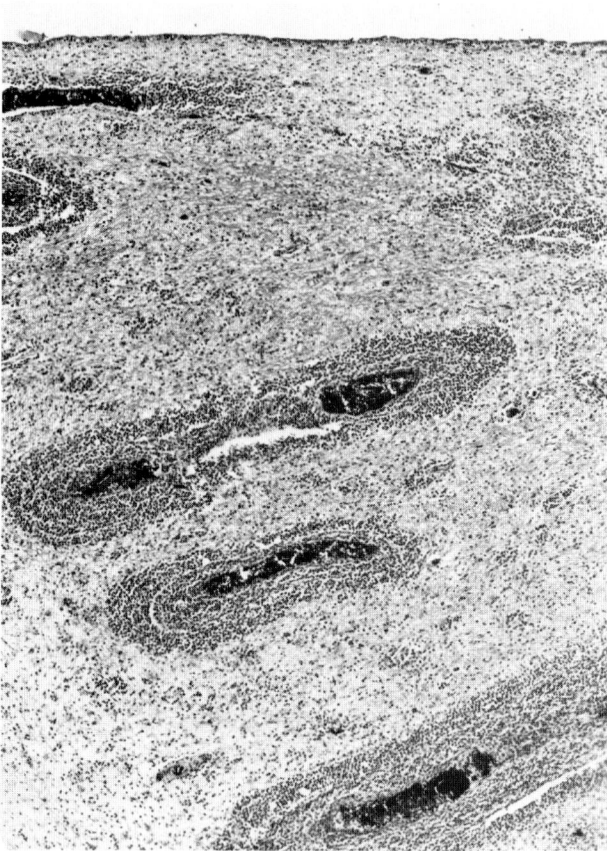

FIGURE 13   Typical appearance of intracranial lymphoma, with thick perivascular cuffs of neoplastic cells that spill out into the parenchyma. (Hematoxylin and eosin, 54×.)

neuritis has been reported by Lipkin et al.,[172] with round cell inflammation in sural nerve biopsies. Two cases of peripheral nerve infection by CMV have also been described,[173] resulting in a Guillain-Barré-like syndrome.

Pediatric Cases

A small number of pediatric AIDS cases with neurological manifestations have been reported;[174-176] the exact incidence of CNS disease in the pediatric age

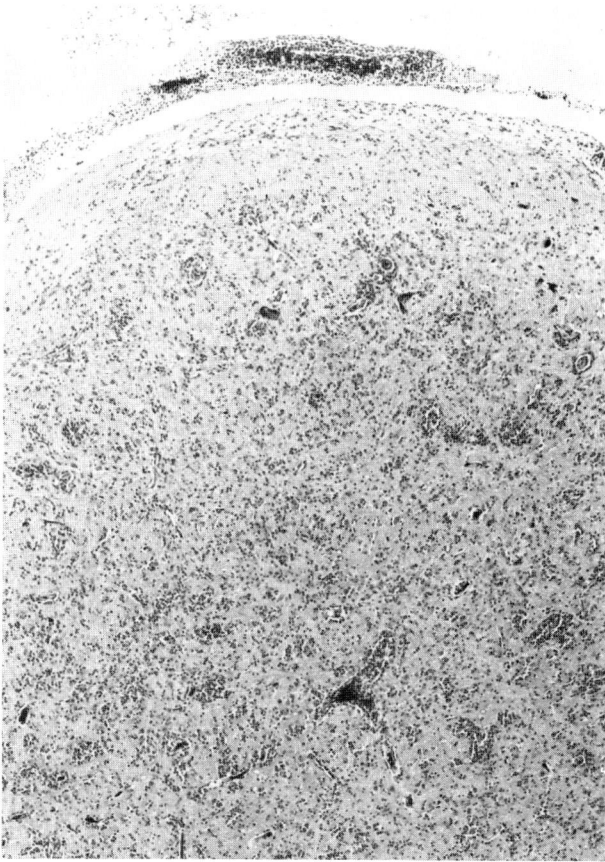

FIGURE 14   More diffuse parenchymal infiltration of lymphoma, with spread into the overlying subarachnoid space. (Hematoxylin and eosin, 54×.)

group, however, is not known.[174] The most common clinical syndrome is a progressive encephalopathy comparable with the SE seen in adults, with a similar neuropathological substrate. In several of these cases, HTLV-III has been demonstrated in the brain.[176] Other findings include long-tract (i.e., corticospinal) degeneration and a calcific vasculopathy of the basal ganglia. Although the number of pediatric cases is small, it has been suggested that opportunistic infections such as toxoplasmosis may be less common in children than in adults.[176]

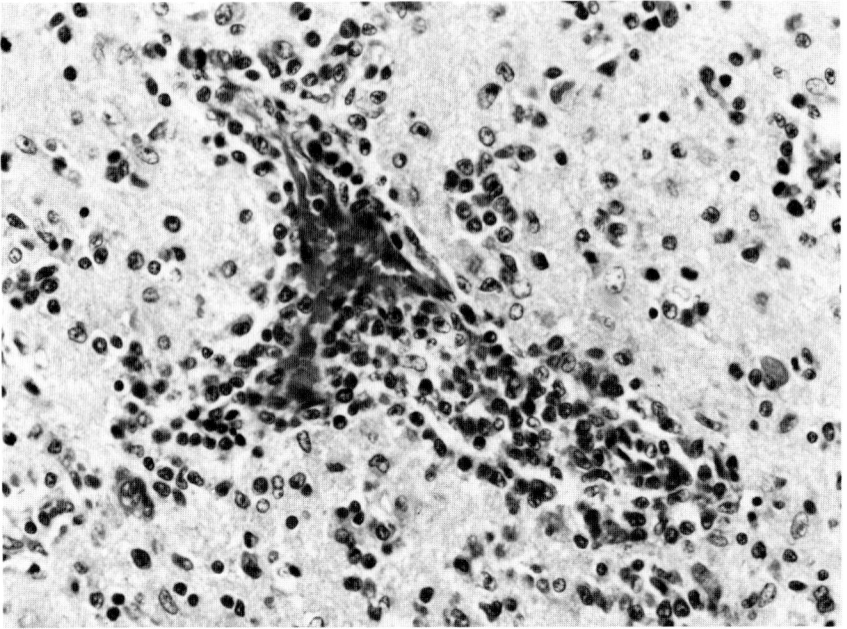

FIGURE 15 At higher power, the perivascular location of the lymphoma cells is easily seen. (Hematoxylin and eosin, 330×.)

References

1. Reichert CM, Kelly VL, Macher AM. Pathologic features of AIDS. In: DeVita VT Jr, Hellman S, Rosenberg SA, eds. AIDS: etiology, diagnosis, treatment and prevention. Philadelphia: JP Lippincott Co, 1985:111–160.
2. Guarda LA, Luna MA, Smith JL Jr, et al. Acquired immune deficiency syndrome: postmortem findings. Am J Clin Pathol 1984; 81:549–557.
3. Hui AN, Koss MN, Meyer PR. Necropsy findings in acquired immunodeficiency syndrome. Hum Pathol 1984; 15:670–676.
4. Reichert CM, O'Leary TJ, Levens DL, Simrell CR, Macher AM. Autopsy pathology in the acquired immune deficiency syndrome. Am J Pathol 1983; 112:357–382.
5. Millard PR. AIDS: histopathological aspects. J Pathol 1984; 143:223–229.
6. Amberson JB, DiCarlo EF, Metroka CE, Koizumi JH, Mouradian JA. Diagnostic pathology in the acquired immunodeficiency syndrome: surgical pathology and cytology experience with 67 patients. Arch Pathol Lab Med 1985; 109:345–351.
7. Ioachim HL, Lerner CW, Tapper ML. The lymphoid lesions associated with the acquired immunodeficiency syndrome. Am J Surg Pathol 1983; 76:543–553.
8. Guarda LA, Butler JJ, Mansel P, et al. Lymphadenopathy in homosexual men. Morbid anatomy with clinical and immunologic correlations. Am J Clin Pathol 1983; 79:559–568.

 9. Domingo J, Chin NW. Lymphadenopathy in a heterogeneous population at risk for the acquired immunodeficiency syndrome—a morphologic study. Am J Clin Pathol 1983; 80:649–654.

10. Brynes RK, Chan WC, Spira TJ, Ewing EP Jr, Chandler FW. Value of lymph node biopsy in unexplained lymphadenopathy in homosexual men. JAMA 1983; 250: 1313–1317.

11. Metroka CE, Cunningham-Rundles S, Pollack MS, et al. Generalized lymphadenopathy in homosexual men. Ann Intern Med 1983; 99:585–591.

12. Ewing EP Jr, Chandler FW, Spira TJ, Brynes RK, Chan WC. Primary lymph node pathology in AIDS and AIDS-related lymphadenopathy. Arch Pathol Lab Med 1985; 109:977–981.

13. Jaffe ES, Clark J, Steis R, et al. Lymph node pathology of HTLV and HTLV-associated neoplasms. Cancer Res 1985; 45(Suppl):4662s–4664s.

14. Lane HC, Masur H, Edgar LC, Whalen G, Rook AL, Fauci AS. Abnormalities of B-cell activation and immunoregulation in patients with the acquired immunodeficiency syndrome. N Engl J Med 1983; 309:453–458.

15. Papadopoulos NM, Lane HC, Costello R, et al. Oligoclonal immunoglobulins in patients with the acquired immunodeficiency syndrome. Clin Immunol Immunopathol 1985; 35:43–46.

16. Biberfeld P, Porwit-Ksiazek A, Bottiger B, Morfeldt-Mansson L, Biberfeld G. Immunohistopathology of lymph nodes in HTLV-III infected homosexuals with persistent adenopathy of AIDS. Cancer Res 1985; 45(Suppl):4665s–4670s.

17. Modlin RL, Meyer PR, Hofman FM, et al. T-lymphocyte subsets in lymph nodes from homosexual men. JAMA 1983; 250:1302–1302.

18. Mangkornkanok-Mark AS, Dong J. Immunoperoxidase evaluation of lymph nodes from acquired immunodeficiency patients. Clin Exp Immunol 1984; 55:581–586.

19. Said JW, Shintaku IP, Teitelbaum A, et al. Distribution of T-cell phenotypic subsets and surface immunoglobulin-bearing lymphocytes in lymph nodes from male homosexuals with persistent generalized adenopathy. Hum Pathol 1984; 15:785–790.

20. Chan WC, Brynes RK, Spira TJ, et al. Lymphocyte subsets in lymph nodes of homosexual men with generalized unexplained lymphadenopathy. Correlation with morphology and blood changes. Arch Pathol Lab Med 1985; 109:133–137.

21. Chen KTK. Multicentric Castleman's disease and Kaposi's sarcoma. Am J Surg Pathol 1984; 8:287–293.

22. Lachant NA, Sun NC, Leong LA, Oseas RS, Prince HE. Multicentric angiofollicular lymph node hyperplasia (Castleman's disease) followed by Kaposi's sarcoma in two homosexual males with the acquired immunodeficiency syndrome (AIDS). Am J Clin Pathol 1985; 83:27–33.

23. Dickson D, Ben-Ezra JM, Reed J, Flax H, Janis R. Multicentric giant lymph node hyperplasia, Kaposi's sarcoma, and lymphoma. Arch Pathol Lab Med 1985; 109: 1013–1018.

24. Keller AR, Hochholzer L, Castleman B. Hyaline-vascular and plasma types of giant lymph node hyperplasia of the mediastinum and other locations. Cancer 1972; 29:670–683.

25. Castella A, Croxson TS, Mildvan D, Witt DH, Zalusky R. The bone marrow in

AIDS. A histologic, hematologic, and microbiologic study. Am J Clin Path 1985; 84:425–432.

26. Abrams DI, Chinn EK, Lewis BJ, Volberding PA, Conant MA, Townsend RM. Hematologic manifestations in homosexual men with Kaposi's sarcoma. Am J Clin Pathol 1984; 81:13–18.

27. Fauci AS. The syndrome of Kaposi's sarcoma and opportunistic infections: an epidemiologically restricted disorder of immunoregulation. Ann Intern Med 1982; 96:777–779. Editorial.

28. Morris L, Distenfeld A, Amorosi E, Karpatkin S. Autoimmune thrombocytopenic purpura in homosexual men. Ann Intern Med 1982; 96:714–717.

29. Murphy MF, Metcalfe P, Waters AH, et al. Immune neutropenia in homosexual men. Lancet 1985; i:217–218. Letter.

30. Savona S, Nardi MA, Lennette ET, Karpatkin S. Thrombocytopenic purpura in narcotics addicts. Ann Intern Med 1985; 102:737–741.

31. Walsh CM, Nardi MA, Karpatkin S. On the mechanism of thrombocytopenic purpura in sexually active homosexual men. N Engl J Med 1984; 311:635–639.

32. Levine AS. Viruses, immune dysregulation, and oncogenesis: interferences regarding the case and evolution of AIDS. In: Friedman-Kien AE, Laubenstein JL, eds. AIDS: the epidemic of Kaposi's sarcoma and opportunistic infections. New York: Masson Publishing, 1984:7–21.

33. Anderson MG, Dixey J, Key P, et al. Persistent lymphadenopathy in homosexual men: a clinical and ultrastructural study. Lancet 1984; i:880–882.

34. Grimley PM, Kang YH, Frederick W, et al. Interferon-related leukocyte inclusions in acquired immune deficiency syndrome: localization in T cells. Am J Clin Pathol 1984; 81:147–155.

35. Ulirsch RC, Jaffe ES. Sjögren's syndrome associated with the AIDS-related complex. Submitted.

36. Gordon JJ, Golbus J, Kurtides ES. Chronic lymphadenopathy and Sjögren's syndrome in a homosexual man. N Engl J Med 1984; 311:1441–1442. Letter.

37. Kovacs J, Hiemenz J, Macher A, et al. Pneumocystis carinii pneumonia: a comparison of clinical features in patients with the acquired immune deficiency syndrome and patients with other immunodeficiencies. Ann Intern Med 1984; 100:663–671.

38. Centers for Disease Control. Update on acquired immune deficiency syndrome (AIDS)—United States. MMWR 1982; 31:507–509.

39. Masur H, Michelis M, Greene J, et al. An outbreak of community-acquired Pneumocystis carinii pneumonia: initial manifestation of cellular immune dysfunction. N Engl J Med 1982; 305:1431–1438.

40. Macher A, Reichert C. The pathologic findings associated with opportunistic infections in AIDS. In: Ebbesen P, Biggar R, Melbye M, eds. AIDS—a basic guide for clinicians. Copenhagen/Philadelphia: Munksgaard/WB Saunders, 1984:113–122.

41. Frenkel J. Pneumocystosis. In: Binford C, Connor D, eds. Pathology of tropical and extraordinary diseases. Washington, DC: Armed Forces Institute of Pathology, 1976:303–307.

42. Macher A, Shelhamer J, MacLowry J, et al. Pneumocystis carinii identified by Gram stain of lung imprints. Ann Intern Med 1983; 99:484–485.

43. Domingo J, Waksal H. Wright's stain in rapid diagnosis of *Pneumocystis carinii*. Am J Clin Pathol 1984; 81:511–514.
44. Current W, Reese N, Erust J, et al. Human cryptosporidiosis in immunocompetent and immunodeficient persons. N Engl J Med 1983; 308:1252–1257.
45. Meisel J, Perera D, Meligro C, et al. Overwhelming water diarrhea, associated with a cryptosporidium in an immunosuppressed patient. Gastroenterology 1976; 70: 1156–1160.
46. Centers for Disease Control. Cryptosporidiosis: assessment of chemotherapy of males with acquired immunodeficiency syndrome (AIDS). MMWR 1982; 31:589–591.
47. Henriksen S, Pohlenz J. Staining of *cryptosporidia* by a modified Ziehl-Neelsen technique. Acta Vet Scand 1981; 22:594–596.
48. Current W. Human cryptosporidiosis. N Engl J Med 1983; 309:1326–1327.
49. Payne P, Lancaster L, Heinzman M, et al. Identification of *cryptosporidium* in patients with acquired immune deficiency syndrome. N Engl J Med 1983; 309: 613–614.
50. Vetterling J, Jervis H, Merrill T, et al. *Cryptosporidium wrairi* sp. from the guinea pig *Cavia porcellus*, with an emendation of the genus. J Protozool 1971; 18:243–247.
51. Lefkowitch J, Krumholz S, Feng-Chen K, et al. Cryptosporidiosis of the human small intestine: a light and electron microscopic study. Hum Pathol 1984; 15:746–752.
52. Mele L, Nadler H, Pappalardo S, et al. *Cryptosporidium*: unusual respiratory tract isolate. (Abstract C96). Presented at the 83rd annual meeting of the American Society of Microbiology, New Orleans, 1983.
53. Forgacs P, Tarshis A, Ma P, et al. Intestinal and bronchial cryptosporidiosis in an immunodeficient homosexual man. Ann Intern Med 1983; 99:793–794.
54. Chiampi N, Sandberg R, Klompus J, et al. Cryptosporidial enteritis and pneumocystis pneumonia in a homosexual man. Hum Pathol 1983; 14:734–737.
55. Markell E, Voge M. Lumen dwelling protozoa—the sporozoans—*Isospora belli*. In: Medical parasitology, 5th ed. Philadelphia: WB Saunders, 1981:68–69.
56. Wong B, Gold J, Brown A, et al. Central nervous system toxoplasmosis in homosexual men and parenteral drug users. Ann Intern Med 1984; 100:36–42.
57. Handler M, Ho V, Whelan M, et al. Intracerebral toxoplasmosis in patients with acquired immune deficiency syndrome. J Neurosurg 1983; 59:994–1001.
58. Pitchenik A, Finch M, Walls K. Evaluation of cerebral mass lesions in acquired immune deficiency syndrome. N Engl J Med 1983; 308:1099.
59. Chan J, Moskowitz L, Olivella J, et al. Toxoplasma encephalitis in recent Haitian entrants. South Med J 1983; 76:1211–1215.
60. Post J, Chan J, Hensley G, et al. Toxoplasma encephalitis in Haitian adults with acquired immune deficiency syndrome: a clinical-pathologic correlation. Am J Roentgenol 1983; 140:861–868.
61. Levy R, Pons V, Rosenblum M. Central nervous system mass lesions in the acquired immuno deficiency syndrome (AIDS). J Neurosurg 1984; 61:9–16.
62. Snider W, Simpson D, Nielson S, Gold JWM, Metroka CE, Posner JB. Neurological complications of acquired immune deficiency syndrome: analysis of 50 patients. Ann Neurol 1983; 14:403–418.

63. Pitchenik A, Fischl M, Dickinson G, et al. Opportunistic infections and Kaposi's sarcoma among Haitians: evidence of a new acquired immunodeficiency state. Ann Intern Med 1983; 98:277–284.
64. Hauser W, Luft B, Conley F, et al. Central nervous system toxoplasmosis in homosexual and heterosexual adults. N Engl J Med 1982; 307:498–499.
65. Horowitz S, Bentson J, Benson D, et al. CNS toxoplasmosis in acquired immune deficiency syndrome. Arch Neurol 1983; 40:649–652.
66. Alonzo R, Heiman-Patterson T, Mancall E. Cerebral toxoplasmosis in acquired immune deficiency syndrome. Arch Neurol 1984; 41:321–323.
67. Luft B, Conley F, Remington J, et al. Outbreak of central nervous system toxoplasmosis in western Europe and North America. Lancet 1983; ii:781–794.
68. Moskowitz LB, Hensley GT, Chan JC, Gregorios J, Conley FK. The neuropathology of acquired immune deficiency syndrome. Arch Pathol Lab Med 1984; 108: 867–872.
69. Dylewski J, Chou S, Merigan T. Absence of detectable IgM antibody during cytomegalovirus disease in patients with AIDS. N Engl J Med 1983; 309:493.
70. Murray J, Felton C, Garay S, et al. Pulmonary complications of the acquired immunodeficiency syndrome. N Engl J Med 1984; 310:1682–1688.
71. Macher A, Reichert S, Strauss S, et al. Death in the AIDS patient: role of cytomegalovirus. N Engl J Med 1983; 309:1454.
72. Knapp A, Horst D, Eliopuolos G, et al. Widespread cytomegalovirus gastroenterocolitis in a patient with acquired immunodeficiency syndrome. Gastroenterology 1983; 85:1399–1402.
73. Rotterdam H, Lerner C, Tapper M. Biopsies of the digestive tract in patients with acquired immunodeficiency syndrome. Lab Invest 1983; 48:72A. (Abstract).
74. Bachman D, Rodrigues M, Chu F, et al. Culture proven CMV retinitis in a homosexual man with acquired immunodeficiency syndrome. Ophthalmology 1982; 89:797–804.
75. Palestine A, Rodrigues M, Macher A, et al. Ophthalmic considerations in acquired immune deficiency syndrome. Ophthalmology 1984; 91:1092–1099.
76. Hawley D, Schaefer J, Schulz D, et al. Cytomegalovirus encephalitis in acquired immunodeficiency syndrome. Am J Clin Pathol 1983; 80:874–877.
77. Horowitz S, Benson D, Gottlieb M, et al. Neurological complications of gay-related immunodeficiency disorder. Ann Neurol 1982; 12:80.
78. Siegal F, Lopez C, Hammer G, et al. Severe acquired immunodeficiency in male homosexuals, manifested by chronic perianal ulcerative herpes simplex lesions. N Engl J Med 1981; 305:1439–1444.
79. Strano A. Herpes group exanthems. In: Binford C, Connor D, eds. Pathology of tropical and extraordinary diseases. Washington, DC: Armed Forces Institute of Pathology, 1976:68–73.
80. Strano A. Progressive multifocal leukoencephalopathy. In: Binford C, Connor D, eds. Pathology of tropical and extraordinary diseases. Washington, DC: Armed Forces Institute of Pathology, 1976:55–57.
81. Miller J, Barrett R, Britton C, et al. Progressive multifocal leukoencephalopathy in a male homosexual with T-cell immune deficiency. N Engl J Med 1982; 307:1436–1438.

82. Bedri J, Weinstein W, DeGregorio P, et al. Progressive multifocal leukoenceph-alopathy in acquired immunodeficiency syndrome (AIDS). N Engl J Med 1983; 309:1455–1457.

83. Edwards J, Lehrer R. Severe candida infections. Clinical perspective, immune defense mechanisms, and current concepts of therapy. Ann Int Med 1978; 88:91–106.

84. Centers for Disease Control. Revision of the case definition of acquired immu-nodeficiency syndrome for national reporting—United States. MMWR 1985; 34:373–375.

85. Binford C, Dooley J. Cryptococcosis. In: Binford C, Connor D, eds. Pathology of tropical and extraordinary diseases. Washington, DC: Armed Forces Institute of Pathology, 1976:572–573.

86. Macher A, Rodrigues M, Kaplan W, et al. Disseminated bilateral chorioretinitis due to *Histoplasma capsulatum* in a patient with the acquired immunodeficiency syndrome. Ophthalmology 1985; 92:1159–1164.

87. Kovacs A, Kovacs J, Overturf G. Disseminated coccidioidomycosis in a patient with acquired immune deficiency syndrome. West J Med 1984; 140:447–449.

88. Abrams D. Disseminated coccidioidomycosis in AIDS. N Engl J Med 1984; 310: 986–987.

89. Sohn C, Schroff R, Kliewer K, et al. Disseminated *Mycobacterium avium intra-cellulare* infection in homosexual men with acquired cell-mediated immunodefi-ciency: a histologic and immunologic study of two cases. Am J Clin Pathol 1983; 79:247–252.

90. Macher A, Kovacs J, Gill V, et al. Bacteremia due to *Mycobacterium avium intracellulare* in the acquired immunodeficiency syndrome. Ann Int Med 1983; 99:782–795.

91. Strom R, Gruninger R. AIDS with *Mycobacterium avium intracellulare* lesions resembling those of Whipple's disease. N Engl J Med 1983; 309:1323–1325.

92. Hymes KB, Greene JB, Marcus A, et al. Kaposi's sarcoma in homosexual men—a report of eight cases. Lancet 1981; ii:598–600.

93. Centers for Disease Control Task Force on Karposi's Sarcoma and Opportunistic Infections. Report. Epidemiologic aspects of the current outbreak of Kaposi's sarcoma and opportunistic infections. N Engl J Med 1982; 306:248–252.

94. Gottlieb GJ, Ragaz A, Vogel JV, et al. A preliminary communication on exclusively disseminated Kaposi's sarcoma in young homosexual men. Am J Dermatopathol 1981; 3:111–114.

95. Safai B. Kaposi's sarcoma and other neoplasms in acquired immunodeficiency syndrome. In: Advances in host defense mechanisms. New York: Raven Press, 1985:59–73.

96. Myskowski PL, Romano JF, Safai B. Kaposi's sarcoma in young homosexual men. Cutis 1983; 29:31–34.

97. Friedman-Kien AE, Laubenstein LJ, Rubenstein P, et al. Disseminated Kaposi's sarcoma in homosexual men. Ann Intern Med 1982; 96:693–697.

98. Gottlieb GJ, Ackerman B. Kaposi's sarcoma: an extensively disseminated form in young homosexual men. Hum Pathol 1982; 13:10–17.

99. Dorfman, RF. Kaposi's sarcoma revisited. Perspect Pathol 1984; 15:1013–1017.

100. Guarda LG, Silva EG, Ordonez HG, et al. Factor VIII in Kaposi's sarcoma. Am J Clin Pathol 1981; 76:197–202.

101. Nadji M, Morales AR, Ziegles-Weissman J, et al. Kaposi's sarcoma: immunohisto- logic evidence for an endothelial origin. Arch Pathol Lab Med 1981; 105:274–278.

102. Akhtar M, Bunuan H, ali MA, et al. Kaposi's sarcoma in renal transplant recipients: ultrastructural and immunoperoxidase study of four cases. Cancer 1984; 53:258– 263.

103. Beckstead JH, Wood GS, Fletcher V. Evidence for the origin of Kaposi's sarcoma from lymphatic endothelium. Am J Pathol 1985; 119:294–300.

104. Silver MA, Macher AM, Reichert CM, et al. Cardiac involvement by Kaposi's sarcoma in acquired immunodeficiency syndrome (AIDS). Am J Cardiol 1984; 53:983–987.

105. Costa J, Rabson AS. Generalized Kaposi's sarcoma is not a neoplasm. Lancet 1983; i:58.

106. Harwood AR, Osoba D, Hofstader SL, et al. Kaposi's sarcoma in recipients of renal transplants. Am J Med 1979; 67:759–765.

107. Stribling J, Weitzner S, Smith GV. Kaposi's sarcoma in renal allograft recipients. Cancer 1978; 42:442–446.

108. Myers BD, Kessler E, Levi J, Pick A, Rosenfeld JB. Kaposi sarcoma in kidney transplant recipients. Arch Intern Med 1974; 133:307–311.

109. Penn I. Kaposi's sarcoma in organ transplant recipients: report of 20 cases. Transplantation 1979; 27:8–11.

110. Grange RW, Jones EW. Kaposi's sarcoma and immunosuppressive therapy: an appraisal. Clin Exp Dermatol 1978; 3:135–146.

111. Klepp O, Dahl O, Stenwig JT. Association of Kaposi's sarcoma and prior immu- nosuppressive therapy: a 5-year material of Kaposi's sarcoma in Norway. Cancer 1978; 42:2626–2630.

112. Hoshaw RA, Schwartz RA. Kaposi's sarcoma after immunosuppressive therapy with prednisone. Arch Dermatol 1980; 116:1280–1282.

113. Ziegler JL, Bragg K, Abrams D, et al. High-grade non-Hodgkin's lymphoma in patients with AIDS. Ann NY Acad Sci 1984; 437:412–419.

114. Ziegler JL; Beckstead JA, Volberding PA, et al. Non-Hodgkin's lymphoma in 90 homosexual men. Relation to generalized lymphadenopathy and the acquired immunodeficiency syndrome. N Engl J Med 1984; 311:565–570.

115. Levine AM, Gill PS, Meyer PR, et al. Retrovirus and malignant lymphoma in homosexual men. JAMA 1985; 254:1921–1925.

116. Steinberg JJ, Bridges N, Feiner HD, Valensi Q. Small intestinal lymphoma in three patients with acquired immune deficiency syndrome. Am J Gastroenterol 1985; 80:21–26.

117. Khojasteh A, Reynolds RD, Mulloy CA. Lymphoreticular malignancies in the setting of acquired immunodeficiency syndrome (AIDS). A potential model for evolution of human lymphoid neoplasms. Mol Med 1985; 82:599–602.

118. Ioachim HL, Cooper MC, Hellman GC. Lymphomas in men at high risk for acquired immune deficiency syndrome (AIDS). A study of 21 cases. Cancer 1985; 56:2831–2842.

119. Petersen JM, Tubbs RR, Savage RA, et al. Small noncleaved B cell Burkitt-like

lymphoma with chromosome t(8;14) translocation and Epstein-Barr virus nu-
clear-associated antigen in a homosexual man with acquired immune deficiency
syndrome. Am J Med 1985; 78:141–148.

120. Magrath I, Erikson I, Whang-Peng J, et al. Synthesis of kappa light chains by cell
lines containing an 8;22 chromosomal translocation derived from a male homosexual with Burkitt's lymphoma. Science 1983; 222:1094–1096.

121. Whang-Peng J, Lee EC, Sieverts H, Magrath IT. Burkitt's lymphoma in AIDS:
cytogenetic study. Blood 1984; 63:818–822.

122. Gyger M, Laverdiere M, Gagnon A, Perreault C, Cousineau S, Forest L. 14q+
abnormality with probable t(8;14)(q24;q32) in a young Haitian immigrant with
acquired immunodeficiency syndrome and concomitant Burkitt's-like lymphoma.
Cancer Genet Cytogenet 1985; 17:283–288.

123. Chagante RSK, Jhanwar SC, Koziner B, et al. Specific translocations characterize
Burkitt's-like lymphoma of homosexual men with acquired immunodeficiency
syndrome. Blood 1983; 61:1269–1278.

124. Croce CM, Tsujimoto Y, Erikson J, Nowell P. Biology of disease: chromosome
translocations and B cell neoplasia. Lab Invest 1984; 51:258–269.

125. Vandermolen LA, Fehir KM, Rice L. Multiple myeloma in a homosexual man with
chronic lymphadenopathy. Arch Intern Med 1985; 145:745–746.

126. Israel AM, Koziner B, Straus DJ. Plasmacytoma and the acquired immunodeficiency syndrome. Ann Intern Med 1984; 101:142–148.

127. Schoeppel SL, Hoppe RT, Dorfman RF, et al. Hodgkin's disease in homosexual
men with generalized lymphadenopathy. Ann Intern Med 1985; 102:68–70.

128. Moore GE, Cook DD. AIDS in association with malignant melanoma and Hodgkin's disease. J Clin Oncol 1985; 3:1437. Letter.

129. Dances A, Odajnyk C, Kriegel RL, et al. Association of Hodgkin's and non-
Hodgkin's lymphomas with the acquired immunodeficiency syndrome. Proc Am
Soc Clin Oncol 1984; 3:61a.

130. Robert NJ, Schneiderman H. Hodgkin's disease and the acquired immunodeficiency syndrome. Ann Intern Med 1984; 101:142–145.

131. Coonley CJ, Straus DJ, Filippa D, Watson R. Hodgkin's disease presenting with
rectal symptoms in a homosexual male. A case report and review of the literature.
Cancer Invest 1984; 2:279–284.

132. Read EJ, Orenstein JM, Chorba TL, et al. Listeria monocytogenes sepsis and small
cell carcinoma of the rectum: an unusual presentation of the acquired immunodeficiency syndrome. Am J Clin Pathol 1985; 83:385–389.

133. Nusbaum NJ. Metastatic small cell carcinoma of the lung in a patient with AIDS. N
Engl J Med 1985; 312:1706. Letter.

134. Moser RJ 3rd, Tenholder MF, Ridenour R. Oat-cell carcinoma in transfusion-
associated acquired immunodeficiency syndrome. Ann Intern Med 1985; 103:478.
Letter.

135. Bordi C, De Vita O, Ferrari C, Altavilla G, Corallini A, Barbanti-Brodano G.
Histologic, immunofluorescence, and ultrastructural study of malignant islet-cell
tumors of the pancreas in hamsters by BK human papovavirus. Am J Pathol 1985;
118:256–265.

136. Takemoto KK, Rabson AS, Mullarkey MF, et al. Isolation of papova virus from

brain tumor and urine of a patient with Wiskott-Aldrich syndrome. J Natl Cancer Inst 1974; 53:1205–1207.

137. Croxson T, Chabon AB, Rorat E, Barash IM. Intraepithelial carcinoma of the anus in homosexual men. Dis Colon Rectum 1984; 27:325–330.

138. Lozada F, Silverman S, Conent M. New outbreak of oral tumors, malignancies and infectious disease strikes young male homosexuals. Can Dent Assoc J 1982; 19:39–45.

139. Conant MA, Volberding P, Fletcher V, et al. Squamous cell carcinoma in sexual partner of Kaposi's sarcoma patient. Lancet 1982; i:286–287.

140. Cooper HS, Patchefsy AJ, Marks G. Cloacogenic carcinoma of the anorectum in homosexual men: an observation of four cases. Dis Colon Rectum 1979; 22:557–561.

141. Vailler B. Anorectal cancer and homosexuality. JAMA 1983; 249:2459–2461.

142. Croxson T, Chabon AB, Rorat E, et al. Intraepithelial carcinoma of the anus in homosexual men. Dis Colon Rectum 1984; 27:325–327.

143. Roseman DS, Ansell JS, Chapman WH. Sexually transmitted diseases and carcinogenesis. Urol Clin North Am 1984; 11:27–43.

144. Purtilo DT, Manolov G, Manolova Y, Harada S, Lipscomb H. Squamous-cell carcinoma, Kaposi's sarcoma and Burkitt's lymphoma are consequences of impaired immune surveillance of ubiquitous viruses in acquired immune deficiency syndrome, allograft recipients and tropical African patients. IARC Sci Publ 1984; 63:749–770.

145. Logothetis CJ, Newell GR, Samuels ML. Testicular cancer in homosexual men with cellular immune deficiency: report of 2 cases. J Urol 1985; 133:484–486.

146. Levy RM, Bradesen DE, Rosenblum ML. Neurological manifestations of the acquired immunodeficiency syndrome (AIDS): experience at UCSF and review of the literature. J Neurosurg 1985; 62:475–495.

147. Jordan BD, Navia BA, Petito C, Cho ES, Price RW. Neurological syndromes complicating AIDS. Front Radiat Ther Oncol 1985; 19:82–87.

148. Lemann W, Sho ES, Nielsen S, Petito C. Neuropathologic (NP) findings in 104 cases of acquired immune deficiency syndrome (AIDS): an autopsy study. J. Neuropathol Exp Neurol 1985; 44:349. Abstract.

149. Moskowitz LB, Hensley GT, Chan JC, Conley FK, Donovan Post M, Gonzalez-Arias SM. Brain biopsies in patients with acquired immune deficiency syndrome. Arch Pathol Lab Med 1984; 108:368–371.

150. Mobley K, Rotterdam HZ, Lerner CW, Tapper ML. Autopsy findings in the acquired immune deficiency syndrome. In: Sommers SC, Rosen PP, Fechner RE, eds. Pathology annual. Part 1, vol. 20. Norwalk: Appleton-Century-Crofts, 1985: 46–65.

151. Urmacher C, Nielsen S. The histopathology of the acquired immune deficiency syndrome. In: Sommers SC, Rosen PP, Fechner RE, eds. Pathology annual. Part 1, vol. 20. Norwalk: Appleton-Century-Crofts, 1985:198–220.

152. Koppel BS, Wormser GP, Tuchman AJ, Maayan S, Hewlett D, Daras M. Central nervous system involvement in patients with acquired immune deficiency syndrome (AIDS). Acta Neurol Scand 1985; 71:337–353.

153. Dolman CL. Microglia. In: Davis RL, Robertson DM, eds. Textbook of neuropathology. Baltimore: Williams and Wilkins, 1985:117–137.

154. Moskowitz LB, Gregorios JB, Hensley GT, Berger JR. Cytomegalovirus induced demyelination associated with acquired immune deficiency syndrome. Arch Pathol Lab Med 1984; 108:873–877.

155. Nielsen SL, Petito CK, Urmacher CD, Posner JB. Subacute encephalitis in acquired immune deficiency syndrome: a postmortem study. Am J Clin Pathol 1984; 82:678–682.

156. Morgello S, Cho L, Nielsen S, Petito C. The pathology of cytomegalovirus (CMV) encephalitis: a review of 30 autopsy cases. J Neuropathol Exp Neurol 1985; 44:350. Abstract.

157. Munoz-Garcia D, Pendlebury WW, Perl DP, Highland R. Subacute encephalitis in AIDS: ultrastructural demonstration of cytomegalovirus in brain. J Neuropathol Exp Neurol 1985; 44:349. Abstract.

158. Wiley CA, Schrier RD, Denaro FJ, Nelson JA, Lampert PW, Oldstone MBA. Localization within the CNS of cytomegalovirus proteins and genome during fulminant infection in an AIDS patient. J Neuropathol Exp Neurol 1985; 44:350. Abstract.

159. Shaw GM, Harper ME, Hahn BH, et al. HTLV-III infection in brains of children and adults with AIDS encephalopathy. Science 1985; 227:177–182.

160. Ho DD, Rota TR, Schooley RT, et al. Isolation of HTLV-III from cerebrospinal fluid and neural tissues of patients with neurologic syndromes related to the acquired immunodeficiency syndrome. N Engl J Med 1985; 313:1493–1497.

161. Resnick L, diMarzo-Veronese F, Schupbach J, et al. Intra-blood-brain barrier synthesis of HTLV-III-specific IgG in patients with neurologic symptoms associated with AIDS or AIDS-related complex. N Engl J Med 1985; 313:1498–1504.

162. Black PH. HTLV-III, AIDS, and the brain. N Engl J Med 1985; 313:1538–1539. Editorial.

163. Petito CK, Navia BA, Cho E-S, Jordan BD, George DC, Price RW. Vacuolar myelopathy resembling subacute combined degeneration in patients with the acquired immunodeficiency syndrome. N Engl J Med 1985; 312:874–879.

164. Goldstick L, Mandybur TI, Bode R. Spinal cord degeneration in AIDS. Neurology 1985; 35:103–106.

165. Edwards RH, Messing R, McKendall RR. Cytomegalovirus meningoencephalitis in a homosexual man with Kaposi's sarcoma: isolation of CMV from CSF cells. Neurology 1985; 35:560–562.

166. Dix RD, Waitzman DM, Follansbee S, et al. Herpes simplex virus type 2 encephalitis in two homosexual men with persistent lymphadenopathy. Ann Neurol 1985; 17:203–206.

167. Tucker T, Dix RD, Katzen C, Davis RL, Schmidley JW. Cytomegalovirus and herpes simplex virus ascending myelitis in a patient with acquired immune deficiency syndrome. Ann Neurol 1985; 18:74–79.

168. Aksamit AJ, Mourrain P, Sever JL, Major EO. Progressive multifocal leukoencephalopathy: investigation of three cases using in situ hybridization with JC virus biotinylated DNA probe. Ann Neurol 1985; 18:490–496.

169. Bernick C, Gregorios JB. Progressive multifocal leukoencephalopathy in a patient with acquired immune deficiency syndrome. Arch Neurol 1984; 41:780–782.
170. Blum LW, Chambers RA, Schwartzman RJ, Streletz LJ. Progressive multifocal leukoencephalopathy in acquired immune deficiency syndrome. Arch Neurol 1985; 42:137–139.
171. Gorin FA, Bale JF, Halks-Miller M, Schwartz RA. Kaposi's sarcoma metastatic to the CNS. Arch Neurol 1985; 42:162–166.
172. Lipkin I, Parry G, Kiprov D, Abrams D. Inflammatory neuropathy in homosexual men with lymphadenopathy. Neurology 1985; 35:1479–1483.
173. Bishopric G, Bruner J, Butler J. Guillain-Barré syndrome with cytomegalovirus infection of peripheral nerves. Arch Pathol Lab Med 1985; 109:1106–1108.
174. Belman AL, Ultmann MH, Horoupian D, et al. Neurological complications in infants and children with acquired immune deficiency syndrome. Ann Neurol 1985; 18:560–566.
175. Epstein LG, Sharer LR, Joshi VV, Fojas MM, Koenigsberger MR, Oleske FM. Progressive encephalopathy in children with acquired immune deficiency syndrome. Ann Neurol 1985; 17:488–496.
176. Sharer LR, Epstein LG, Joshi VV, Rankin LF. Neuropathological observations in children with AIDS and with HTLV-III infection of brain. J Neuropathol Exp Neurol 1985; 44:350. Abstract.

11

Infectious Complications of AIDS

H. Clifford Lane
Anthony S. Fauci
Laboratory of Immunoregulation
National Institute of Allergy
and Infectious Diseases
National Institutes of Health
Bethesda, Maryland

Introduction

The immunosuppression induced by infection with HTLV-III/LAV results in the occurrence of a variety of opportunistic infections in the AIDS patient. Among them are protozoal infections with agents such as *Pneumocystis carinii* and *Toxoplasma gondii*, fungal infections with *Candida albicans* and *Cryptococcus neoformans*, bacterial infections with *Mycobacterium avium-intracellulare* (MAI) and *Salmonella typhimurium*, and viral infections with herpes simplex (HSV), herpes zoster, and cytomegalovirus (CMV).[1-5] As has been pointed out by several authors, those patients with AIDS who manifested an opportunistic infection have immune systems more severely compromised than those patients with only Kaposi's sarcoma.[6-9] This is reflected in the total T4 count for this group of patients (Fig. 1), as well as in their survival statistics. Statistics compiled by the New York City Department of Health

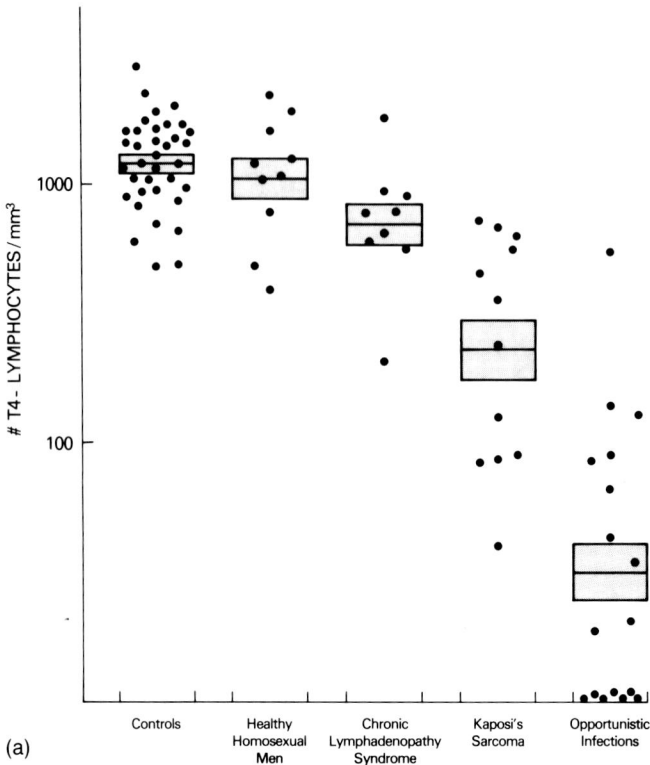

FIGURE 1 (a) Total number of peripheral blood helper/inducer (T4$^+$) lymphocytes in controls and the clinical subpopulations of patients with HTLV-III/LAV disease. Those patients who have experienced an opportunistic infection have the lowest number of T4$^+$-lymphocytes. (b) Representation of this observation in a hypothetical scheme. (From Ref. 9.)

reveal that the median survival for patients with AIDS presenting as *Pneumocystis carinii* pneumonia was 35 weeks and for those patients presenting with any other opportunistic infection, it was 19 weeks. These are in comparison with a median survival of 125 weeks for the AIDS patient presenting only with Kaposi's sarcoma (KS).[10] Kaposi's sarcoma is discussed in several other chapters in this book. The following discussion will address the role the various opportunistic organisms play in producing the myriad of clinical manifestations seen in the patient with AIDS. The reader should also refer to the chapter by Jaffe et al.

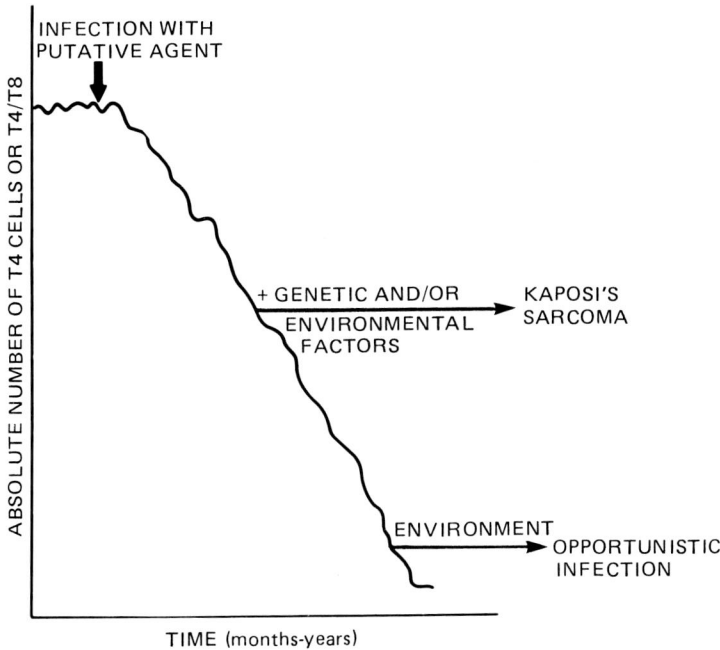

TIME (months-years)

(b)

Pulmonary Infections

The most common pulmonary disease seen in the patient with AIDS is *Pneumocystis carinii* pneumonia (PCP). At the time of report to the Centers for Disease Control (CDC), 59% of patients with AIDS have experienced an episode of PCP.[11] This usually presents as a bilateral interstitial pneumonitis, although the onset can be quite insidious with very few symptoms and essentially normal blood gases. A comparison of the clinical findings of PCP in the non-AIDS patient with PCP in the AIDS patient is given in Table 1. Of note is the longer duration of symptoms and increased incidence of side effects to trimethoprim-sulfamethoxasole in the patients with AIDS. Additionally, fever may not be present and the chest X-ray film may appear normal. Thus, a very high index of suspicion is required to achieve an early diagnosis. Of significance perhaps is the fact that very few patients with AIDS will develop PCP if their peripheral blood absolute T4 count is greater than 200 cell/mm^3 (Fig. 1). Additionally, gallium scanning and pulmonary function testing may be helpful in distinguishing subtle cases of pneumonitis from other conditions.[12]

TABLE 1   *Pneumocystis carinii* Pneumonia: AIDS Versus
Non-Aids

	AIDS	Non-AIDS
Attack per year	35%	0.01–1% (CA,TX)
		22–43% (St. Jude's)
Specific symptoms	Same	Same
Duration of symptoms (median)	28 days	5 days
Signs/laboratory	Subtle	Impressive
X-ray	Subtle	Impressive
Survival	57%	50%
Adverse effects:		
Pentamidine	47%	57%
TMP/SMZ	65%	12%
Relapse/recurrence	20%	0% (adults)
		11% (children)

TMP/SMZ = trimethoprim-sulfamethoxasole.

A diagnosis of PCP requires demonstration of the organism in pulmonary tissue or secretions. Organisms have been detected in sputum, but this has not been a uniformly reliable test. Likewise, the serological tests for antigen or antibody are not currently clinically helpful. The diagnostic procedure of choice for detecting *Pneumocystis carinii* is bronchoalveolar lavage with transbronchial biopsy. This procedure will yield a positive result in over 90% of cases. Lung biopsies of AIDS patients with PCP generally show large numbers of *Pneumocystis* cysts and impressive mononuclear cell infiltrate and intraalveolar exudate [(Fig. 2a,b) (Fig. 2b—see Plate I, facing p. 192)].

The standard therapy for PCP in patients with AIDS is either trimethoprim-sulfamethoxasole (cotrimoxazole) or pentamidine isoethionate. Clinical improvement is usually not seen until about 5 to 7 days after the initiation of therapy. At the present time, there are not data to support the use of one of these agents over the other, nor are there data to support their use in combination. In contrast to other patient groups, AIDS patients treated with cotrimoxazole have an extremely high rate of adverse drug reactions. These range from mild fever and skin rash to exfoliative dermatitis, bone marrow suppression, and hepatitis. Side effects of pentamidine include nephrotoxicity, granulocytpoenia, and hyperglycemia.[13] Thus, there is a need for additional agents for treatment of PCP. Among the experimental agents currently being evaluated are dapsone, DFMO, and a methotrexate analog, trimetrexate.[14]

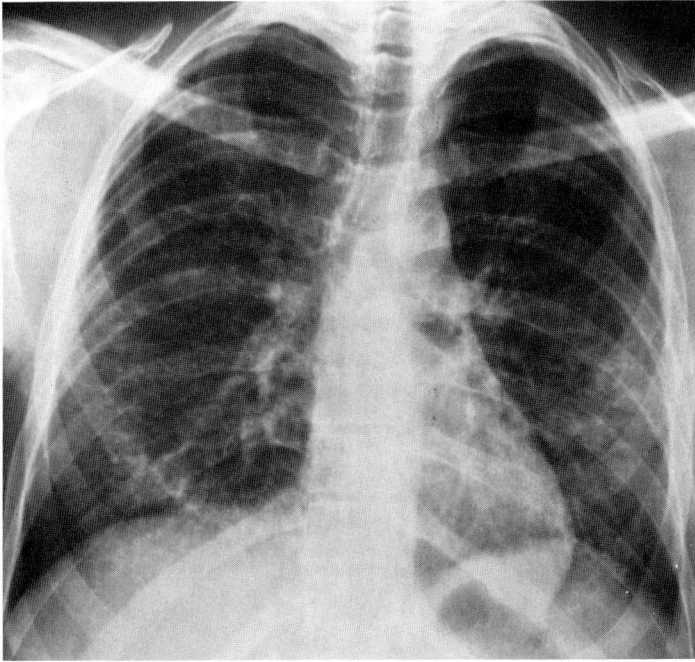

FIGURE 2a   Radiographic findings of *Pneumocystis carinii* pneumonia (PCP) in an AIDS patient.

Pneumocystis carinii pneumonia recurs in at least 20% of AIDS patients. This high rate of recurrence when compared with that in other immunosuppressed adults has led many to believe that prolonged and/or prophylactic therapy is required in the patient with AIDS who has experienced an episode of PCP or who appears at high risk of PCP by virtue of a low number of helper/inducer T-lymphocytes. While 2 weeks is the standard course of therapy for the non-AIDS patient with PCP, most clinicians treat AIDS patients for a minimum of 3 weeks. It generally takes 3 to 6 weeks of therapy to result in clearing of organisms and inflammation.[15] It remains unresolved whether or not continuation of therapy until bronchoalveolar lavage and biopsy are negative will result in better overall survival or decreased rate of relapse. Daily administration of cotrimoxazole has been an effective prophylactic regimen to decrease the incidence of PCP in children with acute leukemia.[16] The high rate of adverse reactions to this drug in the AIDS patient makes this approach impractical in the AIDS patient population. A variety of prophylactic regimens are being tried in AIDS patients, including twice a week cotrimoxazole and once a week fansidar. It is currently unclear which, if any, of these strategies will prove to be of benefit to the patient with AIDS.

Cytomegalovirus (CMV) is the second leading cause of pneumonitis in AIDS, accounting for one-third of all deaths due to respiratory failure.[17] Cytomegalovirus infection is very common in homosexual men with AIDS. At the National Institutes of Health (NIH), 26 of the first 27 homosexual AIDS patients studied were excreting CMV from either blood, throat, or urine, and all were seropositive for CMV. The primary infection with CMV when symptomatic is often associated with fever, malaise, and lymphadenopathy. Following primary infection, the virus assumes a latent state that may reactivate during periods of immunosuppression, such as is seen in AIDS. A variety of clinical syndromes attributable to CMV may occur in the AIDS patient. Among them are pneumonitis, esophagitis, colitis, and retinitis. Cytomegalovirus infection produces a necrotizing pneumonitis that is often fatal. The pneumonitis caused by CMV is generally bilateral and often clinically indistinguishable from PCP [(Fig. 3a,b) (Fig. 3b—see Plate I, facing p. 192)]. Diagnosis is based on transbronchial or open lung biopsy. Infection with CMV is characterized by intranuclear or intracytoplasmic inclusion bodies. Due to the high percentage of AIDS patients with positive throat, urine, or blood cultures for CMV, it should be stressed that a positive biopsy culture for CMV in the absence of an appropriate histological picture is not sufficient for a diagnosis of CMV pneumonia. The recent availability of an acyclic nucleotide known as 9-(1-3-dihydroxy-2-propoxymethyl guanine (DHPG), for treatment of CMV infection has improved the short-term outlook for patients with this disease.[18]

Among other opportunistic pathogens that have been reported to cause pulmonary disease in patients with AIDS are MAI, *Mycobacterium tuberculosis, Cryptococcus neoformans,* and *Legionella pneumophila.* Aspergillus has been reported to cause pneumonia in AIDS patients, but thus far, this has been seen predominantly in the setting of neutropenia. Patients with AIDS have also been reported to have an increased incidence of pneumonias due to standard bacterial infections. This latter finding may be a reflection of qualitative abnormalities of the B-cell limb of the immune response.[19]

In addition to these well-recognized infectious causes of pulmonary disease in patients with AIDS, inflammatory lung disease occurs in a significant percentage of patients in the absence of an obvious cause. These idiopathic interstitial pneumonitides, which are particularly common in the pediatric patient with AIDS (see the chapter by Parks and Scott), account for approximately 10% of all the pneumonias which occur in AIDS patients.[21] It has been suggested that at least some of these may be due to direct infection of the lung with the causative agent of AIDS, HTLV-III/LAV. There is no effective therapy for this particular condition, although corticosteroids may provide a degree of temporary symptomatic relief.

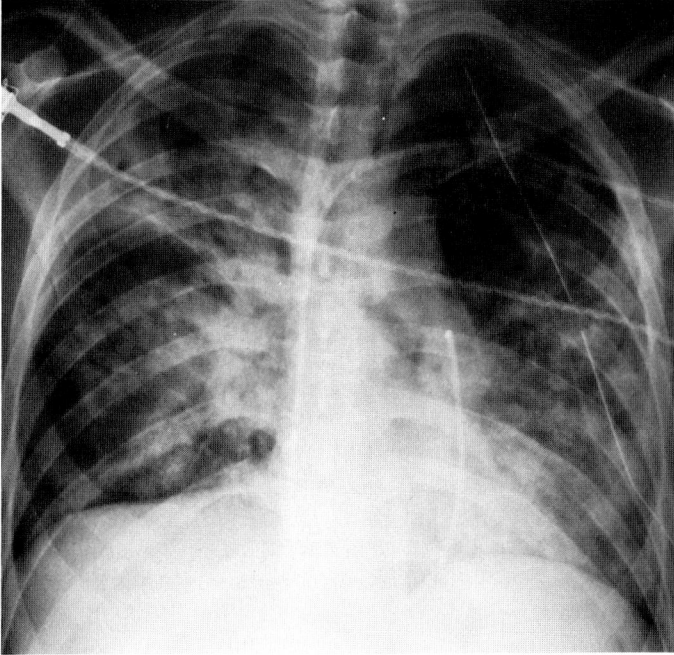

FIGURE 3a Radiographic findings of cytomegalovirus (CMV) pneumonia in an AIDS patient.

The final category of pulmonary involvement in AIDS is neoplastic. Kaposi's sarcoma affects the lung in approximately 30% of patients with AIDS and Kaposi's sarcoma. The diagnosis is difficult to make on the small fragments of tissue obtained at bronchoscopy, and open lung biopsy is often required. In contrast to PCP, KS involving the lung is often associated with pleural effusions. These are often hemorrhagic and reflect direct involvement of the pleura with tumor. Cytological examination of pleural fluid is usually negative. Aside from the frequent presence of pleural fluid, the radiographic appearance of KS of the lung is virtually indistinguishable from that of the other causes of pulmonary disease in AIDS.[22]

Central Nervous System Infections

Next to pulmonary infections, central nervous system (CNS) infections probably constitute the greatest threat to the life of the AIDS patient, and these are also discussed in several chapters in this book. In one autopsy series,[17] respiratory failure accounted for death in 56% of all AIDS patients, while CNS disease was second, accounting for 26% of deaths. In one large series of 318 patients,[23] 39% had some sort of neurological complaint. The multitude of neurological syndromes that have been described in this group reflects the wide array of organisms that have been implicated as causes of CNS disease.

Toxoplasmosis is the leading cause of CNS disease in this patient group, accounting for approximately one-third of all lesions.[23] This disease often presents as CNS mass lesions, although more subtle presentations such as headache or mild encephalopathy may occur. Spinal fluid examination is usually nondiagnostic and often normal. While serological diagnosis is often of value in the non-AIDS patient with toxoplasmosis, antibody levels and subclass response are of little value in the patient with AIDS due to the immunoregulatory defects at the level of the B cell in AIDS. Computerized tomography (CT) scanning with contrast will reveal ring-enhancing or hypo-dense masses in approximately 75% of patients with CNS toxoplasmosis (Fig. 4).[24] As is the case for most of the opportunistic infections seen in patients with AIDS, the diagnostic procedure of choice is biopsy of the affected site when this is anatomically feasible. Treatment is far from satisfactory. The standard therapy of sulfadiazine and pyrimethamine is associated with a high incidence of bone marrow suppression. This can sometimes be temporized by the use of folinic acid, but often results in premature cessation of therapy. Extended therapy is the rule in this infection, and at least 2 to 4 months of therapy are recommended. Relapse is common following discontinuation, and some experts recommend chronic therapy for as long as possible. In patients unable to tolerate sulfadiazine and pyrimethamine, clindamycin or spiramycin have been suggested for use based upon animal data or anecdotal data in humans.[25] Recently, a new dihydrofolate reductase inhibitor, trimetrexate, has been found to have both in vitro and in vivo activity against *Toxoplasma gondii,* and this agent is now being tested in clinical trials.

Most of the other opportunistic pathogens that cause CNS disease are seen much less frequently in AIDS patients. *Cryptococcus neoformans* is probably the most common CNS pathogen after *Toxoplasma gondii,* accounting for approximately 15% of CNS disease. Of 27 AIDS patients with cryptococcal disease, it was the initial opportunistic infection in 14.[26] This probably reflects the high degree of pathogenicity inherent in this organism. In contrast to non-AIDS patients with cryptococcal disease, AIDS patients may have minimal clinical findings, and spinal fluid analysis may be close to normal. Patients generally present with headache, nausea, and changes in mental status. The diagnosis is made by demonstrating cryptococcal antigen in spinal fluid or culturing the organism. About 50% of AIDS patients with cryptococcal disease respond to therapy with amphotericin with or without 5-flucytosine (FC);

PLATE I
(*Chapter 11*)

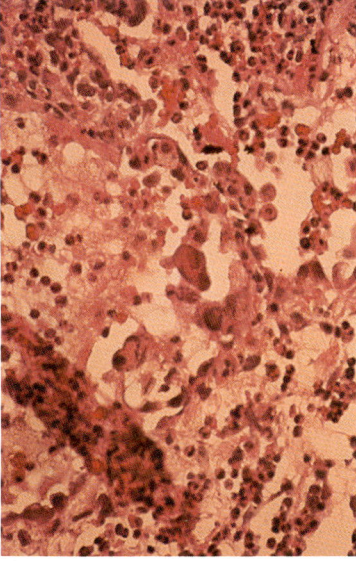

FIGURE 3b Histological appearance of cytomegalovirus (CMV) pneumonia in an AIDS patient.

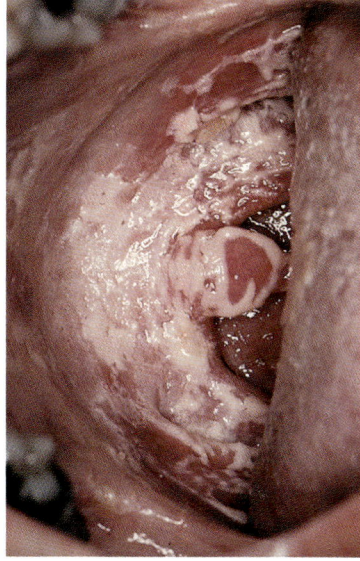

FIGURE 7a Oropharyngeal candidiasis in an AIDS patient.

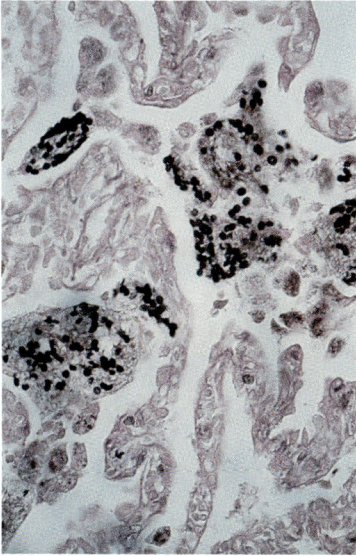

FIGURE 2b Histological appearance of *Pneumocystis carinii* pneumonia (PCP) in an AIDS patient.

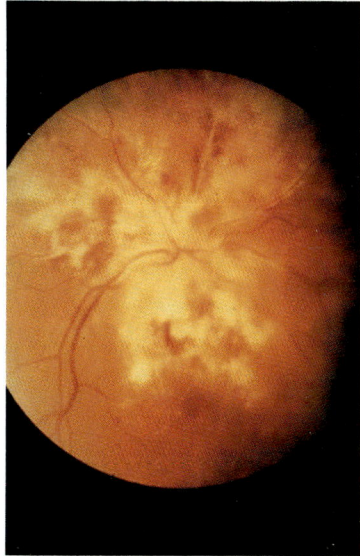

FIGURE 6 Funduscopic appearance of cytomegalovirus (CMV) retinitis in an AIDS patient. Hemorrhage and exudate are the characteristic findings.

PLATE II
(*Chapters 11 and 13*)

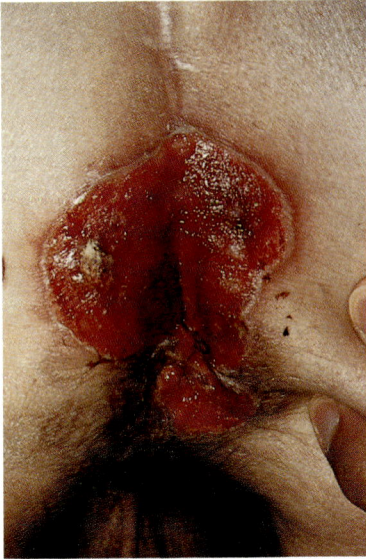

FIGURE 8 Severe, erosive perianal herpes simplex virus (HSV) in an AIDS patient (Chap. 11).

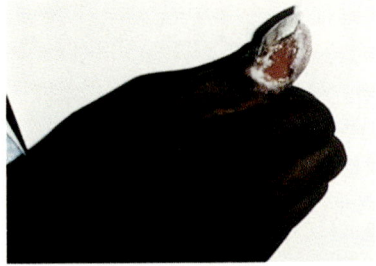

FIGURE 9 Herpetic whitlow in an AIDS patient before and after a 2-week course of oral acyclovir (Chap. 11).

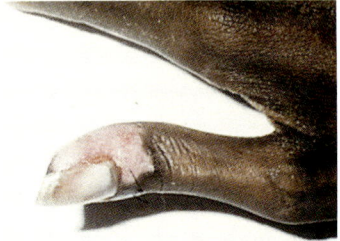

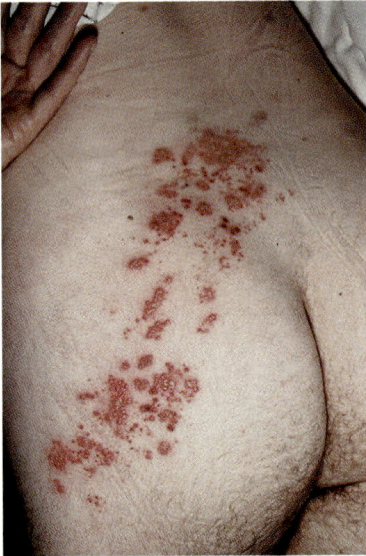

FIGURE 10 Localized herpes zoster in an AIDS patient (Chap. 11).

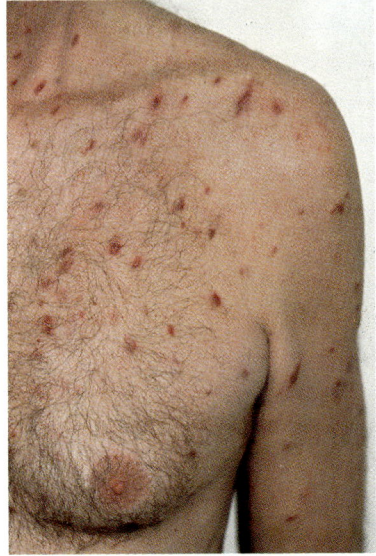

FIGURE 1 Kaposi's sarcoma in an AIDS patient (Chap. 13).

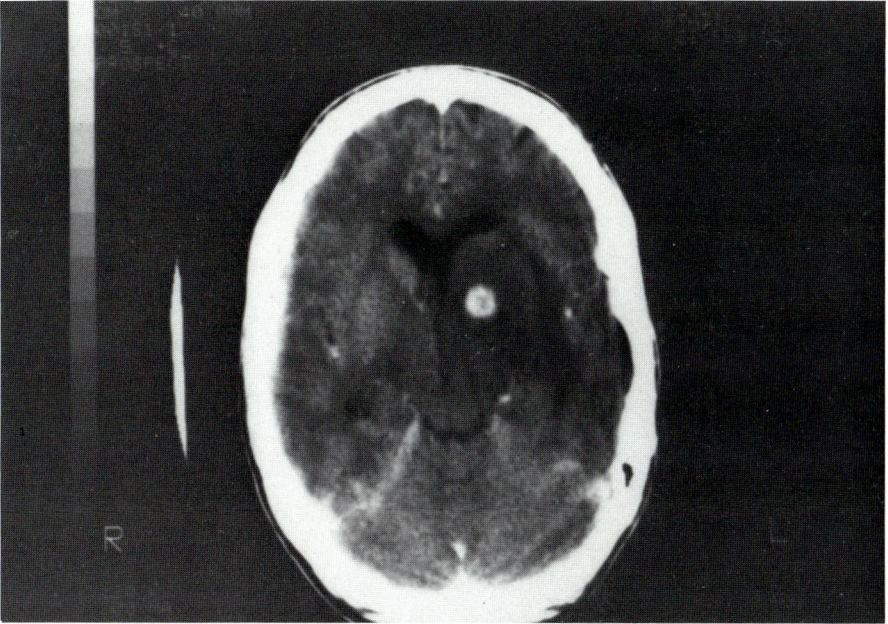

FIGURE 4 CT scan of an AIDS patient with cerebral toxoplasmosis demonstrating a ring-enhanced lesion.

however, the rate of relapse after 2 or 3 grams of amphotericin is at least 60%. The use of 5-FC in these patients is often limited by its bone marrow toxicity.

In addition to protozoal and fungal infections, infections of the CNS of the patient with AIDS have been reported with a variety of viruses. Among the clinical syndromes that have been described are meningoencephalitis with CMV, progressive multifocal encephalopathy presumably due to JC virus or SV-40, and most recently direct infection of the CNS with the AIDS retrovirus. This latter syndrome is being recognized with an increasing frequency because the earlier reports of unexplained neuropsychiatric deterioration in this patient group were coupled with reports of isolation of the AIDS retrovirus from tissues and fluid of the CNS. It now appears that the CNS may, in fact, be a major reservoir for HTLV-III/LAV infection. The virus has been demonstrated by in situ hybridization both in giant cells and glial cells of the brain. Clinically, patients with this syndrome present with a progressive dementia, which may or may not be associated with focal defects. CT scanning generally reveals cortical thinning with ventricular dilatation (Fig. 5). Spinal fluid examination typically shows mild aseptic meningitis with pleocytosis and elevated protein. There is no treatment for this problem, and the patients may

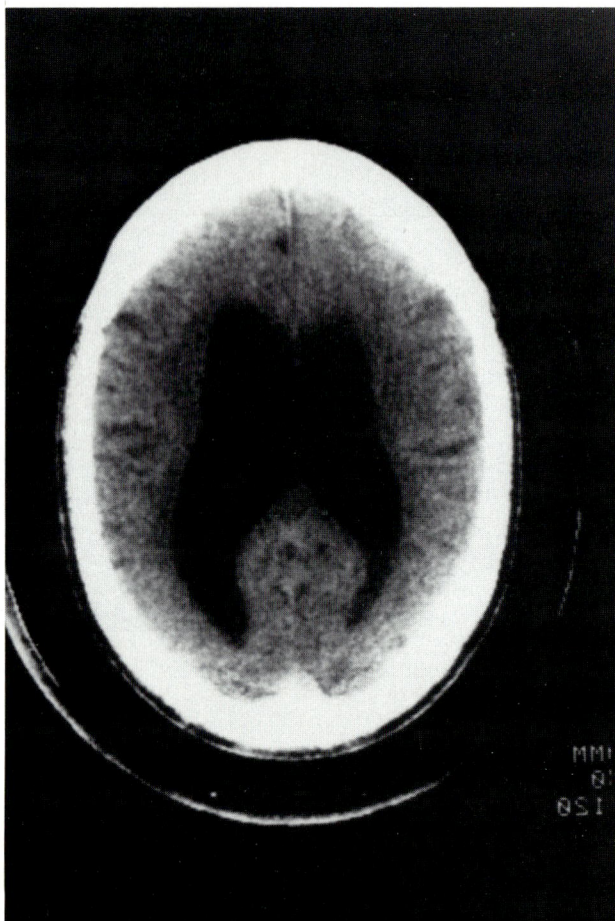

FIGURE 5 CT scan of an AIDS patient with AIDS encephalopathy demonstrating cortical thinning and ventricular dilatation.

deteriorate into a vegetative state. In addition to this chronic degenerative picture, a syndrome of acute, transient encephalopathy coincident with sero-conversion for HTLV-III/LAV has also been reported.[27,28]

A variety of other processes may involve the CNS. Among the other infectious causes of CNS disease in the patient with AIDS are HSV, varicella-zoster, *Candida albicans,* MAI, *Mycobacterium tuberculosis,* and *Treponema pallidum.* Included within the differential diagnosis of CNS disease are neo-plasms. The most common CNS neoplasm in this group is lymphoma, which may be limited to the CNS or occur as part of a more extensive process. These are almost always of B-lymphocyte origin and appear histologically with either a large cell or immunoblastic pattern. Rarely does Kaposi's sarcoma within the CNS appear as a cerebrovascular accident. Lymphomas of the CNS are discussed in other chapters of this book.

Although not definitively associated with any known infectious etiologies, a variety of peripheral and cranial nerve syndromes have been reported to occur in patients with AIDS. These include Guillian-Barré-like syndromes, stocking glove-type mixed motor and sensory neuropathies, and Bell's palsies.

Retinitis is a particularly severe complication of AIDS. The two main etiologies are CMV and toxoplasmosis. In addition, AIDS patients often develop cotton-wool spots in the retina, which do not interfere with sight and may spontaneously resolve. Evidence of active infection with CMV, as determined by positive cultures of throat washings, urine, or blood, is present in over 90% of all patients with AIDS.[4] This DNA virus may persist indefinitely in a latent form in the immunocompetent host; however, it tends to reactivate in individuals with cellular immunodeficiencies. Perhaps the most severe complication of CMV reactivation is the development of retinitis.[29] This usually presents as a visual field defect or as the development of "floaters" across the visual field. On funduscopic examination, one sees the presence of hemorrhage and exudate, often along the course of retinal vessels [Fig. 6 (see Plate I, facing p. 192)]. The retinitis of CMV may be unilateral or bilateral, is usually seen in the setting of CMV viremia, is necrotizing, results in permanent loss of vision in affected areas, and often progresses to total blindness. The recent introduction of DHPG (discussed previously) to the therapeutic armamentarium against this agent has been of great value in delaying the devastating effects of CMV retinitis. Retinitis due to CMV can be particularly difficult to distinguish from that due to toxoplasmosis. Patients with CMV retinitis often tend to be more immunosuppressed than those with toxoplasmosis, and as mentioned earlier, those with CMV retinitis usually have positive blood cultures for CMV. In a difficult case, tissue for histopathological examination may be required.

Gastrointestinal Infections

Although generally not life-threatening, infections of the gastrointestinal tract are a significant cause of morbidity for the patient with AIDS. Multiple infectious agents have been implicated in a variety of disease conditions from the oral cavity to the rectum.

One of the most common gastrointestinal infections in the patient with AIDS or AIDS-related complex (ARC) is *Candida albicans*. Oral *Candida* may be the initial manifestation of immunological deficiency in the patient with HTLV-III/LAV disease. In one study, half of 18 individuals at risk for AIDS who developed oral candidiasis developed AIDS within a median time of 3 months.[30] Oropharyngeal candidiasis may be quite severe and extensive or subtle and only evident on careful examination of the labial-gingival border [Fig. 7a (see Plate I, facing p. 192)]. The infection can extend to the esophagus or occur there independent of oral involvement. *Candida* esophagitis may present with substernal burning or discomfort, and occasionally causes difficulty in swallowing. A barium swallow performed in the patient with esophagitis will often reveal mucosal erosions (Fig. 7b). However, esophagoscopy with biopsy is required to differentiate esophagitis due to *Candida* from that due to CMV, HSV, or Kaposi's sarcoma. Because all of these are potentially treatable entities, making an accurate diagnosis is of substantial importance. *Candida* infections of the gastroinestinal tract are usually easy to treat. Mild cases often respond to topical therapy with nystatin or clotrimazole, while more extensive cases require systemic therapy with ketoconazole. In severe cases, low dose intravenous therapy with amphotericin may be required. It is important to point out that *Candida* infections are rarely eradicated completely, and, thus, periodic therapy is usually required for an indefinite period in the patient with oral *Candida*. Due to the potential serious complications of esophagitis, including perforation or hemorrhage, systemic therapy is indicated for the initial treatment. Ketoconazole or amphotericin is usually effective for this disease. In the patient who has experienced an episode of *Candida* esophagitis, chronic therapy with ketoconazole is usually required to keep the disease under control.

The *Herpesviruses* CMV or HSV may also cause esophagitis in the patient with AIDS. Although indistinguishable from *Candida* on clinical or radiographic grounds, the gross findings at esophagoscopy of erosion and ulceration without a thick white exudate are usually confirmed by positive viral cultures or histology revealing inclusion bodies. Specific therapy exists for HSV in the form of acyclovir, and for CMV in the form of DHPG. However, as mentioned earlier, these infections tend to recur, and repeated courses of therapy are often needed.

Diarrhea is a major cause of morbidity for the patient with AIDS. A large number of pathogens have been isolated from the intestinal tracts of these patients. Among them are standard protozoa, such as giardia and amoeba, unusual protozoa, such as cryptosporidia and isospora, and enteric bacteria, such as *Salmonella typhimurium* and *Campylobacter fetus*.[31]

There is no evidence that amoebiasis and giardiasis are more severe in AIDS patients than in other patient populations. In addition, there does not appear to be any predisposition for these organisms to invade the bowel wall in AIDS patients. *Cryptosporidium* is a protozoan which, prior to 1976, was felt to be a

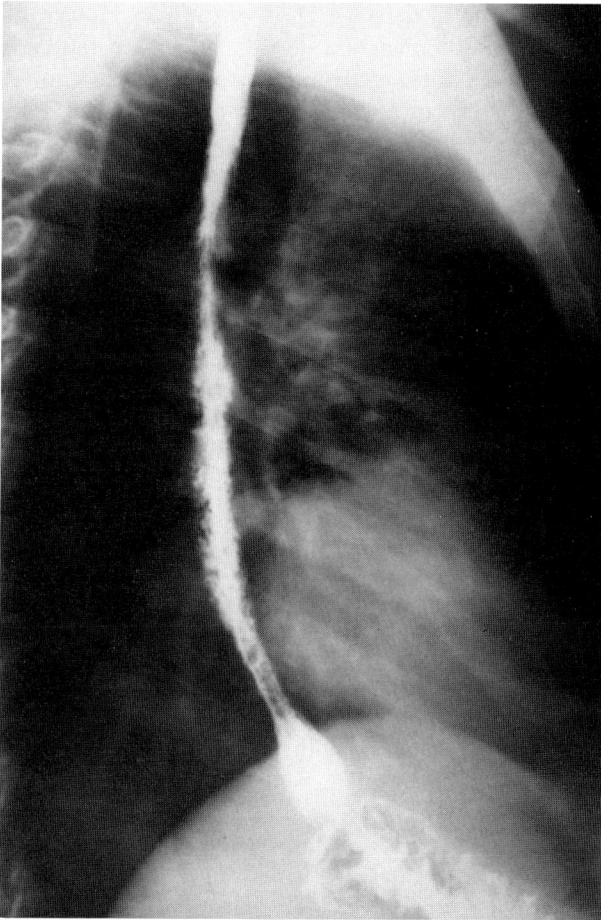

FIGURE 7b Barium swallow in an AIDS patient with *Candida* esophagitis demonstrating multiple mucosal irregularities.

cause of diarrhea only in domestic animals. It is commonly found in calves, pigs, goats, and lambs. It may also infect household pets such as cats and dogs. Pathologically, it is usually found in the intestinal tract closely apposed to the microvillus border of the intestinal epithelium. In AIDS patients, intestinal infection with *Cryptosporidium* has manifested as profound voluminous watery diarrhea occasionally associated with abdominal cramps. Patients may put out 10 to 15 liters of diarrhea per day, which may result in weight loss, malnutrition, and obtundation. In contrast to *E. histolytica* and *G. lamblia* which can be

directly observed in stool specimens, demonstration of *Cryptosporidium* requires special staining of the stool specimen or a sugar flotation preparation of
the stool specimen with Giemsa, modified methylene blue, or acid-fast stain. In
addition to being found in stool, cryptosporidia have also been isolated from
sputum, pleural fluid, stomach, and gall bladder. Therapy for cryptosporidia
enteritis is mainly supportive, although there are anecdotal reports that spiramycin, a macrolide antibiotic, has been of value.[32-34] *Isospora belli* is closely
related to *Cryptosporidium* and has been reported as a cause of intractable
diarrhea in patients with AIDS. It can also be detected by acid-fast staining of
stool specimens. Anecdotal reports suggest that prolonged therapy with sulfa-
methoxazole-trimethoprim may be of benefit.[35]

Salmonella typhimurium and *Campylobacter fetus* have been reported to
cause intestinal infection in association with bacteremia in patients with AIDS.[36,37]
These infections tend to be recurrent, and chronic therapy is usually required.
Other bacteria that have been found to cause intestinal disease in AIDS are MAI
and *Shigella* species.[38]

Aside from protozoa and bacteria, viruses and, in particular, CMV may
cause significant intestinal disease in the patient with AIDS. Cytomegalovirus
colitis may result in profound watery diarrhea. It can be diagnosed endo-
scopically with biopsy and histological examination of colonic tissue. As in the
case of CMV retinitis, patients with CMV colitis generally have positive blood
cultures for the virus. DHPG has been effective in treating this problem.[18]

Painful perirectal lesions may occur as a result of recurrent HSV infection.
While recurrent HSV generally presents as painful vesicles and erythema in
the immunocompetent individual, in the AIDS patient, it often results in a
severe erosive lesion that is extremely painful [Fig. 8 (see Plate II, facing p.
193)]. Any AIDS patient with rectal pain or a rectal discharge should be
examined carefully for the presence of a herpetic ulcer. The diagnosis is made
by examining scrapings of the ulcer for multinucleated giant cells, or culturing
the base of the ulcer for HSV. Cultures usually turn positive within 48 hours.
Treatment with systemic acyclovir, either intravenously or orally, is quite
effective in suppressing this infection. Topical acyclovir is probably of minimal
value. Included in the differential diagnosis for painful perirectal lesions in the
patient with AIDS are gonorrhea and Kaposi's sarcoma.

Cutaneous Infections

As mentioned previously, HSV may cause erosive perirectal lesions. It may
also cause mucocutaneous eruptions in the area of the mouth and cutaneous
lesions, especially of the digits, in the form of herpetic whitlow. Although
these lesions generally respond to short courses of systemic acyclovir, they

tend to recur and repeated courses of therapy become the rule [Fig. 9 (see Plate II, facing p. 193)]. Diagnosis is made by culturing or demonstrating multinucleated giant cells on scrapings.

Reactivation of herpes zoster is common in patients with AIDS and in patients with less severe forms of HTLV-III/LAV infection. The disease usually occurs in a dermatomal distribution as shingles [Fig. 10 (see Plate II, facing p. 193)], but may undergo cutaneous dissemination. Visceral dissemination with varicella-zoster has not been reported in patients with AIDS. Intravenous acyclovir is effective for the patient with cutaneous dissemination, although chronic therapy may become necessary to prevent further episodes of dissemination. Disseminated disease may occur in the absence of shingles.

A variety of other skin infections may occur in patients with AIDS, including septic emboli from bacteremias, septic phlebitis, onychomycoses, and molluscum contagiosum.

Disseminated Infections

A variety of microorganisms cause disseminated infection in patients with AIDS without major organ involvement. Among them are MAI, CMV, Epstein-Barr virus (EBV), and *Histoplasma capsulatum*.

MAI is a group II atypical mycobacterium, which is an ubiquitous environmental organism found in dust, dirt, domestic animals, and dairy products. It had been rarely reported as a cause of disseminated disease in humans prior to AIDS.[39] It has been isolated from as many as 50% of all patients with AIDS at some time during their course.[4] This organism has been isolated from bone marrow, liver, lung, spleen, and blood. In tissues infected with MAI, granulomas and histiocytes may not be present despite large numbers of acid-fast organisms. Although infected patients may exhibit fever, fatigue, weight loss, and debility, it is often hard to sort out the contribution of MAI to these symptoms from that of other agents such as CMV and EBV. Even though organisms may be present in huge quantities in liver, spleen, or lymph nodes, their direct effect on organ function is unclear. Pulmonary infection with MAI is usually sparse, and it has rarely been implicated as a cause of significant pneumonitis. A clinical syndrome similar to Whipple's disease has been reported to occur in association with lymph node and bowel wall infection with MAI.[38] MAI is most commonly diagnosed by blood culture or culture and staining of bone marrow, lymph node, or other biopsy specimens. It should be emphasized, however, that the precise contribution of MAI to the clinical syndromes seen in AIDS is unclear at the present time. This, coupled with the lack of effective therapy for the organism, has led most investigators *not* to treat patients with MAI infection unless a serious clinical syndrome, such as fever and weight loss, is present in the absence of any other recognizable cause. In that instance, a variety of combination therapies have been proposed, which generally include ansamycin, clofazimine, isoniazid, and amikacin.

Mycobacterium tuberculosis is a common infection in AIDS patients from developing countries and from other groups with an increased incidence of tuberculosis.[40] In patients with AIDS, *M. tuberculosis* usually presents as disseminated or localized extrapulmonary disease. Granulomas may or may not be present. Due to its relatively high degree of pathogenicity, disseminated infection with *M. tuberculosis* is often the first sign of AIDS in patients from developing countries. In most instances, this is felt to represent the reactivation of a latent disease. Treatment of *M. tuberculosis* in patients with AIDS follows the same guidelines as standard treatment for *M. tuberculosis* and is usually initially successful.

Infection with *Histoplasma capsulatum* has been reported in patients with AIDS who have resided in areas endemic for this fungus. Clinical manifestations are similar to those of the nonimmunosuppressed patient with disseminated histoplasmosis and include fever, weight loss, and bone marrow suppression. Despite prolonged therapy with amphotericin, this infection has been difficult to eradicate.[41-42]

CMV and EBV can be isolated from about 90% of patients with AIDS.[4] These DNA viruses may be responsible for a variety of clinical conditions. As mentioned, CMV may cause pneumonitis, retinitis, esophagitis, and colitis. In addition, some investigators feel it may be responsible for some of the undiagnosed syndromes of fever, weight loss, and fatigue seen in AIDS. DHPG appears to have at least a temporizing effect on organ dysfunction clearly due to CMV infection.[18] EBV is commonly found in throat washings from patients with AIDS, and EBV-positive B-cell lines can easily be generated from the peripheral blood mononuclear cells of patients with AIDS.[43] Although no definite clinical syndromes have been described in AIDS patients as a result of EBV infection, there is a high degree of suspicion that EBV may play an etiological role in many of the B-cell lymphomas seen in these patients. (For example, see the chapters by Levine et al. and Groopman.)

Disseminated infections with other organisms commonly seen in immunosuppressed patients, such as aspergillus, listeria, and *Candida albicans,* have been rarely reported in AIDS patients. Most examples of disseminated infections with these organisms in AIDS patients have been in the setting of neutropenia, and provide insight as to the relative roles of the lymphoid and phagocytic arms of the immune system in host defense.

Conclusions

The occurrence of multiple infectious diseases in the patient with AIDS signifies an immune system that has lost the ability to defend the host against a variety of environmental organisms. The unique nature of the immune defect that develops as a result of infection with HTLV-III/LAV is reflected in the fact that while many standard opportunistic infections such as PCP occur commonly in this group, several others such as listeriosis do not. While therapies exist for many of the infectious complications such patients develop, these therapies do nothing for the underlying immune defect of this syndrome and, thus, in an effort to prevent recurrences, prolonged or repeated courses of therapy are generally required. Until such time as effective therapies are available that will reverse the underlying immune defect seen in these patients, either through inactivating or suppressing the etiological retroviral agent or by directly boosting the immune system, patients will be prone to chronic, recurrent, and often fatal infections.

References

1. Gottleib MS, Schroff R, Schanker HM, et al. Pneumocystis carinii pneumonia and mucosal candidiasis in previously healthy homosexual men: evidence for a new acquired cellular immunodeficiency. N Engl J Med 1981; 305:1425.
2. Masur H, Michelis MA, Greene JB, et al. An outbreak of community-acquired Pneumocystis carinii pneumonia: initial manifestation of cellular immune dysfunction. N Engl J Med 1981; 305:1436.
3. Siegal FP, Lopez C, Hammer GS, et al. Severe acquired immunodeficiency in homosexual males, manifested by chronic perianal ulcerative herpes simplex lesions. N Engl J Med 1981; 305:1439.
4. Fauci AS, Macher A, Longo DL, Lane HC, Masur H, Gelmann EP. Acquired immunodeficiency syndrome: epidemiologic, clinical, immunologic, and therapeutic considerations. Ann Intern Med 1984; 100:92.
5. Gold JWM, Armstrong D. Infectious complications of the acquired immune deficiency syndrome. Ann NY Acad Sci 1984; 437:383.
6. Shroff RW, Gottlieb MS, Prince HE, Chai LL, Fahey JL. Immunological studies of homosexual men with immunodeficiency and Kaposi's sarcoma. Clin Immunol Immunopathol 1983; 27:300.
7. Ammann AJ, Abrams D, Conant M, et al. Acquired immune dysfunction in homosexual men: immunologic profiles. Clin Immunol Immunopathol 1983; 27:315.
8. Stahl RE, Friedman-Kien AE, Dubin R, Marmor M, Zolla-Pazner S. Immunologic abnormalities in homosexual men: relationship to Kaposi's sarcoma. Am J Med 1982; 73:171.
9. Lane HC, Masur H, Gelmann EP, et al. Immunologic profiles define clinical subpopulations of patients with the acquired immunodeficiency syndrome. Am J Med 1985; 78:417.
10. Rivin BE, Monroe JM, Hubschman BP, Thomas PA. AIDS outcome: a first follow-up. N Engl J Med 1984; 311:857.
11. Centers for Disease Control. Acquired immunodeficiency syndrome (AIDS) update—United States. MMWR 1983; 32:309.

12. Levin M, McLeod R, Young Q, et al. Pneumocystis pneumonia: importance of gallium scan for early diagnosis and description of a new immunoperoxidase technique to demonstrate Pneumocystis carinii. Am Rev Resp Dis 1983; 128:182.
13. Kovacs JA, Hiemenz JW, Macher AM, et al. Pneumocystis carinii pneumonia: a comparison between patients with acquired immunodeficiency syndrome and patients with other immunodeficiencies. Ann Intern Med 1984; 100:663.
14. Fauci AS, Masur H, Gelmann EP, Markham PD, Hahn B, Lane HC. The acquired immunodeficiency syndrome: an update. Ann Intern Med 1985; 102:800.
15. Shelhamer JH, Ognibene FP, Macher AM, et al. Persistence of Pneumocystis carinii in lung tissue of acquired immunodeficiency syndrome patients treated for pneumocystis pneumonia. Am Rev Respir Dis 1984; 130:1161.
16. Hughes WT, Kuhn S, Chaudhary S, et al. Successful chemoprophylaxis for Pneumocystis carinii pneumonitis. N Engl J Med 1977; 297:1419.
17. Moskowitz L, Hensley GT, Chan JC, Adams K. Immediate causes of death in acquired immunodeficiency syndrome. Arch Pathol Lab Med 1985; 109:735.
18. Masur H, Lane HC, Palestine A, et al. Effect of 9-(1,3-dihydroxy-2-propoxymethyl) guanine on serious cytomegalovirus disease in 8 immunosuppressed homosexual men. Ann Intern Med 1986; 104:41.
19. Lane HC, Masur HM, Whalen G, Rook AH, Fauci AS. Abnormalities of B cell activation and immunoregulation in patients with the acquired immunodeficiency syndrome. N Engl J Med 1983; 309:453.
20. Polsky B, Gold JW, Whimbey E, Dryjanski J, Brown AE, Schiffman G, Armstrong D. Bacterial pneumonia in patients with the acquired immunodeficiency syndrome. Ann Intern Med 1986; 104:38.
21. Stover DE, White DA, Romano PA, Gellene RA, Robeson WA. Spectrum of pulmonary diseases associated with the acquired immune deficiency syndrome. Am J Med 1985; 78:429.
22. Ognibene FP, Steis RG, Macher AM, et al. Kaposi's sarcoma causing pulmonary infiltrates and respiratory failure in the acquired immunodeficiency syndrome. Ann Intern Med 1985; 102:471.
23. Levy RM, Bredesen PE, Rosenblum ML. Neurologic manifestations of the acquired immunodeficiency syndrome (AIDS): experience of UCSF and review of the literature. J Neurosurg 1985; 62:475.
24. Post MJ, Chan JC, Hensley GT, Hoffman TA, Moskowitz LB, Lippman S. Toxoplasma encephalitis in Haitian adults with acquired immunodeficiency syndrome: a clinical-pathological CT correlation. Am J Radiol 1983: 140:861.
25. Masur H, Lane HC. The acquired immunodeficiency syndrome. In Remington JS, Schwartz MS, ed. Current clinical topics in infectious diseases. volume 6. New York: McGraw-Hill, 1985.
26. Kovacs JA, Kovacs AA, Polis M, et al. Cryptococcosis in the acquired immunodeficiency syndrome. Ann Intern Med 1985; 103:533.
27. Ho DD, Rota TR, Schooley RT, Kaplan JC, Allan JD, Resnick L, Felsenstein D, Andrews CA, Hirsch MS. Isolation of HTLV-III from cerebrospinal fluid and neural tissues of patients with neurologic syndromes related to the acquired immunodeficiency syndrome. N Engl J Med 1985; 313:1493.
28. Resnick L, diMarzo-Veronese F, Schüpbach J, et al. Intra-blood-brain barrier syn-

thesis of HTLV-III-specific IgG in patients with neurologic symptoms associated with AIDS or AIDS-related complex. N Engl J Med 1985; 313:1498.

29. Palestine AG, Rodgrigues MM, Macher AM, Chan CC, Lane HC, Fauci AS, Masur H, Longo D, Reichert CM, Stein R, Rook AH, Nussenblatt RB. Ophthalmic involvement in acquired immunodeficiency syndrome. Ophthalmology 1984; 91:1092.

30. Klein RS, et al. Oral candidiasis in high-risk patients as the initial manifestation of the acquired immune deficiency syndrome. N Engl J Med 1984; 311:354.

31. Sworkin B, Wormser GP, Rosenthal WS, Heier SK, Braunstein M, Weiss L, Jankowski R, Levy D, Weiselberg S. Gastrointestinal manifestations of the acquired immunodeficiency syndrome: a review of 22 cases. Am J Gastroenterol 1985; 80:774.

32. Current WL, Reese NC, Ernst JV, Bailey WS, Heyman MB, Weinstein WM. Human cryptosporidiosis in immunocompetent and immunodeficient persons. Studies of an outbreak and experimental transmission. N Engl J Med 1983; 308:1252.

33. Soave R, Danner RL, Honig CL, Ma P, Hart CC, Nash T, Roberts RB. Cryptosporidiosis in homosexual men. Ann Intern Med 984; 100:504.

34. Portnoy D, Whiteside ME, Buckley E, MacLeod CL. Treatment of intestinal cryptosporidiosis with spiramycin. Ann Intern Med 1984; 101:202.

35. Whiteside ME, Barkin JS, May RG, Weiss SD, Fischl MA, MacLeod CL. Enteric coccidiosis among patients with the acquired immunodeficiency syndrome. Am J Trop Med Hyg 1984; 33:1065.

36. Galser JB, Morton-Kute L, Berger SR, Weber J, Siegal FP, Lopex C, Robbins W, Landesman SH. Recurrent Salmonella typhimurium bacteremia associated with the acquired immunodeficiency syndrome. Ann Intern Med 1985; 102:189.

37. Costel EE, Wheeler AP, Gregg CR. Campylobacter fetus ssp fetus cholecystitis and relapsing bacteremia in a patient with acquired immunodeficiency syndrome. South Med J 1984; 77:927.

38. Roth RI, Owen RL, Keren DF, Volberding PA. Intestinal infection with Mycobacterium avium in acquired immune deficiency syndrome (AIDS). Histological and clinical comparison with Whipple's disease. Dig Dis Sci 1985; 30:497.

39. Macher AM, Kovacs JA, Gill V, et al. Bacteremia due to Mycobacterium avium-intracellulare in the acquired immunodeficiency syndrome. Ann Intern Med 1983; 99:782.

40. Pitchenik AE, Cole C, Russell BW, Fisch MA, Spira TJ, Snider DE Jr. Tuberculosis, atypical mycobacteriosis, and the acquired immunodeficiency syndrome among Haitian and non-Haitian patients in south Florida. Ann Intern Med 1984; 101:641.

41. Wheat LJ, Slama TG, Zeckel ML. Histoplasmosis in the acquired immune deficiency syndrome. Am J Med 1985; 78:203.

42. Bonner JR, Alexander WJ, Dismukes WE, App W, Griffin FM, Little R, Shin MS. Disseminated histoplasmosis in patients with the acquired immune deficiency syndrome. Arch Intern Med 1984; 144:2178.

43. Birx DL, Redfield RR, Tosato G. Defective regulation of Epstein-Barr infection in patients with acquired immunodeficiency syndrome (AIDS) or AIDS-related disorders. N Engl J Med 1986; 314:874.

.

12

Kaposi's Sarcoma: An Overview of Classical and Epidemic Forms

Bijan Safai
Memorial Sloan-Kettering Cancer Center
and Cornell University Medical College
New York, New York

Introduction

Kaposi's sarcoma (KS) represents a potential model for a virally associated human tumor. Prior to 1981, KS was considered a rare tumor that occurred in cluster distribution. A sudden increase in the number of KS cases along with *Pneumocystis carinii* pneumonia (PCP) and other opportunistic infections was observed among the victims of the epidemic of acquired immune deficiency syndrome (AIDS). Initially, the cases were seen in New York and California, but now they have been reported from most large cities in the United States and many other countries. The first reports were exclusively among homosexual men and intravenous drug abusers. However, the disease is now being observed among Haitians, hemophiliacs, and even in some children with AIDS.

In this new epidemic form, KS presents with a more aggressive course involving skin, gastroinestinal tract, lymph nodes, and other organs.[1] The epidemic form of KS has a similar course to lymphadenopathic KS seen in African children. While opportunistic infections (OI) have been the major cause of death in this epidemic, patients have been seen in whom KS has spread rapidly to vital organs such as lung, liver, and spleen. Much interest has been generated in the study of KS since the epidemic of AIDS. It is anticipated that the renewal of interest in KS will stimulate more investigative work and will provide a better insight into this interesting tumor.

History

Moritz Kaposi was born on October 23, 1827 in the regional trade center of Kaposvar on the river Kapos in southern Hungary. He graduated from Vienna University as a Doctor of Medicine in 1861, a Doctor of Surgery in 1862, and Master of Obstetrics in 1865. Dr. Kaposi became an associate professor in 1866 and later a professor of dermatology in 1875. He became the chairman of the Department of Dermatology, replacing Dr. Ferdinand Hebra, his father-in-law.

Dr. Kaposi first described the disease as "idiopathic, multiple pigmented sarcomas of the skin" in 1872.[2] At the suggestion of Koebner, the disease was later named "Kaposi's sarcoma." Dr. Kaposi, however, preferred "sarcoma idiopathicum multiplex hemorrhagicum," a name that he believed more accurately described the condition. Within the next 15 years, the entity was recognized in many countries, and its characteristics were well appreciated. Kaposi described the disseminated form of the disease in 1887, and de Amicis described involvement of the tumor in a 5-year-old child in 1882. Hallenberger[3] described a case involving an African patient in 1914. However, the prevalence of the disease in Africa was not appreciated until 20 years later, when Smith and Elmes[4] reviewed a series of 500 tumors in which 10 cases (or 2%) were diagnosed as Kaposi's sarcoma. Over the next three decades, several other reviews of Kaposi's sarcoma in Africa appeared, culminating in 1961 in a conference on Kaposi's sarcoma held in Kampala, Uganda. The presentations were later published in a monograph by Ackerman and Murray[5] in 1962.

In June 1981, an increased occurrence of KS and *Pneumocystis carinii* pneumonia was observed in homosexual men. Subsequently, other opportunistic infections were found in this population of patients, and the disease complex was renamed "acquired immunodeficiency syndrome" or AIDS. This syndrome is widely expanding in number and heterogeneity of the patient population, and at the time of writing, there are over 20,000 cases reported by the Centers of Disease Control (CDC). Approximately 25% of all reported cases of AIDS have manifested with KS. Some recent observations, however, indicate that the number of KS AIDS cases is decreasing. Cases of KS AIDS have been reported in heterosexuals, Haitians, intravenous drug abusers, hemophiliacs, spouses of AIDS patients, and children with AIDS.[6]

These patients are centered mostly in New York City, San Francisco, and Los Angeles, but many other reports continue to accrue from other cities in the United States, Europe, and South America.[7]

Epidemiology

Incidence

Kaposi's sarcoma is considered to be a rare tumor except in certain endemic regions. In the United States, the incidence is well below 1%. Reviewing a 38-year experience at the Mayo Clinic, Reynolds et al.[8] reported only 70 cases (or 0.06%) of tumors diagnosed at that institution. Dorn and Cutler[9] and Oettle[10] estimate an even lower incidence of 0.02% in the United States.

Kaposi's sarcoma in Africa has shown a very sharp geographical localization. The areas are predominantly hill and open Savannah bush country at an altitude of 1200 to 1500 meters in Zaire, Kenya, and Tanzania. However, even within this endemic region, native blacks are far more frequently affected than nonblacks. Scattered cases from around the world have been reported from Western Europe, Armenia, India, China, and Japan, but are distinctly not as frequent in those areas as it is in North America.

KS has been also observed with increasing incidence among renal transplant recipients.[11,6] An increased occurrence of KS has been recently recognized among homosexual men in New York and California.[12-14] KS in this new population is part of the epidemic of AIDS.[15-18]

KS cases in the epidemic of AIDS have been seen more often among homosexual men than among IV drug abusers or other risk groups. KS has been seen in hemophiliacs with AIDS, Haitian patients, and some children with AIDS. Table I summarizes the reported cases of KS in the epidemic of AIDS by the Centers for Disease Control. KS is more often seen among New York AIDS cases than those from Florida. The cases of KS in homosexuals have been reported mostly from New York City and San Francisco, cities with large homosexual populations.

Sex, Age, and Racial Distribution

Most investigators[8,9,19,20] report a strong male predominance (10 to 15 males to 1 female) in the African variety. A lower male to female ratio of 3 to 1 was noted in a review of cases of KS in Memoiral Sloan-Kettering Cancer Center.[21] Of interest is the reversal of the sex ratio among the white population of South Africa and Nigeria.[22-24] This type, as seen in children and young adults, has

TABLE 1   Incidence of KS in the Epidemic of Aids

Disease Group[a]	Adult/Adolescent		Pediatric	
	Cases (%)	Known Deaths (%)	Cases (%)	Known Deaths (96)
Both KS and PCP	1045 (6)	689 (66)	4 (1)	4 (100)
KS without PCP	3352 (18)	1355 (40)	6 (2)	6 (100)
PCP without KS	10765 (58)	5807 (54)	146 (53)	102 (70)
OI without KS or PCP	3448 (19)	1964 (57)	117 (43)	51 (44)

[a]KS = Kaposi's sarcoma; OI = opportunistic infection; PCP = *Pneumocystis carinii* pneumonia.
Source: Acquired Immunodeficiency Syndrome (AIDS) Weekly Surveillance Report, Centers for Disease Control, March 31, 1986.

equal sex distribution. In the epidemic of AIDS, KS is mostly seen in male homosexuals. Female cases are very infrequent, and are either intravenous drug abusers or Haitians.

The average age of non-African KS is 63 years, and the highest incidence is seen in the sixth through eighth decade of life. The epidemic KS is seen in young patients with an average age of 39 years.[6] The African KS, as analyzed by Davies and Lothe,[25] shows peak incidence in the first decade, rare cases in the second decade, and then a progressive incidence throughout adult life.

It has long been argued whether or not the North American Kaposi's sarcoma is characterized by a geographical localization along racial lines. The majority of patients in America have ancestry going back to Eastern Europe or Italy or are Jewish. Rothman[19] has used this finding to argue in favor of a racial predisposition to developing KS. Bluefarb,[26] on the other hand, presented data showing that the geographical origin of the patients is most important because the vast majority of patients are directly of Eastern European or Italian extraction. It seems that the greatest concentration of cases occurring in North America is in the descendents of immigrants from these European regions. KS has been reported in two persons with pure Eskimo heritage.[27] In the epidemic of AIDS, KS is seen more frequently among white than black patients.[6]

Clinical Manifestation and Course of the Disease

KS is generally believed to be multifocal, and manifests initially with single or, more frequently, multiple red to violaceous macules, papules, and/or nodules.

With time, there is a progression from the macules and patch stage to the plaques and nodule stage. The lesions may coalesce to form large plaques or tumors, which may become eroded, ulcerated, or fungating. New lesions may develop along the superficial vein. Initially, the lesions may appear unilateral, but with progression, bilateral involvement is generally seen. In the older literature,[20] the lower limb, usually the foot or ankle, was the site of initial involvement (75% of cases). The hand or forearm was reported as the initial stage in about 5% of cases, and the remainder of cases had the first lesion on the head and trunk. Solitary nodules on the penis,[20] ear,[28] mouth,[29] eyelid,[29] conjuctiva,[30] and nose[31] have been reported as the sites of initial manifestation.

Several authors have reported patients complaining of pruritis of the affected areas,[28,32] and there is even a report of pruritis preceding the appearances of the lesions.[33] However, Bluefarb[26] considered both of these presentations to be distinctly unusual, and in the patients examined by us, pruritis has not been a notable feature.

It is thought that the development of new lesions is not the result of metastases from a primary lesion, but rather of multifocal origin, a point that was recognized by Kaposi himself.[2] Metastases, while reported in aggressive forms of disease, are considered quite rare.

In the epidemic of AIDS, KS lesions appear to be elongated and oval-shaped and follow the lines of cleavage as seen in pityriasis rosea. In contrast to the cutaneous lesions of the classical KS, the lesions in the epidemic KS tend to be smaller, pink to purple in color, and located on the upper trunk and head and neck areas.[18] Frequent involvement of mucous membranes, lymph nodes, and/or gastrointestinal tract (G) is one of the characteristics of the epidemic form of KS. Violaceous plaques and nodules may be seen in the oral mucosa or GI tract. Cases have been reported in whom the disease has initially manifested in the lymph nodes or GI tract. The majority of cases will eventually develop widespread KS. The GI tract is the most common extra-cutaneous site, but lesions in the lung, liver, pancreas, adrenal gland, spleen, testis, and larynx have been reported.[34,35] These patients also manifest with systemic complaints of fever, weight loss, malaise, anorexia, and diarrhea.[36]

Internal organ and lymph node involvement is less frequent in classical KS as compared with AIDS KS. Involvement of internal organs may reveal itself by a patient complaining of GI hemorrhage or diarrhea and leading to weight loss and emaciation. Visceral involvement is the pattern most commonly seen in African children in whom lymphadenopathy is the main clinical feature. The lymphadenopathic KS cases in Africa are mostly seen in the first decade of life and rarely in the second decade.[10] An increasing incidence of other forms (nodular, florid, infiltrative) of KS is reported throughout adult life in Africa. Involvement of internal organs is probably more frequent than clinically appreciated, with estimates ranging from 10 to 70% of patients showing internal involvement.[37,38] The most common site is the bowel, which is most reliably diagnosed by endoscopy because the lesions may not be protuberant to cause radiological defects. Other sites less frequently involved are the adrenals, pericardium, lymph nodes, and liver.

In Kaposi's original description[2] the course of the disease was stated to be rapidly fatal within 2 or 3 years. However, in a later publication on the subject,[39] he modified this view with the recognition that most European cases were quite protracted. It is now well appreciated that the course of KS ranges from slow indolent to rapid and fulminant with dissemination. In the classical KS, the course of the disease is usually indolent, with the slow development of an increasing number of lesions. The average survival time in the North American series is reported to be 8 to 13 years; however, survival up to 50 years and cases of spontaneous regression of the tumors are also reported.[8,10,20,24,40-42]

In Africa, the nodular form has a chronic indolent course with prolonged survival. A worse prognosis is seen among patients with the infiltrative type of disease. The florid type usually occurs in patients over the age of 50 years, with the acceleration of the disease after years of apparent quiescence. Lymphadenopathic KS, which is seen in African children and young adults, has a very poor prognosis and, on autopsy, remarkably little visceral involvement is found.[43-45]

The course of KS in the North American and European patient is chronic and progressive, but most patients do not die as a result of KS. They may succumb to death due to a second primary malignancy or one of the other diseases that befall the elderly.[18]

KS in renal transplant recipients is reported to be moderately aggressive and, in some cases, regression of the KS is seen following decrease or discontinuation of the immunosuppressive therapy.[11,46,47] The course of the disease in the epidemic KS appears to be aggressive, with dissemination and rapid spread. The patients, however, die mostly of opportunistic infections and rarely due to dissemination of KS. The average survival of epidemic KS cases is thus far reported to be 18 months.[6] In the epidemic cases of KS, the number of the lesions and the amount of tumor mass vary considerably. In addition, the course of the disease and the prognosis do not appear to be related to the extent of the tumor. The only exception is in cases where the lung is involved by KS tumor, representing a poor prognosis. In our series of KS AIDS, we have, on one hand, seen cases where the disease manifests with extensive tumor load at the early stage of the disease, with an average surival of 18 to 24 months. On the other hand, there are patients whose lesions are few and observed only in the late stage of the disease, indicating that the extent of the tumor is not, in most cases, related to the course or the prognosis of the disease. We have also seen a small number of KS AIDS cases who have very

TABLE 2   Kaposi's Sarcoma Features

	Classical KS	AIDS KS
Mean age (yr)	63	39
Sex ratio	10:1	Mostly men
Distribution	Africa, USA, Europe	USA, Europe, Haiti
Skin lesions	Lower extremities	Head, neck, trunk
Lymphadenopathy	Rare (except in African children)	Frequent
Gastrointestinal	Rare	Frequent
Biologic behavior	Slow and indolent	Aggressive and fulminant
Associated diseases	Lymphoma and leukemias	Opportunistic infections
Immune deficiency	Borderline	Severe and progressive
HLA-DR5 frequency	Increased	Increased

few skin lesions, and their disease is stable with minimal or no progression of the disease. These individuals usually have a normal or moderately altered immunological profile.

In some patients, spontaneous regression of one or more nodules of KS has been seen; however, cases of spontaneous regression of all lesions have also been noted.[48] Table 2 summarizes some of the features of classical and epidemic KS.

Histopathology

Histopathological features of KS tumor are characteristic and include interweaving bands of spindle cells and vascular structures embedded in a network of reticular and collagen fibers. The disease process appears to start in the dermis. The vascular component appears as cleft-like spaces between the spindle cells or delicate capillaries. The spindle cells may show a wide range of nuclear pleomorphism. The histological features of KS vary according to the characteristics and quantity of the vascular component, spindle cells, fibrosis, and nuclear pleomorphism in the tumor. A helpful microscopic feature is the presence of extravasated red blood cells and hemosiderin between the spindle cells. Phagocytosis of red blood cells by interspersed macrophages may be prominent.

An inflammatory infiltrate composed of lymphocytes, histiocytes, and plasma cells is present in varying degrees. It is important to keep in mind the chronological changes that occur in the development of KS.[33] Early macular lesions are subtle, with the presence of abnormal and dilated vessels surrounding the normal superficial vasculature. The inflammatory infiltrate may be sparse, and is usually mixed with the presence of plasma cells around the new vessels. Neutrophils are absent, and nuclear atypia and mitoses are rare.

The plaque lesions show more extensive involvement with neoplastic proliferation from the superficial to the deep dermis and, at times, into the adipose tissue. The infiltrate is more prominent than that described for the macular lesion, with the addition of more spindle cells coursing between the collagen bundles and more extravasated red blood cells. Phagocytized hemosiderin is more conspicuous, but nuclear atypia and mitoses can still be subtle.

The nodules show a marked increase in the spindle cell population, with more extravasation of red blood cells, nuclear atypia, pleomorphism, and mitoses. Staining for iron to demonstrate hemosiderin is of diagnostic importance, and this may be seen within the spindle cells.[49] The spindle cells produce little collagen, but do produce significant reticulum fibers; a Foot stain for reticulum will aid in their recognition. The histological features of the epidemic KS have been reported to be similar to those of classical KS.[43,18]

Involvement of the lymph nodes shows replacement of the normal architecture with irregular vascular spaces, fascicles of spindle cells, extravasated red blood cells, and plasma cells in varying degrees.

Associated Diseases

A close association between KS and other primary malignancies has been reported. Moertel[50] reviewed the literature relating the development of second neoplasms among patients with lymphoreticular tumors, and found 51 of 565 developed KS, an incidence of 9%, which is markedly in excess of the proportion of KS generally seen in American patients. In another series, only 2 cases of KS among 4475 cases of lymphoreticular neoplasms were noted.[51] The occurrence of a lymphoreticular neoplasm developing in patients with KS has been seen in 5 cases among 70 patients with KS in one study[8] and 9 of 63 patients in another.[52] In a recent study reviewing a period from 1949 to 1975 at Memorial Sloan-Kettering Cancer Center, 92 patients with KS were followed, among whom 34 (or 37%) developed a second primary malignancy.[21,53] Of these KS patients, 59% had a second primary malignancy involving the lymphoreticular system, whereas only 8% of all patients with primary malignancy other than KS developed a second cancer involving the lymphoreticular system. Other malignancies reported in association with KS from the latter study included neoplasms of the GI tract (two cases), skin (four cases), breast (two cases), and urinary tract (one case). In contrast to that study, only a few KS AIDS cases have shown development of second primary cancer, namely lymphoreticular malignancies.

Several reports have suggested that reduced immunity may play a role in the development and course of KS. The occurrence of KS in a patient with systemic lupus erythematosus during immunosuppressive therapy was reported.[54] An increased incidence of KS has also been reported in patients with disorders of the immune system such as immunodeficiencies, plasma cell dyscrasia, thymoma, or polymyositis.[14,55-58] Also reported are cases of renal transplant recipients who developed KS during the course of immunosuppressive therapy. The KS nodules regressed when therapy was tapered down or discontinued.[47] In KS AIDS cases, the presence of progressive and profound immune deficiency, autoantibodies, and disorders such as thrombocytpoenic purpura has been reported. Master et al.[59] reported a severe impairment of delayed hypersensitivity reactions to dinitrochlorobenzene in patients with the florid type of KS. In contrast, normal responsiveness was observed by these authors in patients with the more benign nodular form of KS. Correlation between the clinical morphology of the disease and cell-mediated immunity has been described by Taylor et al.[60-62] It has been shown that the patients with the aggressive form of KS had lowered blastogenic responsiveness as compared with that in the indolent disease.

In the epidemic form of KS, progressive and severe immune deficiency is the hallmark of the disease.[15-18] The immune deficiency usually manifests with:

1. Decreased white blood cell count and progressive lymphopenia
2. Imbalance of T-lymphocyte subsets, with reversal of the ratio of T-helper/T-suppressor cells (It is important to note that there is an absolute decrease in the helper T-cell population in addition to the lack of function of this T-cell subtype.)
3. Decreased responsiveness to mitogens and antigens and allogenic stimulation
4. Decreased level of production of interferon and interleukin-2 by the peripheral blood cells of these patients
5. High levels of circulating immune complexes
6. Polyclonal activation of B cells
7. Hypergammaglobulinemia
8. Presence of acid-labile interferon in serum

It is speculated that due to this immune dysfunction, the victims of AIDS have developed disseminated and aggressive KS, fatal opportunistic infections, or both. These observations might be taken as evidence relating the immune dysfunction with the pathogenesis of KS. Whether an initial viral infection

causes the development of KS, or rather the development of an immunodeficiency state precedes multiple viral infections as well as KS is unclear. Among
the large population of KS AIDS cases that we have followed over the past 4
years, there is a small group of patients with KS AIDS who have stable disease
and have not progressed to develop widespread KS or OI. Most of these
individuals have normal immune parameters and have remained immunologically stable. The development of KS in these individuals thus raises the
question of whether the presence of immune deficiency is a prerequisite for
the development of this tumor. It is conceivable that the development of KS is
related to the viral infection with HTLV-III/LAV, but not with the immune
deficiency (Safai et al., unpublished data).

Histogenesis

There has been a long-standing controversy as to the cell of origin of KS. Based
on histochemical studies, various cells of origin were proposed, such as Schwann
cell,[63] multipotential primitive mesenchymal cell,[64] endothelial or perithelial
cells of small vessels, or malignant deviation of vascular cells.[49] There was also a
variability in the staining of the spindle cells versus the perivascular cells.[65,66]
This variability was seen in the acid phosphatase that was positive in the spindle
cells and absent in the perivascular cells, and alkaline phosphatase which
showed the reverse. Although cholinesterase was absent from all cells, pseudo-
cholinesterase activity was seen in the spindle cells.[63] Subsequent electron
microscopic studies, as described previously, showed a morphological appearance more consistent with vascular tissue origin. More recently, immunohistochemical studies detected factor VIII-related antigens in KS tissue.[67,68]
There was a variability in the intensity of staining, with the cells lining the
vascular lumina showing a more intense reaction as opposed to the spindle cells
that showed a positive reaction but to a lesser extent. Similar reactions to factor
VIII-related antigens were seen in classical as well as AIDS-associated KS.[68]

The etiology of KS is still unknown. The most widely accepted view is a
multifactorial cause involving possible infectious agents and genetic and environmental factors. The infrequency of familial cases negates a simple Mendelian dominant or recessive inheritance. On the other hand, studies of major
histocompatability antigens have demonstrated increased frequency of HLA-
DR5 in classical KS.[69]

In the epidemic of AIDS, an increased frequency of HLA-DR5 in Jewish
and Italian patients and an increased frequency of HLA-DR2 in Northern
European patients with KS AIDS[70] were initially observed. However, as the
number of tested patients has increased, the frequency of HLA-DR5 has decreased. While these observations suggest a possible predisposing role for the

genetic host factors, it does not necessarily prove a requirement of HLA-DR5 or DR2 for KS to develop. The environmental factors suspected in the case of African KS and AIDS KS include repeated antigenic stimulations such as those of parasitic infections or life style factors. However, in cases of renal transplant recipients and the classical KS, it is unclear what factors may be involved. An important association has been observed, although the cause and effect relationship is not established, between cytomegalovirus (CMV) and KS. Elevated levels of CMV titers in KS sera, presence of CMV-DNA sequences, and CMV antigens within KS tumor tissues have been reported.[71] It seems very likely that the presence of a certain degree of immune dysbalance, repeated antigenic stimulation, and persistent CMV infection in a genetically predisposed individual may result in development of KS. CMV has been quite prevalent among homosexual men for sometime, but increased incidence of KS is quite recent in this group. This indicates that while CMV may play a role as a co-factors, it is unlikely to play an etiological role. One may also speculate that infection with HTLV-III/LAV may cause release of mediator(s), which in turn may result in proliferation of endothelial cells and formation of KS tumor. Some of these issues are discussed in the accompanying chapter by Gelmann and Broder.

Acknowledgments

This chapter was supported in part by U.S. Public Health Service Grants CA-31643, CA-23766, CA-10599, CA-34995 and CA-34822 from the National Institutes of Health, and the Ancell Fund.

References

1. Safai B. Kaposi's sarcoma. Curr Iss Dermatol 1984; 1:3.
2. Kaposi M. Idiopathisches multiples Pigmensarkom der Haut. Arch Derm Syph 1872; 4:265–273.
3. Hallenberger O. Multiple angiosarkome der Haut bein einem Kammerunneger. Arch Schiffs Trop Hgy 1914; 18:647.
4. Smith EC, Elmes BGT. Malignant disease in the natives of Nigeria. An analysis of 500 tumors. Ann Trop Med Parasitol 1934; 28:461.
5. Ackerman LV, Murray JF. Symposium on Kaposi's sarcoma. Basel: S. Karger, 1963.
6. Haverkos HW, Currant JW. The current outbreak of Kaposi's sarcoma and opportunistic infections. CA-A Cancer J Clin 1982; 32:330.
7. Thomsen HK, Jacobsen M, Malchow-Moller A. Lancet 1981; ii:688.
8. Reynolds WA, Winkelmann RK, Soule EH. Kaposi's sarcoma. Medicine 1965; 44:419.

9. Dorn HF, Cutler SJ. Morbidity from cancer in the United States. Part I. Variation in incidence by age, sex, marital status and geographic region. Washington, DC: Public Health Monograph, No 29, 1955:121.

10. Oettle AG. Geographical and racial differences in the frequency of KS as evidence of environmental or genetic causes. Acta Un Int Cancer 1962; 18:330.

11. Harwood A, Osoba D, Hofstader S, Goldstien M, Cardella C, Holecek M, Kunynetz R, Giammarca R. Kaposi's sarcoma in recipients of renal transplants. Am J Med 1979; 67:759–765.

12. Centers for Disease Control. Kaposi's sarcoma and Pneumocystis pneumonia among homosexual men—New York City and California. MMWR 1981; 30:305–3089.

13. Curran J. AIDS—two years later. N Engl J Med 1983; 309:609–611.

14. Myskowski PL, Romano JF, Safai B. Kaposi's sarcoma in young homosexual men. Cutis 1982; 29:31.

15. Gottlieb M, Schroff R, Schanker H, Weisman J, Fran P, Wolf R, Saxon A. Pneumocystis carinii pneumonia and mucosal candiasis in previously health homosexual men. N Engl J Med 1981; 305:1425–1431.

16. Masur H, Michelis M, Greene J, Onorato I, Stouwe R, Holzman R, Wormser G, Brettman L, Lange M, Murray H, Cunningham-Rundles S. An outbreak of community-acquired pneumocystis carinii pneumonia. N Engl J Med 1981; 305:1431–1438.

17. Siegel F, Lopez C, Hammer G, Brown A, Kornfeld S, Gold J, Hassett J, Hirschman S, Cunningham-Rundles C, Adelsberg B, Parham D, Siegal M, Cunningham-Rundles S, Armstrong D. Severe acquired immunodeficiency in male homosexuals, manifested by chronic perianal ulcerative herpes simplex lesions. N Engl J Med 181; 305:1439–1444.

18. Urmacher C, Myskowski P, Ochoa M, Kris M, Safai B. Outbreak of Kaposi's sarcoma in young homosexual men. Am J Med 1982; 72:569–575.

19. Rothman S. Remarks on sex, age and racial distribution of Kaposi's sarcoma and on possible pathogenic factors. Acta Un Int Cancer 1962; 18:322.

20. Lothe F. Kaposi's sarcoma in Ugandan Africans. Acta Pathol Microbiol Scand 1963; 161(Suppl):1.

21. Safai B, Mike V, Giraldo G, Beth E, Good RA. Association of Kaposi's sarcoma with second primary malignancies: possible etiopathogenic implications. Cancer 1980; 45:1472.

22. Rothman S. Medical research in Africa. Arch Dermatol 1962; 85:311.

23. Oettle AG. Geographic and racial differences in frequency of Kaposi's sarcoma as evidence of environmental or genetic causes. In: Ref. 4, p. 330.

24. Palmer PES. Haemangiosarcoma of Kaposi. Acta Radiol Rev 1972; 12:640 (Suppl 316, p. 6).

25. Davies JNP, Lothe F. Kaposi's sarcoma in African children. In: Ref. 4, p. 81.

26. Bluefarb SM. Kaposi's sarcoma. Springfield, Ill: Charles C. Thomas, 1957.

27. Mikkelsen F, Hojgaard-Nielsen N, Hart-Gansen J. Kaposi's sarcoma in polar eskimos. Acta Derm Venereol (Stockholm) 1977; 56:539–541.

28. Symmers D. Kaposi's sarcoma. Arch Pathol 1941; 32:764.

29. McLaren DS. Kaposi's sarcoma of the eyelids of an African child. Arch Ophthalmol 1960; 63:859.

30. Mortada A. Conjunctival regressing Kaposi's sarcoma. Br J Ophthalmol 1967; 51: 275.
31. Hansson CJ. Kaposi's sarcoma. Clinical and radiotherapeutic studies on 23 patients. Acta Radiol (Stockh) 1940; 21:457.
32. Meyers DS, Jacobson VC. Multiple hemorrhagic sarcoma of Kaposi. Am J Pathol 1927; 3:321.
33. Dorffel J. Histogenesis of multiple idiopathic hemorrhagic sarcoma of Kaposi. Arch Derm Syph 1932; 26:608.
34. Holecek MJ, Harwood AR. Radiotherapy of Kaposi's sarcoma. Cancer 1978; 41: 1733–1738.
35. Friedman-Kien AE. Disseminated Kaposi's sarcoma syndrome in young homosexual men. J Am Acad Dermatol 1981; 5:468–471.
36. Centers for Disease Control. Epidemiologic aspects of the current outbreak of Kaposi's sarcoma and opportunistic infections. N Engl J Med 1982; 306:248–252.
37. Ecklund RE, Valaitis J. Kaposi's sarcoma of lymph nodes. Arch Pathol 1962; 74:224.
38. Cox FX, Helwig EB. Kaposi's sarcoma. Cancer 1959; 12:289.
39. Kaposi M. Zur nomeclatur des idiopathischen Pigmentsarkom Kaposi. Arch Derm Syph (Berl) 1894; 29:164.
40. Taylor JF, Templeton AC, Vogel CL, Ziegler JC, Kyalwazi SK. Kaposi's sarcoma in Uganda: a clinico-pathological study. Int J Cancer 1971; 8:122.
41. Rothman S. Some clinical aspects of Kaposi's sarcoma in the European and North American populations. Acta Un Int Cancer 1962; 18:364.
42. Keen P. The clinical features of Kaposi's sarcoma in the South African Bantu. Acta Un Int Cancer 1962; 18:380.
43. Gottlieb GJ, Ackerman AB. Kaposi's sarcoma: an extensively disseminated form in young homosexual men. Hum Pathol 1982; 13:882.
44. Dutz W, Stout AP. Kaposi's sarcoma in infants and children. Cancer 1960; 13:684.
45. Lothe F, Murray JF. Kaposi's sarcoma: autopsy findings in the African. In: Ref. 4, p. 116.
46. Law I. Kaposi's sarcoma and plasma cell dyscrasia. JAMA 1974; 2291329–1331.
47. Myers B, Kessler E, Kepi J, Pick A, Rosenfeld J, Tikvah P. Kaposi's sarcoma in kidney transplant recipients. Arch Intern Med 1974; 133:307–311.
48. Templeton AC. Kaposi's sarcoma. In: Andrade, Gumport, Popkin, Rees, eds. Cancer of the skin, vol. 2. Philadelphia: WB Saunders, 1976:1183.
49. Hashimoto K, Lever WF. Kaposi's sarcoma. Histologic and electron microscopic studies. J Inv Derm 1964; 43:539.
50. Moertel CG. Multiple primary malignant neoplasms. vol. 7. Recent results in cancer research. Berlin: Springer-Verlag, 1966.
51. Moertel CG, Hagedorn AB. Leukemia or lymphoma and coexistent primary malignant lesion. A review of the literature and a study of 120 cases. Blood 1957; 12:788.
52. O'Brien PH, Brasfield R. Kaposi's sarcoma. Cancer 1966; 19:1497.
53. Safai B, Good RA. Kaposi's sarcoma. A review and recent developments. Clin Bull 1980; 10:62.
54. Klein MB, Pereira FA, Kantor I. Kaposi's sarcoma complicating systemic lupus erythematosus treated with immunosuppression. Arch Dermatol 1974; 110:602.

55. Kapadia SB, Krause JR. Kaposi's sarcoma after long-term alkylating agent therapy for multiple myeloma. South Med J 1977; 70:1011.

56. Mazzaferri EL, Penn GM. Kaposi's sarcoma associated with multiple myeloma. Report of a patient and review of the literature. Arch Int Med 1968; 122:521.

57. Dantzig PI. Kaposi's sarcoma and polymyositis. Arch Dermatol 1974; 110:605.

58. Ettinger DS, Humphrey RL, Skinner MD. Kaposi's sarcoma associated with multiple myeloma. Johns Hopkins Med J 1975; 137:88.

59. Master S, Taylor J, Kyalwazi S, Ziegler J. Immunological studies in Kaposi's sarcoma in Uganda. Br Med J 1970; 1:600–602.

60. Taylor J, Junge U, Wolfe L, Deinhardt F, Kyalwazi S. Lymphocyte transformation in patients with Kaposi's sarcoma. Int J Cancer 1971; 8:468–474.

61. Taylor J. Lymphocyte transformation in Kaposi's sarcoma. Lancet 1973; i:833–884.

62. Taylor J, Ziegler J. Delayed cutaneous hypersensitivity reactions in patients with Kaposi's sarcoma. Br J Cancer 1974; 30:312–318.

63. Becker BJP. The histogenesis of Kaposi's sarcoma. Acta Un Int Cancer 1962; 18:477.

64. Mustkallis KK, Leponen E, Roekellis J. Histochemistry of Kaposi's sarcoma. I. Hydrolases and phosphorylases. J Exp Mol Pathol 1963; 2:303.

65. Camain R, Quenum A. Histopathologie et histogenese de la maladie de Kaposi. In: Ackerman LF, Murray JF, eds. Symposium on Kaposi's sarcoma. New York: Hafner Publishing, 1963;140–146.

66. Dorfman RF. Kaposi's sarcoma: the contribution of enzyme histochemistry to the identification of cell types. Acta Un Int Cancer 1862; 18:464.

67. Nadji MD, Morales AR, Aiegler-Weissman J, et al. Kaposi's sarcoma: immunological evidence for an endothelial origin. Arch Pathol Lab Med 1981; 105:274.

68. Guarda LG, Silva EG, Ordonez NG, et al. Factor VIII in Kaposi's sarcoma. Am J Clin Pathol 1981; 76:197.

69. Pollack MS, Safai B, Myskowski PL, Gold J, Pandey J, Dupont B. Frequency of HLA and Gm immunogenetic markers in Kaposi's sarcoma. Tissue Antigens 1983; 21:1–8.

70. Pollack MS, Safai B, Dupont B. HLA-DR5 and DR2 are susceptibility factors for acquired immunodeficiency syndrome with Kaposi's sarcoma in different ethnic subpopulations. Disease Markers 1983; 1:135–139.

71. Giraldo G, Beth E, Huang E. Kaposi's sarcoma and its relationship to cytomegalovirus. III. CMV, DNA and CMV early antigens in Kaposi's sarcoma. Int J Cancer 1980; 26:23–29.

13

Kaposi's Sarcoma in the Setting of the AIDS Pandemic

Edward P. Gelmann
Samuel Broder
Clinical Oncology Program
National Cancer Institute
National Institutes of Health
Bethesda, Maryland

Kaposi's sarcoma (KS) is one of the indicia of HTLV-III/LAV infection, and falls into the category of opportunistic neoplasms (discussed in several chapters of this book) that helped to define the disease now called AIDS. Kaposi's sarcoma is a neoplasm manifested primarily by multiple vascular nodules in the skin and other organs [Fig.1 (see Plate II, facing p. 193)]. The disease is multifocal, with a course that may range from indolent regional disease to fulminant disseminated neoplasia. Although this definition of Kaposi's sarcoma has not changed for decades, the advent of the acquired immunodeficiency syndrome (AIDS) has transformed what was once a rarity in the United States into something commonplace. AIDS has also changed the epidemiological and clinical considerations of KS in Africa. Kaposi's sarcoma was first described by the Austrian dermatologist Moritz Kaposi (pseudonym) in 1872. The occurrence of the disorder is restricted to four well-defined groups, in each of which KS appears to follow a different clinical course.

It is noteworthy that despite the abundant supply of clinical samples and autopsy tissues, there have been no reports of success in establishing KS cells in permanent culture or as a heterograft in the nude mouse. The lack of a laboratory model for KS has undoubtedly delayed the progress of our understanding this enigmatic and morbid neoplasm.

African Kaposi's Sarcoma (Before the Advent of AIDS)

Kaposi's sarcoma has been commonest in Africa where its heterogeneous geographic distribution is centered in Zaire, a country where Kaposi's sarcoma represents approximately 10% of all malignancies.[1,2] Although the disease is not seen in the desert regions of northern Africa, there is a gradual decline in incidence, moving south from Zaire, such that in South Africa Kaposi's sarcoma represents 1.1% of all malignancies. Because of difficulties inherent in surveying large samples of Africans, the available data are largely based on the rate of Kaposi's sarcoma as a proportion of other malignancies observed in the same area over the same interval of time. Epidemiological surveys using this measure of the incidence of this disease have consistently shown that cases in Africa tend to cluster near the equator. The relative rates observed in this area are much higher than the 0.06% rate in the United States. In Zaire, for example, 12.8% of all malignancies are Kaposi's sarcoma, and in Uganda the figure is 4.2%.[1] The disease is not distributed randomly in these countries, but apparently occurs in zones of very high frequency. Eastern Zaire and the western edges of Uganda and Tanzania seem to be areas where the relative incidence of Kaposi's sarcoma is highest. Occurrence of the disease declines steadily to the north and west of this area, so that in Tunisia the rate is 0.04%, comparable with that in the United States. The reason for these geographic differences in the prevalence of KS is not clear, but it seems that the variations are a reflection of some unknown environmental influence.[2] It is worth noting that there is considerable geographic overlap between areas endemic for KS and areas endemic for Burkitt's lymphoma. A genetic contribution to the apparent susceptibility of people living in the "hot spots" is possible, however, since most cases occur in African blacks. The disease is a rarity in African whites. African KS (prior to the onset of AIDS-related KS) affected males more frequently than females by a 10:1 ratio and tended to be a neoplasm of younger adult populations. In Tanzania, for example, Slavin and associates[3] found the highest incidence in the fourth decade, and 7% of cases were in children less than 16 years of age. Clinical features of the disease in Africa are quite variable. Taylor and associates[4] divided African cases of Kaposi's sarcoma into four subtypes based primarily on clinical features. The nodular form is similar to the classic type seen in the United States. It accounts for about one-quarter of all cases, and occurs in adults. Generally, nodules or plaques of tumor develop on the lower extremity distal to the knee, usually in association with nonpitting edema. The tumors generally remain limited to the dermis; extracutaneous disease or extension to adjacent bone is unusual. Occasionally patients note spontaneous resolution of lesions, and most have stable disease for many years.

Florid Kaposi's sarcoma occurs in 40% of African cases and presents as an exophytic, fungating mass. These tumors either develop de novo or evolve from nodular lesions by growth of tumor through the epidermis. The resulting mass weeps serous fluid and usually becomes infected. The tumor also grows deep into the tissues, invades the underlying bone in most cases, and produces considerable pain and limitation of motion of the affected limb. Despite the locally aggressive nature of the tumor, it rarely metastasizes other than to regional draining lymph nodes. Local therapy is generally indicated because of the destructive nature of florid KS

Infiltrative Kaposi's sarcoma accounts for about 15% of all cases. This starts in the dermis, extends to and invades deeper structures, and infiltrates the affected hand or foot diffusely. A dense fibroblastic reaction accompanies the growth of this tumor. The tumor and fibroblastic reaction result in diffuse swelling and a woody induration of the involved limb. Distant spread beyond the site of the primary lesion is distinctly unusual; morbidity results nearly exclusively from localized disease. Response to therapy in this form of Kaposi's sarcoma is poor.

The remaining 20% of cases present with disseminated lymph node involvement with or without associated cutaneous disease. Most cases of this lymphadenopathic form of the disease occur in children less than 16 years of age.[4-6] Cervical and inguinal nodes are most frequently and extensively affected, though most superficial and deep nodal groups may be involved. Other sites of involvement include the lacrimal and parotid glands and the eyelids, resulting in a form of Mickulicz syndrome. Visceral involvement may occur. This form of Kaposi's sarcoma follows a fulminant course if not treated, with death occurring within a year in most cases. These children can be successfully treated wtih a combination of actinomycin-D, vincristine, and DTIC.[6]

Classical Kaposi's Sarcoma

In Europe and North America, classical Kaposi's sarcoma is a rare tumor (0.29 per 100,000), characteristically appearing in middle-aged men of Mediterranean extraction.[7] In this setting, it appears usually as an indolent, lower-extremity dermal neoplasm. Investigators at the Mayo Clinic were able to collect a series of only 70 patients over a 38-year period,[8] and malignancies seen at the University of Chicago over a 15-year period.[9] Men were affected much more commonly than women. The male:female ratio in most reviews ranges between 10:1 and 15:1. Most of the cases occurred in Italian men, with other ethnic groups (Russians, Jews, and Poles) comprising the majority of the remaining cases.[10] The disease in the United States occurs in mid to late life. In cases seen at the Armed Forces Institute of Pathology and the Mayo Clinic, 83% of the patients were 40 years of age and older.[8,11]

The rarity of juvenile Kaposi's sarcoma other than in Africa is emphasized by the study of Dutz and Stout, who reviewed the world's literature on this disease in 1960. Of the 1256 cases reviewed, 40 occurred in children less than 15 years of age, and 45% of these were in African children.

In most cases, the neoplasm starts as a nodule or plaque (with a purple or red hue) on the lower extremities. The disease usually has an indolent clinical course. The tumor may not significantly affect life expectancy, and is often palliated with radiotherapy. In the Mayo Clinic series, 88% of initial lesions appeared on the skin of the leg distal to the knee, and lower extremity lesions eventually developed in all patients sometime during the course of this disease. Noncutaneous disease was found in only 3% of patients prior to the development of skin disease. If left untreated, skin lesions occasionally underwent spontaneous regression but, more commonly, progressed locally and eventually spread to other cutaneous sites. With local progression of skin disease, about 10% of patients will develop extensive induration and subcutaneous extension of the neoplasm.

Visceral disease develops in about 10% of patients either at presentation or, more commonly, during the course of the disease. In a series of cases made up exclusively of patients from the United States,[8,11] visceral disease most commonly involved the gastrointestinal tract, the lungs, and the heart. Lesions in these organs were similar in appearance to those in the skin, and caused clinical manifestations as a result of either extensive local growth or hemorrhage. Perforation of the small intestine due to localized Kaposi's sarcoma has also been reported.[13] Heart involvement, reported in several cases,[14,15] has resulted in acute pericardial tamponade and death. Involvement of other visceral organs and the brain has been reported, but is rare.[16] Lymph node involvement, when present, usually occurs in nodes draining an affected lower extremity, but may be generalized.[8,11]

About half of the patients with classic Kaposi's sarcoma in several series remained alive, with up to 15 years of observation from the time of diagnosis. Between 15% and 25% of patients die as a direct result of Kaposi's sarcoma, usually because of progressive gastrointestinal or pulmonary involvement. Of those who die as a result of Kaposi's sarcoma, most have died within 3 years of the diagnosis, although occasionally patients die of the disease only after many years of its slow progression. The remaining 25% of patients die of causes unrelated to Kaposi's sarcoma.

An inordinate number of second malignancies develop in patients with Kaposi's sarcoma, and death due to these tumors accounts for a significant portion of the deaths in groups of Kaposi's patients. In a study of 92 cases of Kaposi's sarcoma seen at Memorial Sloan-Kettering Cancer Center, Safai and associates[17] found that 37% of all patients had a second primary malignancy diagnosed before (35%), coincident with (24%), or after (41%) the diagnosis of Kaposi's sarcoma. In 58% of these cases, the second primary malignancy was of the lymphoreticular system. This compares with an 8% incidence of second malignancies of the lymphoreticular system in patients with other forms seen in New York over the same period of time. Of 72 patients diagnosed as having Kaposi's sarcoma in the absence of a second malignancy and then followed by this study, nine subsequently developed a lymphoreticular malignancy. This corresponds to an observed annual rate of roughly 1600 cases per 100,000 patients, at least 20 times higher than the general population. For first tumors other than Kaposi's sarcoma, except for malignant lymphomas, the likelihood of developing a malignancy of the lymphoreticular system is not increased above the rate expected for the general population. Moertel and associates[18] have also observed an association of Kaposi's sarcoma and lymphoreticular malignancies. Some of these issues are discussed in the accompanying chapter by Safai.

Kaposi's Sarcoma Associated with Immunosuppressive Drug Therapy

Kaposi's sarcoma is seen in association with the use of immunosuppressive drugs such as azathioprine and corticosteriods. Approximately 50 cases have been reported with demonstrated association.[19-36] The underlying conditions for which these drugs were given have generally required prolonged immunosuppression and include rheumatoid arthritis, asthma, systemic lupus erythematosus, pemphigus vulgaris, bullous pemphigoid, autoimmune hemolytic anemia, idiopathic thrombocytopenia purpura, and renal allograft transplantation. The mean duration of immunosuppressive therapy prior to the first occurrence of Kaposi's sarcoma in these patients was 8.5 months. The most frequent and best studied association has been with renal transplantation.[19] The Denver Transplant Tumor Registry has found 630 malignancies among renal transplant recipients and, of those, 20 (3.2%) have been Kaposi's sarcoma. Among cancers that occur in this setting, this represents a proportion of Kaposi's sarcoma 50 times higher than the expected proportion (0.06%) for this type of tumor. Since the smaller figure was derived from a cancer patient population not receiving immunosuppressive drugs, it appears Kaposi's sarcoma is one malignancy whose particular development is favored by a perturbation of the immune system associated with immunosuppressive drugs and perhaps antigenic challenge.

The Kaposi's sarcoma that develops in patients receiving immunosuppressive drugs has several features that distinguish it from the classic form of the disease; 25% of the patients are less than 40 years of age at the time of diagnosis and females are more frequently affected, though the male:female ratio is still 1.8:1. The disease seems to be more aggressive than the classic form, with 29% of patients developing visceral or nodal involvement. Most of these patients (68% of the reported cases), however, are of Jewish or Mediterranean extraction. Treatment of Kaposi's sarcoma in this group of patients is not particularly useful, but it is of interest that in many patients, the KS responds favorably to a discontinuation or a reduction in dosages of the immunosuppressive drugs. Of 9 patients treated this way (and not given any other therapy), 6 had complete responses, 1 had a partial response, and 2 had no response.[19,30,31] The duration of their responses was not reported in most cases, but two complete responders were still disease-free more than 19 to 24 months after the dosages of their immunosuppressive drugs were reduced.[30]

Kaposi's Sarcoma in AIDS Patients

Kaposi's sarcoma is an epiphenomenon of the acquired immunodeficiency syndrome. Unlike the classic presentation, Kaposi's sarcoma in the acquired immunodeficiency syndrome may present as skin or lymph node involvement anywhere on the body. The histological characteristics of these lesions are indistinguishable from that in classic Kaposi's sarcoma and tend to have an angiomatous appearance. Patients often have progressive disease culminating in multiple organ involvement, particularly of the gastrointestinal tract and pulmonary parenchyma. At autopsy, the histological characteristics of these disseminated lesions show that the neoplasm appears to have taken on a more aggressive angiosarcomatous pattern with spindle cell proliferation.

Kaposi's sarcoma is unevenly distributed among risk group subsets of the poulation with the acquired immunodeficiency syndrome. Gay men have 46% incidence of Kaposi's sarcoma at their initial diagnosis of acquired immunodeficiency syndrome. In evaluating this figure, one should keep in mind that Kaposi's sarcoma (in certain age groups) is one of the diagnostic criteria of AIDS in its own right. Among AIDS patients who are heterosexual males with a history of intravenous drug use, the incidence of KS is 3.8%.[37] This statistic suggests that gay men with acquired immunodeficiency syndrome are exposed to additional factors that have a causative role in Kaposi's sarcoma. One such factor may be cytomegalovirus infection. Male homosexuals have 94% positive serological characteristics for cytomegalovirus as compared with 66% for intravenous drug users. Because of the ubiquity of cytomegalovirus, etiological considerations can not be made on the basis of seroepidemiology. Boldogh and colleagues[38] have studied African patients with Kaposi's sarcoma as well as tissue samples of Kaposi's sarcoma cultured in vitro, and found cytomegalovirus infections prevalent in the patients and cytomegalovirus nucleic acid widely present both in tumor specimens and the cultured cells. Cytomegalovirus has also been shown by in situ nucleic acid hybridization of histological sections to be present in Kaposi's sarcoma cells, but not in the surrounding dermis.[39] Moreover, cytomegalovirus has the capacity for cell transformation by virtue of the transformation of hamster cells in vitro and, more recently, by the demonstration that subgenomic fragments of cytomegalovirus DNA can transform NIH/3T3 fibroblasts and hamster embryo cells in vitro after DNA-mediated gene transfer.[40,41] The role of cytomegalovirus in the cause of Kaposi's sarcoma has not yet been clarified, but mounting circumstantial evidence continues to support an etiological association between the virus and the neoplasm. Questions have also been raised concerning the possibility of a direct etiological role for HTLV-III/LAV in Kaposi's sarcoma. However, sero-epidemiological studies of African patients with classic Kaposi's sarcoma have failed to show an increased level of seropositivity to HTLV-III.[42] Moreover, molecular hybridization of Kaposi's sarcoma tissue DNA with cloned HTLV-III genomic probe has failed to show evidence of virus infection.

Kaposi's sarcoma in AIDS patients differs markedly in many respects from the disease classically seen in North America and Europe prior to the AIDS pandemic. In many respects, it tends to resemble the lymphadenopathic form of the disease seen in young African patients before the outbreak of AIDS.

The disease in gay male AIDS patients tends to be aggressive, with frequent involvement of mucosal surfaces (a careful oral cavity examination is essential in these patients), visceral organs, and lymph nodes as well as skin.[43,44] The cutaneous tumors range from pink to deep purple, and frequently have a surrounding halo of brown pigmentation. Occasionally, patients develop what appear to be multiple subcutaneous ecchymoses in the absence of thrombocytopenia or a history of trauma. The tumors are usually nodular, but macules, patches, and plaques are also seen. Involvement of most skin surfaces occurs, including the palms, soles, and genitalia. There is no characteristic initial site of involvement or pattern of spread. The epidermis overlying the tumor typically remains intact, but occasionally, particularly in dependent areas, it becomes infiltrated by tumor that results in its disruption. A sero-sanguineous drainage then develops and local infection occurs.

Internal organ involvement is common; for example, of 19 patients seen at

New York University, 16 had skin involvement, 13 had nodal involvement, 12 had gastrointestinal tract involvement, 3 had splenic involvement, and 1 had lung involvement. At autopsy, nearly all AIDS patients with Kaposi's sarcoma followed in the Medicine Branch at the National Cancer Institute were found to have internal organ involvement. In addition to involvement of sites already listed, involvement of the upper airway, heart, diaphragm, pancreas, liver, urinary bladder, gallbladder, and epididymis has been seen.

Although internal organ involvement is frequent, overt clinical manifestations of the visceral KS occur in a comparatively small subset of the patients early in their course. Most patients with nodal involvement note only asymptomatic swelling of nodes, especially in the cervical and inguinal areas. The nodes are firm, usually up to 1 to 2 cm in diameter, movable, nontender, and not fixed to one another. Biopsy of clinically suspicious nodes is essential to distinguish nodal Kaposi's sarcoma from the lymphadenopathy due to follicular hyperplasia frequently seen in AIDS patients.

Gastrointestinal involvement occurs in up to 50% of patients, but most patients remain asymptomatic. Diffuse abdominal pain of varying intensity has been observed in these patients, but it is difficult to prove that the pain is related to neoplastic involvement of the gut. Massive upper gastrointestinal tract bleeding is rare. Occult blood loss is only slightly more common. Occasionally, patients develop very extensive gastrointestinal tract involvement, with growth of the tumor along the plane of the mucosa rather than into the gut lumen. Functional impairment as a result of which growth may cause a syndrome consisting of severe, persistent, watery diarrhea and hypoalbuminemia suggestive of a protein-losing enteropathy.

Pulmonary involvement with KS may be a major clinical problem and presents a diagnostic dilemma. The tumor infiltrates the interstitial space, causing a spectrum of clinical manifestations. Some patients have no symptoms and are noted to have pulmonary involvement only at autopsy. Others have massive intraalveolar hemorrhage and ventilatory failure.[45] Involvement of the upper airway may result in pain and obstruction. Involvement of the heart, liver, urinary bladder, gallbladder, pancreas, and epididymis may be observed at autopsy, and additionally result in no symptoms.

Although it is clear the AIDS-associated Kaposi's sarcoma is often an aggressive disease, death due directly to this complication of AIDS does not occur in the majority of cases. About 30% of the patients with AIDS and concomitant Kaposi's sarcoma followed at the National Cancer Institute died as a direct result of Kaposi's sarcoma. A new staging classification has been proposed to delineate more clearly the prognostic subgroups of KS.[46] However, since the immune status of the patient has more influence on prognosis than does the burden of KS, it is unclear what significance this staging classification will have in management and therapy decisions.[47]

Although therapeutic approaches for Kaposi's sarcoma in Africa have been well established, the potential difficulties presented by the underlying immuno-suppression in the acquired immunodeficiency syndrome have stimulted clini-cians to search for other therapeutic approaches. Immune modulator therapy, represented most prominently by treatment with parenteral alpha-interferon, has been an area of intense clinical experimentation. Several groups have published results of therapeutic trials using alpha-interferon therapy for Ka-posi's sarcoma in the acquired immunodeficiency syndrome. Investigators from Memorial Sloan-Kettering[48] and the University of California in San Francisco[49] reported an approximate 40% response rate for Kaposi's sarcoma lesions after alpha-interferon therapy. At the National Cancer Institute (NCI), results were not as encouraging.[50] However, analysis of the data showed that the probability of a favorable response to the alpha-interferon as an antitumor agent was increased by a more favorable pretherapy immune status manifested by higher levels of T4$^+$ cells and the absence of a previous or concurrent opportunistic infection.

Upon examination the immune status of patients included in the three trials,[48,50] it can be seen that 60 to 80% of responders had T4/T8 ratios greater than 0.4. Most of all patients treated at Memorial Sloan-Kettering and the University of California in San Francisco Medical Center had T4/T8 ratios greater than or equal to 0.4; however, only 25% of the patients in the NCI trial began therapy with as good an immune profile. Taken together, these data show that 30 to 40% of selected patients with Kaposi's sarcoma will respond to moderate parenteral doses of alpha-interferon. An independent analysis of therapeutic trials of KS patients arrived at a number of conclusions.[51] This response rate categorizes Kaposi's sarcoma as one of the most responsive solid tumor for which interferon therapy has been attempted. Unfortunately, the original role intended for alpha-interferon as a potential immune modulator in the acquired immunodeficiency syndrome has not been fulfilled. No signifi-cant effect was seen for improvement of immune function, and there was no alteration of ongoing cytomegalovirus infections so common in these pa-tients.[49,50]

Kaposi's sarcoma is a radioresponsive neoplasm, and in patients with clas-sic Kaposi's sarcoma limited to the skin, electron-beam irradiation therapy is successful in controlling the disease.[52] The Radiation Oncology Branch of the National Cancer Institute studied the efficacy of electron-beam irradiation therapy in AIDS patients with Kaposi's sarcoma. Although it was clear that AIDS-associated Kaposi's sarcoma was radioresponsive and the dose-response curve was similar to that in patients with classic KS, the duration of response was usually less than 4 months. In several patients with impending upper airway obstruction due to extensive laryngeal Kaposi's sarcoma, local irradia-tion therapy resulted in prompt regression of the disease in each case.

Because of its efficacy in cases of African KS and despite fears of immunosuppressive effects, cytotoxic chemotherapy has been used to treat KS associated with AIDS. Based on the results of therapeutic trials in Uganda for the treatment of KS with chemotherapy,[36,53-62] both single-agent and combination regimens have been devised for the treatment of KS in AIDS patients.

Two single-agent regimens have been reported in the literature. One employed etoposide (150 mg/m^2 daily for 3 days every 28 days) to treat early-stage KS.[63] The overall response rate was 76%, but the median response duration was only 9 months. Volberding and co-workers[64] treated 38 patients with vinblastine (4 to 8 mg/week, titrated to the total leukocyte count). In this trial only 26% of patients had an objective response, and 50% had stable disease. The latter trial accrued patients with both early-stage and advanced disease, which may explain part of the discrepancy between the results of the two single-agent trials.

Combination chemotherapy regimens have also been described for the treatment of advanced stage KS in AIDS. The ABV regimen (doxorubicin, 40 mg/m^2 on day 1; bleomycin, 15 U on days 1 and 15; and vinblastine 6 mg/m^2 on day 1) was used by Laubenstein and co-workers[63] to treat 31 patients with disseminated KS. The overall response rate was 84%, and the median duration of response was 8 months. At the National Cancer Institute, a regimen of two noncross-resistant chemotherapy regimens, ABV/ADV, was employed in disseminated KS patients. The drugs administered were adriamycin (20 mg/m^2), vinblastine 4 mg/m^2), and bleomycin (15 U) all on day 1, actinomycin D (1 mg/m^2), vincristine (1.4 mg/m^2), and DTIC (375 mg/m^2), all on day 8, and bleomycin (15 U) on day 15. The overall response rate was 78%, but the duration of response was less than 5 months (Gelmann et al., submitted for publication).

Whereas there was no doubt about the efficacy of chemotherapy for the short-term management of KS in AIDS patients, there was considerable concern about chemotherapy potentiation of opportunistic infections. A randomized trial was conducted comparing recombinant alpha-interferon and chemotherapy (ABV/ADV with the 15 bleomycin omitted) in advanced KS. A crossover provision was included in the trial for those patients who failed initial therapy. Eighteen patients accrued on the trial accumulated 32 months on interferon therapy with six intratherapy opportunistic infections, and 50 months on chemotheapy with five intratherapy opportunistic infections (Gelmann et al., submitted for publication). Treatment response did not differ from previous results with interferon and chemotherapy.

Thus it appears that combination chemotherapy may be used safely for short-term treatment of severe KS in AIDS patients. Also, patients may be maintained on single-agent chemotherapy for prolonged periods of time. None of the therapeutic modalities used for KS in AIDS patients have produced disease-free remission rates for more than a few months. Since there is no evidence that effective treatment of KS prolongs survival of AIDS patients, the management of KS should be directed at palliating morbid lesions and controlling severe pulmonary and gastrointestinal disease.

Conclusions and Prospects

The advent of the AIDS epidemic has brought with it an explosion in the incidence of Kaposi's sarcoma in North America. Since KS is not equally prevalent in all individuals at high risk for AIDS, but rather has a marked predominance among male homosexuals, there appears to be co-factors affecting the development of KS in the setting of of AIDS. Also, the proportion of Kaposi's sarcoma in gay men with HTLV-III/LAV infection (the risk group with the largest number of cases) may be decreasing compared with the number of cases of *Pneumocystis* pneumonia. In the subset of these patients, KS causes substantial and life threatening morbidity. For these patients, despite the nature of their underlying immunodeficiency, we must provide rational and, hopefully, effective therapy for management of this neoplasm. Moreover, it is unclear whether in AIDS patients who have had chronic KS, the lesions would disappear automatically if new therapies were able to reverse the immunodeficiency. The experience with the transplantation patient whose KS resolves when his or her immunosuppressive therapy is stopped at the first appearance of a KS lesion may not be directly applicable to the AIDS patient who has extensive KS. In any event, it would appear that a definitive therapy for KS in the setting of AIDS will depend on the development of effective strategies for restoring the immunological capacity of the patient with AIDS and suppressing the retrovirus that is responsible for the disease in the first place. Some of these issues are discussed in the chapter by Yarchoan and Broder.

References

1. Hutt MS. The epidemiology of Kaposi's sarcoma. Antibiot Chemother 1981; 28:3–8.
2. Oettle AG. Geographical and racial differences in the frequency of Kaposi's sarcoma as evidence of environmental or genetic causes, Acta Un Int Cancer 1962; 18:330.
3. Slavin G, Cameron HM, Singh H. Kaposi's sarcoma in mainland Tanzania. A report of 117 cases. Br J Cancer 1969; 23:349.
4. Taylor JF, Templeton AC, Vogel C, et al. Kaposi's sarcoma in Uganda: a clinico-pathological study. Int J Cancer 1971; 8:122.
5. Bhana D, Templeton AC, Master SP, et al. Kaposi's sarcoma of lymph nodes, Br J Cancer 1970; 24:464.

6. Olweny CLM, Kaddumukasa A, Atine L, et al. Childhood Kaposi's sarcoma: clinical features and therapy. Br J Cancer 1976; 33:555.

7. Bigger RJ, Horn J, Fraumeni JF, Greene MH, Goedert JJ. Incidence of Kaposi's sarcoma and mycosis fungoides in the United States including Puerto Rico. J Natl Cancer Inst 1984; 73:89–94.

8. Reynolds WA, Winkelmann RK, Soule EH. Kaposi's sarcoma: a clinicopathologic study with particular reference to its relationship to the reticuloendothelial system. Medicine 1965; 44:419.

9. Rothman S. Remarks on sex, age and racial distribution of Kaposi's sarcoma and on possible pathogenetic factors. Acta Un Int Cancer 1962; 18:326.

10. Dorffel J. Histogenesis of multiple idiopathic hemorrhagic sarcoma of Kaposi. Arch Derm Syph 1932; 26:608.

11. Cox FH, Helwig EB. Kaposi's sarcoma. Cancer 1959; 12:289.

12. Dutz W, Stout AP. Kaposi's sarcoma in infants and children. Cancer 1960; 13:684.

13. Mitchell N, Feder LA: Kaposi's sarcoma with secondary involvement of the jejunum, perforation and peritonitis. Ann Intern Med 1949; 31:324.

14. Weller GL. The clinical aspects of cardiac involvement (right auricular tumor) in idiopathic hemorrhagic sarcoma (Kaposi's disease). Ann Intern Med 1940; 14:314.

15. Choisser RM, Ramsey EM. Angioreticuloendothelioma (Kaposi's disease) of the heart. Am J Pathol 1939; 15:155.

16. Rwomushana RJW, Bailey LC, Kyalwazi SK. Kaposi's sarcoma of the brain. Cancer 1975; 36:1127.

17. Safai B, Mike V, Giraldo G, et al. Association of Kaposi's sarcoma with secondary primary malignancies. Cancer 1980; 45:1472.

18. Moertel CG, Hagedorn AB. Leukemia or lymphoma and coexistent primary malignant lesions: a review of the literature and a study of 120 cases. Blood 1957; 12:788.

19. Penn I. Kaposi's sarcoma in organ transplant recipients. Transplantation 1979; 278.

20. Gange RW, Jones EW. Kaposi's sarcoma and immunosuppressive therapy: an appraisal. Clin Exp Dermatol 1978; 3:135.

21. Hoshaw RA, Schwartz RA. Kaposi's sarcoma after immunosuppressive therapy with prednisone. Arch Dermatol 1980; 116:1280.

22. McGinn JT, Rieca JJ, Currin F. Kaposi's sarcoma following allergic angiitis. Ann Intern Med 1955; 42:921.

23. Zemek L, Strom L, Gordon G, et al. Hemolytic anemia with Kaposi's sarcoma. JAMA 1964; 187:144.

24. Martensson J, Henrikson H. Immuno-hemolytic anemia in Kaposi's sarcoma with visceral involvement only. Act Med Scand 1954; 150:175.

25. Turnbull A, Almeyda J. Idiopathic thrombocytopenia purpura and Kaposi's sarcoma. Proc R Soc Med 1970; 63:603.

26. Rosenmann E. Kaposi's sarcoma in a patient with pemphigus vulgaris. Isr J Med Sci 1966; 2:269.

27. Tye MJ. Bullous pemphigoid and Kaposi's sarcoma. Arch Dermatol 1970; 101:690.

28. Klein MB, Pereira FA, Kantor I. Kaposi's sarcoma complicating systemic lupus erythematosis treated with immunosuppression. Arch Dermatol 1974; 110:602.

29. Klepp O, Dahl O, Stenwig JT. Association of Kaposi's sarcoma and prior immunosuppressive therapy. Cancer 1978; 42:2626.

30. Myers BD, Kessler E, Levi J, et al. Kaposi's sarcoma in kidney transplant recipients. Arch Intern Med 1974; 133;307.
31. Harwood AR, Osoba D, Hofstader SL. Kaposi's sarcoma in renal transplants. Am J Med 1979; 67:759.
32. Stribling J, Weitzner S, Smith GV. Kaposi's sarcoma in renal allograft recipients. Cancer 1978; 42:442.
33. Nissenkorn I, Servadio C. Kaposi's sarcoma in a patient with a renal transplant. Int Surg 1977; 62:163.
34. Rudolph RI. Kaposi's sarcoma after renal transplantation. Arch Dermatol 1977; 113:1307.
35. Straehley CJ, Santos JI, Downey DM, et al. Kaposi's sarcoma in a renal transplant recipient. Arch Pathol 1975; 99:611.
36. Haim S, Shafrir A, Better OS, et al. Kaposi's sarcoma in association with immunosuppressive therapy. Isr J Med Sci 1972; 8:1933.
37. DeJarlais DC, Marmor M, Thomas P, Chamberland M, Zolla-Pazner S, Spencer DJ. Kaposi's sarcoma among four different AIDS risk groups. N Engl J Med 1984; 310:1119.
38. Boldogh I, Beth E, Huang E-S, Kyalwazi SK, Giraldo G. Kaposi's sarcoma: IV detection of CMV DNA, CMV RNA and CMNA in tumor biopsies. Int J Cancer 1981; 28:469–474.
39. Genolgio CM, McDougall JK. The relationship of cytomegalovirus to Kaposi's sarcoma. In: Friedman-Kein AE, Laubenstein LJ, eds. AIDS. The epidemic of Kaposi's sarcoma and opportunistic infections. New York: Masson Publishing, 1984:329–336.
40. Nelson JA, Fleckenstein B, Galloway DA, McDougall JK. Transformation of NIH 3T3 cells with cloned fragments of human cytomegalovirus strain AD169. J Virol 1982; 43:83–91.
41. Clanton DJ, Jariwalla RJ, Kress C, Rosenthal IJ. Neoplastic transformation by a cloned human cytomegalovirus gene fragment uniquely homologous to one of the transforming regions of herpes simplex virus type 2. Proc Natl Acad Sci USA 1983; 80:3826–3830.
42. Biggar RJ, Melbye M, Kestems I, et al. Kaposi's sarcoma in Zaire is not associated with HTLV-III infection. N Engl J Med 1984; 311:1051.
43. Friedman-Kien AE, Laubenstein LJ, Rubenstein P, et al. Disseminated Kaposi's sarcoma in homosexual men. Ann Intern Med 1982; 96:693.
44. Hymes KB, Greene JB, Marcus A, et al. Kaposi's sarcoma in homosexual men: a report of eight cases. Lancet 1981; ii:598.
45. Ognibene F, Steis R, Macher A, Liotta L, Gelmann E, Pass H, Lane C, Fauci A, Parrillo J, Masur H, Shelhamer J. Kaposi's sarcoma causing pulmonary infiltrates and respiratory failure in the acquired immunodeficiency syndrome. Ann Intern Med 1985; 102:471–475.
46. Krigel RL, Laubenstein LJ, Muggia FM, et al. Kaposi's sarcoma: a new staging classification. Cancer Treat Rep 1983; 67:531–535.
47. Taylor J, Afrasiabi R, Fahey J, et al. A prognostically significant classification of immune changes in AIDS with Kaposi's sarcoma. Blood 1986; 67:666–671.
48. Krown SE, Real FX, Cunningham-Rundles S, et al. Preliminary observations on the

effect of recominant leukocyte A interferon in homosexual men with Kaposi's sarcoma. N Engl J Med 1983; 308:671–676.

49. Groopman JE, Gottlieb MS, Goodman J, et al. Recombinant alpha-2 interferon therapy for Kaposi's sarcoma associated with the acquired immunodeficiency syndrome. Ann Intern Med 1984; 100:671–676.

50. Gelmann EP, Preble OT, Steis R, Lane HC, Rook AH, Wesley M, Jacob J, Fauci A, Masur H, Longo D. Human lymphoblastoid interferon treatment of Kaposi's sarcoma in AIDS: clinical response and prognostic parameters. Am J Med 1985; 78:737–741.

51. Vadhan-Raj S, Wong G, Grecco C, Cunningham-Rundles S, Krim M, Real FX, Oettgen HF, Krown S. Immunologic variables and prediction of prognosis in patients with Kaposi's sarcoma and the acquired immunodeficiency syndrome. Cancer Res 1986; 46:417–428.

52. Nisce LZ, Safai B, Poussin-Rosillo H. Once weekly total and subtotal skin electron beam therapy for Kaposi's sarcoma. Cancer 1981; 47:640.

53. Vogel CL, Templeton CJ, Templeton AC, et al. Treatment of Kaposi's sarcoma with actinomycin-D and cyclophosphamide: results of a randomized clinical trial. Int J Cancer 1971; 8:136.

54. Vogel CL, Primack A, Dhru D, et al. Treatment of Kaposi's sarcoma with a combination of actinomycin D and vincristine. Cancer 1973; 31:1382.

55. Olweny CLM, Toya T, Katongole-Mbidde E, et al. Treatment of Kaposi's sarcoma by a combination of actinomycin-D, vincristine and imidazole carboxamide (NSC-45388): results of a randomized clinical trial. Br J Cancer 1974; 14:649.

56. Kyalwazi SK, Bhana D, Master SP. Actinomycin D in malignant Kaposi's sarcoma. East Afr Med J 1971; 48:16.

57. Scott WP, Voight JA. Kaposi's sarcoma: management with vincaleucoblastine. Cancer 1966; 19:557.

58. Tucker SB, Winkelmann RK. Treatment of Kaposi's sarcoma with vinblastine. Arch Dermatol 1976; 112:958.

59. Solan AJ, Greenwald ES, Silvay O. Long-term complete remissions of Kaposi's sarcoma with vinblastine therapy. Cancer 1981; 47:637.

60. Olweny CLM, Masaba JP, Sikyewunda W, et al. Treatment of Kaposi's sarcoma with ICRF-159 (NSC-129943). Cancer Treat Rep 1976; 60:111.

61. Olweny CLM, Katongole-Mbidde E, Toya T, et al. Phase II studies with adriamycin. In: Adriamycin Review, EROTC International Symposium, part IV. Ghent: European Press, 1975.

62. Vogel CL, Clements D, Wanume AK, et al. Phase II clinical trials of BCNU (NSC 409962) and bleomycin (NSC 125066) in the treatment of Kaposi's sarcoma. Cancer Chemother Rep 1973; 57:325.

63. Laubenstein LJ, Krigel RL, Odajnyk CM, et al. Treatment of epidemic Kaposi's sarcoma with etoposide or a combination of doxorubicin, bleomycin, and vinblastine (ABCV). J Clin Oncol 1984; 2:1115–1118.

64. Volberding PA, Abrams DI, Conant M, et al. Vinblastine therapy for Kaposi's sarcoma in the acquired immunodeficiency syndrome. Ann Intern Med 1985; 103:335–338.

14

AIDS-Related Malignant B-Cell Lymphomas

Alexandra M. Levine
Parkash S. Gill
Suraiya Rasheed
University of Southern California
School of Medicine
Los Angeles, California

Introduction

Approximately 2 years after the first recognition of patients with the classic acquired immunodeficiency syndrome (AIDS), various investigators began to note the development of malignant lymphoma in those same population groups at risk for AIDS. Initial reports by Ziegler et al.,[1] Levine et al.,[2] and others[3] described the occurrence of rather unusual lymphomas in homosexual men, but the precise relationship between these malignancies and AIDS remained largely unknown. A multicenter collaborative study,[4] describing 90 cases of malignant lymphoma in homosexual men from Los Angeles, San Francisco, New York, and Houston, further validated the potential relationship between AIDS and the development of lymphoma, as did a report from the University of Southern California Cancer Surveillance Program, which is a population-based cancer registry for Los Angeles County. The data indicated quite clearly that a statistically significant increase in B-cell immunoblastic sarcoma and small noncleaved lymphoma (either Burkitt or Burkitt-like) had occurred in never-married males in Los Angeles County since 1981. No such increase had occurred in married males, married females, or never-married females.[5] It was likely then, that the spectrum of AIDS did include malignant lymphoma. Problematically, however, it did not seem appropriate to designate any homosexual man with lymphoma as having AIDS, and the precise characteristics of those lymphomas associated with the AIDS epidemic remained to be defined.

Since 1982, we have cared for 44 homosexual men with malignant lymphoma, whose initial diagnosis was made in our institution. From a careful evaluation of the clinical, pathological, immunological, and virological features of disease in these patients, we have been able to elucidate those factors that serve to define the AIDS-related lymphomas.[6] Furthermore, in recognition of the relationship between lymphoma and AIDS, the definition of classic AIDS was revised by the Centers for Disease Control in June 1985 to include high-grade B-cell lymphoma in AIDS-risk group members who have been exposed to human T-lymphotropic virus III (HTLV-III)/lymphadenopathy-associated virus (LAV).[7] The precise nature of AIDS-related lymphomas will be discussed here.

Past Medical History

Approximately one-third of homosexual patients who develop lymphoma have a history of classic AIDS, with opportunistic infection or Kaposi's sarcoma either prior to or simultaneous with the diagnosis of lymphoma. It is important to recognize that an individual who is diagnosed initially with lymphoma is "allowed" or may be expected to develop unusual opportunistic infections or even Kaposi's sarcoma in the course of their underlying lymphomatous disease. Thus, the diagnosis of AIDS in a patient previously diagnosed with lymphoma would not be appropriate based on the guidelines set forth by the CDC.[8] With these factors in mind, it is nonetheless apparent that approximately 30% of homosexual men who develop lymphoma will have had diseases that would be diagnosed as classic AIDS prior to the initial diagnosis of lymphoma. In our series, for example, eight patients had histories of opportunistic infection and/or Kaposi's sarcoma prior to the onset of lymphoma. Two additional patients were diagnosed simultaneously with Kaposi's sarcoma and lymphoma, one had lymphoma and systematic cytomegalovirus infection, one had onset of lymphoma and *Edwardoella tarde* infection, while a fifth patient was diagnosed simultaneously with immunoblastic sarcoma, Kaposi's sarcoma, acute cytomegalovirus infection, and *Pneumocystis carinii* pneumonia.[9] Thus, a total of 13 (30%) had prior or simultaneous evidence of AIDS.

Epidemiological History

The epidemiological factors present in our patients were quite similar to what has previously been described in patients with classic AIDS.[8] Two patients had history of intravenous heroin abuse without homosexuality. The remaining 42 patients were homosexual or bisexual, and all had engaged in anonymous sexual contact. All of these 42 patients had some history of receptive anal intercourse, and the majority had practiced promiscuous sexual activity, with an average of 108 different life-time male sexual partners. All but four admitted to the use of various "recreational" street drugs, including amyl nitrate, cocaine, amphetamines, and marijuana in the majority. Three patients had used intravenous heroin in addition to their homosexual exposure.

Pathological Characteristics of Disease

The pathological spectrum of lymphomatous disease found in these patients was quite interesting and unusual. Thirty-seven patients (84%) had high-grade lymphomas[10] including small noncleaved lymphomas, either Burkitt or Burkitt-like in 23 (52%), and B-cell immunoblastic sarcoma in 14 (32%). Seven patients had low-grade lymphomas, including small-cleaved cell lymphomas in four and plasmacytoid lymphocytic lymphomas in two. One of these presented with a prolymphocytic leukemia of B-cell type. Morphologically, all 44 cases were consistent with B-lymphoid origin. Immunoglobulin phenotype studies were performed in 35 cases,[11] and confirmed the B-cell nature in 33. Twenty-seven cases were monoclonal by surface and/or intracytoplasmic immunoglobulin light chain staining. One additional case marked with IgG, while three other cases stained with the LN-1 antibody. Two cases stained with both kappa and lambda light chains.

Thus, a spectrum of B-cell lymphomatous disease was seen in our patients, ranging from low-grade disorders to B-prolymphocytic leukemia to very high-grade malignancies. Moreover, the distribution of pathological types of disease was quite distinct from what has previously been reported in routine series of lymphomas. For example, in a series of 425 cases of lymphoma reported from our institution in 1978,[11] the incidence of B-IBS was only 3.5%, while small noncleaved (SNC) lymphoma comprised 6.8% of the total group. Likewise, the National Cancer Institute (NCI)-sponsored study of 1175 cases of lymphoma from four institutions[10] revealed small noncleaved lymphoma in 5% of all cases, while immunoblastic lymphoma (which would include both T- and B-cell disease) was found in 7.9%. The small-cleaved cell type was most commonly encountered, diagnosed in 29.4% of the NCI series[10] and in 28% of the series reported by Lukes et al.[11] In contrast, the pathological spectrum of disease seen in our AIDS-related lymphomas was most distinct, with 84% presenting with high-grade lymphomas, and only 15% diagnosed with the more commonly expected low grade disease. This unusual pathological spectrum of disease is a distinguishing feature of the AIDS-related lymphomas.[2,6]

Clinical Manifestations

The mean age of our 44 patients was 39 years (range 20 to 65 years). There were 33 Caucasians, two blacks, and nine Hispanics. Systemic "B" symptoms[12] were quite common, present at diagnosis in 35 cases (80%). Aside from fever, night sweats, and/or significant weight loss, another common symptom at diagnosis was malaise, which was described as profound in 21 cases.

At staging evaluation, extranodal disease was present in 39 patients (89%), including six with localized extranodal disease (central nervous system in five, and anus in one) and 33 with disseminated stage IV involvement. The vast majority of these patients presented with multiple sites of extranodal disease, including involvement of bone marrow in 13, central nervous system in six, rectum in five, heart in four, liver in five, kidney in five, adrenals in two, colon in three, small bowel in five, and stomach, lung, bladder, skin, subcutaneous tissues, bone, and mandible in one patient each.

Only five patients in the series (11%) had disease limited to nodal sites at presentation. This distribution of initial stage in our patients is most unusual when compared with that in previous series of patients with non-Hodgkin's lymphoma. Thus, in a series of 405 patients with newly diagnosed lymphoma,[13] disease limited to lymph nodes alone (stage I, II, or III) was found in 61%, while only six patients (1%) were found to have localized extranodal disease (stage IE) at presentation. In contrast, only 11% of our current patients presented with lymphoma confined to nodal sites. This characteristic of widely disseminated disease at diagnosis will serve as yet another distinctive feature of the AIDS-related lymphomas.[6]

Several aspects of the disseminated nature of these lymphomas warrant further discussion. First, the specific sites of extranodal involvement are quite unique in this patient population. Five current patients presented with stage IV disease including lymphoma in the rectal area.[14] One additional patient presented with localized disease of the anus. In a previous series from our institution,[15] malignant lymphoma of the rectum or anus was described in eight patients whose diagnosis was made over a 10-year period. In the current series, we report six such cases, all diagnosed within the past 2 years. Initial involvement of the heart by lymphoma was also a most unusual finding in our current patients. Lymphomatous disease within the myocardium was documented in four patients, whose initial symptoms included chest pain and cardiac failure closely mimicking the symptoms and signs of acute myocardial infarction. Two-dimensional echocardiography proved to be the most helpful diagnostic tool in these patients, with actual mass lesions demonstrated within the ventricular wall.[16] Kidney involvement was also most impressive in our series, with multiple bilateral lesions defined on computerized axial tomography (CT), and proven to be lymphoma by CT-directed percutaneous renal biopsies. Of note, none of these five patients had actual renal dysfunction at diagnosis. One patient presented with isolated involvement of the mandible in a manner identical to the classic presentation of Burkitt's lymphoma in Africa.[17] Interestingly, the pathological diagnosis in this patient was a B-cell immunoblastic sarcoma.

Central nervous system (CNS) involvement by lymphoma at diagnosis was also quite unusual in our current series. Six patients presented with multiple sites of extranodal disease, including the CNS, while an additional five had isolated disease within the brain. Thus, a total of 11 patients (25%) had CNS involvement at initial diagnosis. In a prior series,[18] initial CNS disease had been reported in 8.6% of patients with diffuse histiocytic lymphoma and in 12% with diffuse undifferentiated lymphoma, which included the categories of immunoblastic sarcoma and small noncleaved lymphoma, respectively. It is important to recognize the varied clinical manifestations of CNS disease in these patients, ranging from the finding of abnormal cells upon lumbar puncture in patients who are entirely asymptomatic to the abrupt onset of seizures or other focal neurological abnormalities.[19] Furthermore, several of these patients first presented with very subtle changes in personality or behavior as the only indication of underlying lymphomatous disease within the brain.

Immunological Studies

The majority of our patients were abnormal immunologically at initial presentation. The mean absolute lymphocyte count in the peripheral blood was 1452/dl (range 84 to 6293/dl). The mean absolute T4-"helper" cells were 355/dl (range 16 to 1927/dl), with a mean absolute T8-"suppressor" cell count of 647/dl (range 32 to 2270/dl). The mean ratio of T4:T8 cells was 0.65 (range 0.03 to 3.5; normal = 0.9 to 2.9). Only 10 patients had a normal T4:T8 ratio, and two of these had low-grade pathological types of disease.

Serum protein electrophophoresis and quantitative immunoglobulins were performed on 26 patients. The mean gamma fraction was 1.64 gm/dl (range 0.9 to 7.4 gm/dl; normal = 0.7 to 1.7gm/dl). The mean quantitative IgG was 1682 mg/dl (range 687 to 7710 mg/dl; normal = 600 to 2000 mg/dl). Mean IgM was 357 mg/dl (range 77 to 1120 mg/dl; normal = 40 to 250 mg/dl). Mean IgA was 303 mg/dl (range 60 to 651 mg/dl; normal = 50 to 400 mg/dl). One patient with prolymphocytic leukemia had a serum monoclonal IgM paraprotein; all other precipitin arcs were normal in configuration.

Analysis for HTLV-III/LAV

Using sera from 36 current patients (all members of populations at risk for AIDS), antibodies directed against HTLV-III/LAV were studied using an enzyme-linked immunosorbent assay.[20] As demonstrated in Table 1, antibodies to HTLV-III were detected in 24 (67%) of our 36 patients. When looking specifically at the 29 patients with high grade types of lymphoma (B-immunoblastic sarcoma or small noncleaved lymphoma), HTLV-III-related antibodies were detected in 22 (76%). In the seven patients with low-grade lymphoma, only two (29%) had antibody against HTLV-III.

Interestingly, six patients who were repeatedly negative for HTLV-III/LAV antibodies were found to be culture-positive for the retrovirus in peripheral blood lymphocytes when cultured in the presence of interleukin-2 and assayed for reverse transcriptase activity using an exogeneous template primer (poly rA, oligo dT) in the presence of magnesium.[21] Four of these patients had high-grade types of lymphoma, while two had low-grade disease.

When looking at all evidence of retrovirus infection, including either antibody or direct viral culture, 30 (83%) of 36 patients had been exposed to the virus, including 26 (90%) of 29 with high-grade lymphomas and four (57%) of seven with low-grade disease.

The serological information regarding HTLV-III/LAV was compared with results obtained from three control groups. Group 1 controls consisted of 40 asymptomatic heterosexuals selected at random from health care professionals who work with AIDS patients or AIDS specimens in the laboratory at the University of Southern California School of Medicine. None of these 40 individuals were found to have antibody against HTLV-III/LAV. Group 2 controls consisted of 11 heterosexual patients (seven women and four men) with no known risk factor for AIDS, who had been diagnosed at our institution since 1980 with the same types of high-grade lymphoma as our homosexual patients (B-cell immunoblastic sarcoma or small noncleaved lymphoma). Serum samples from Group 2 controls were obtained at the time of diagnosis and had been stored at $-20°C$. As shown in Table 1, one of these patients (9%) was positive for HTLV-III antibody (p < 0.001 compared with current patients

TABLE 1 Results of Analysis for HTLV-III/LAV from 36 Patients

	Antibody against HTLV-III/LAV	Positive culture for HTLV-III/LAV	Total: evidence of infection with HTLV-III/LAV
Current patients (n = 36)	24/36 (67%)	6	30/36 (83%)
Current patients with high grade lymphoma (B-IBS or SNC) (n = 29)	22/29 (76%)	4	26/29 (90%)
Current patients with low grade lymphoma (SC;P-L; B-Prolym) (n = 7)	2/7 (29%)	2	4/7 (57%)
Group 1 Control: asymptomatic heterosexual health care workers (n = 40)	0/40 (0%)	ND	(0%)
Group 2 Control: heterosexual patients with B-IBS or SNC, diagnosed in 1980s (n = 11)	1/11 (9%)	ND	(9%)
Group 3 Control: asymptomatic, well homosexual men (n = 31)	17/31 (55%)	ND	(55%)

B-IBS = B-cell immunoblastic sarcoma; SNC = small noncleaved lymphoma; SC = small-cleaved lymphoma; P-L = plasmacytoid lymphocytic lymphoma; B-prolym = B-prolymphocytic leukemia.

having high grade lymphoma). Group 3 controls consisted of 31 asymptomatic homosexual men living in Los Angeles County, who were clinically well, had normal physical examinations, and had no history of any current illness. Seventeen of these men (55%) had antibodies against HTLV-III/LAV, which was, again, significantly different from that in our current patients with high-grade lymphoma.

The potential etiological relationship between HTLV-III/LAV and malignant B-cell lymphomas may also be seen by our ability to isolate retrovirus directly from B-cell lymphoma tissue in nine of the current patients; retrovirus was also demonstrated by electron microscopy in these cases.[22] To determine the specificity of the viral antigens isolated from these cases, we prepared immunoblots of the proteins (Western blots) from the virus-productive cultures. Comparison of the bands obtained using patients' sera with those obtained using HTLV-III or LAV reference sera indicated several differences in the number and intensities of the antigen-antibody reactions, although definite cross-reactivity with HTLV-III and LAV antibodies was present.

Analysis for Epstein-Barr Virus

Serum antibodies against the Epstein-Barr virus (EBV) were tested in 28 patients.[23] All patients tested had sustained prior EBV infections, and the majority had antibody patterns and titers within the range of healthy seropositive individuals. Only six patients showed evidence of possible reactivation, with increases in either EB-viral capsid antigen (VCA), antirestricted portion of the early antigen (anti-R), or both.

By Southern blot analysis, lymphoma tissue from eight patients was studied for presence of EBV genome within tumor cell DNA. Of five high-grade cases, four were positive, containing from five to 50 EBV genome equivalents per cell. Of three low-grade lymphoma cases, all were negtive for EBV genome.

Response to Treatment, Course of Disease and Survival

Two patients in the series were diagnosed with lymphoma only at the time of autopsy, and two patients died within 2 weeks of presentation. Five additional patients with low-grade lymphoma and asymptomatic disease were left initially untreated. Fourteen patients were treated with a variety of multiagent chemotherapeutic regimens on no specific protocol. The remaining 21 patients with high-grade disease were treated prospectively using one of two successive regimens. The first 10 patients (Group I) received the M-BACOD regimen.[24] Complete remission was attained in six (60%). In spite of the use of high-dose methotrexate, relapse within the central nervous system occurred in two of these patients, and median survival for the group was only 11 months. In an attempt to improve these results, a novel regimen was designed,[25] including two cycles of induction with high dose cytosine arabinoside on day 1 (3 g/m^2 given every 12 hours four times) and with vincristine, bleomycin, and prednisone administered on days 8 and 15. Cyclophosphamide (1500 mg/m^2) was given on day 22, while high dose methotrexate (2 g/m^2) was administered on day 36. This was followed by cranial irradiation, intrathecal methotrexate, and subsequent consolidation with etoposide alternating with the CHOP regimen.[26] Eleven patients were treated using this regimen (Group 2), with complete remission attained in only four (36%). In spite of the cranial irradiation, intrathecal methotrexate, and use of high-dose cytosine arabinoside and methotrexate, central nervous system relapse occurred in three of these patients, all of whom subsequently died. The median survival for Group 2 patients was only 5 months. Toxicity was more severe in Group 2, with a higher incidence of systemic infection, a lower nadir granulocyte count, and a lower nadir platelet count.

Eight patients developed opportunistic infections while being treated for lymphoma. These included *Pneumocystis carinii* pneumonia in four, *Mycobacterium avium* and cryptosporidiosis in one, cryptosporidiosis alone in one, pulmonary aspergillosis in one, and *Candida* retinitis in one.

Two patients with low-grade disease were treated with suramin, a potent competitive inhibitor of reverse transcriptase which is necessary for retroviral replication.[27,28] One patient experienced disease progression as well as *Candida* retinitis while on the drug.. The second patient with stage IV small-cleaved lymphoma (involving bone marrow and lymph nodes) as well as biopsy-proven Kaposi's sarcoma attained a pathologically documented complete remission of the lymphoma and Kaposi's sarcoma after 6 weeks of Suramin therapy. This patient remains in complete remission on weekly Suramin 8 months from initial onset of treatment.[29]

The median survival of 42 patients in this series is 6 months; the two patients whose lymphoma was discovered at autopsy were eliminated from this survival analysis. At the current time, 27 (61%) of 44 patients have died, with no stable plateau phase evident in the remaining patients. Twenty of the 27 patients have died because of lymphoma, with extensive multisystem disease documented in those who were taken to autopsy.

Potential Pathogenesis

The potential etiological relationship between HTLV-III/LAV and B-cell lymphoma is not yet understood. Because we have isolated these retroviruses directly from monoclonal B-cell tumors, it is evident that this virus is capable of propagation in B lymphocytes.[22] We have also shown that all of our current patients have had prior infection with Epstein-Barr virus, and similar to endemic Burkitt's lymphoma, EBV genome has been demonstrated in four of five current high grade lymphoma cases. The adaptation of LAV to grow in EBV-transformed B lymphocytes has been documented in vitro.[30] It is possible that prior infection with EBV may predispose these infected B cells to HTLV-III/LAV infection. Since the unique life cycle of retroviruses depends on the replication of integrated provirus with the cellular DNA, the presence of hyperplastic and hyperactive B cells may offer a proliferative advantage,[31] as well as a suitable cellular milieu for the transcription and translation of proviral DNA in these individuals.

The potential etiological relationship between HTLV-III/LAV and malignant lymphoma in our patients is further strengthened by the recent evidence that simian AIDS (SAIDS) is caused by a retrovirus that is related, although distinct, from HTLV-III/LAV.[32] If injected into normal monkeys, this virus may cause malignant lymphoma of the same high-grade pathological types as described in our current series of patients.[33]

Summary

The malignant lymphomas associated with the current outbreak of AIDS are quite unique, pathologically and clinically. They may be best defined as high-grade B-cell lymphomas that present in disseminated fashion in unusual extranodal sites such as the central nervous system or rectum. They are associated with a reversal in the T4:T8 ratio in the peripheral blood, as well as exposure to HTLV-III/LAV and distant exposure to Epstein-Barr virus. Results of treatment using standard intensive multiagent chemotherapy have been disappointing, with median survival of less than 1 year in treated patients. Central nervous system relapse may occur in spite of attempts at prophylactic therapy to this sanctuary site. The precise mechanism of development of lymphoma in these patients remains to be defined.

Acknowledgments

This work was supported in part by Public Health Service Grant CA 36301-01A1, and Contract NO1-A1-62509, awarded by the National Cancer Institute, National Institutes of Health. The authors gratefully acknowledge the help of Werner Henle, M.D., Division of Virology; Joseph Stokes, Jr., Research Institute of Philadelphia in performing serological work related to Epstein-Barr virus; and George Klein, M.D., Karolinska Institute, Stockholm, Sweden for Southern blot analysis of Epstein-Barr virus in lymphoma tissue. Rebecca Skibinski provided secretarial assistance, while Azita Shoshani and Lily Chang provided technical assistance.

References

1. Ziegler JL, Drew WL, Miner RC, et al. Outbreak of Burkitt-like lymphoma in homosexual men. Lancet 1982; i:631–633.
2. Levine AM, Meyer PR, Begandy MK, et al. Development of B-cell lymphoma in homosexual men: clinical and immunologic findings. Ann Intern Med 1984; 100:7–13.

3. Snider WD, Simpson DM, Aronyk KE, Nielsen SL. Primary lymphoma of the nervous system associated with acquired immunodeficiency syndrome. N Engl J Med 1983; 308:45. Letter.

4. Ziegler JL, Beckstead JA, Volberding PA, et al. Non-Hodgkin's lymphoma in 90 homosexual men: relationship to generalized lymphadenopathy and acquired immunodeficiency syndrome (AIDS). N Engl J Med 1984; 311:565–570.

5. Ross RK, Dworsky RL, Paganini-Hill A, Levine AM, Mack T. Non-Hodgkin's lymphomas in never married men in Los Angeles. Br J Cancer 1985; 52:785–797.

6. Levine AM, Gill PS, Meyer PR, et al. Retrovirus and malignant lymphoma in homosexual men. JAMA 1985; 254:1921–1925.

7. Revision of the case definition of acquired immunodeficiency syndrome for national reporting—United States. MMWR 1985; 34:25.

8. Follow-up on Kaposi's sarcoma and Pneumocystis pneumonia. MMWR 1981; 30:409–410.

9. Burkes RL, Gal AA, Stewart ML, Gill PS, Abo W, Levine AM. Simultaneous occurrence of Pneumocystis carinii pneumonia, cytomegalovirus infection, Kaposi's sarcoma and B-immunoblastic sarcoma in homosexual men. JAMA 1985; 253:3425–3427.

10. Non-Hodgkin's lymphoma pathologic classification project: National Cancer Institute sponsored study of classifications of non-Hodgkin's lymphomas: summary and description of a working formulation for clinical usage. Cancer 1982; 49:2112–2235.

11. Lukes RJ, Parker JW, Taylor CR, Tindle BH, Cramer AD, Lincoln TL. Immunologic approach to non-Hodgkin's lymphomas and related leukemias. Analysis of the results of multiparameter studies of 425 cases. Semin Hematol 1978; 15:322–351.

12. Carbone PP, Kaplan HS, Musshoff K, et al. Report of the Committee on Hodgkin's Disease Staging Classification. Cancer Res 1971; 31:1860–1861.

13. Jones SE, Fuks Z, Bull M, et al. Non-Hodgkin's lymphomas IV. Clinicopathologic correlation in 405 cases. Cancer 1973; 31:806–823.

14. Burkes RL, Meyer PR, Gill PS, et al. Rectal lymphoma in homosexual men. Arch Intern Med 1986; 146:913–915.

15. Vanden Heule B, Taylor CR, Terry R, Lukes RJ. Presentation of malignant lymphoma in the rectum. Cancer 1982; 49:2602–2607.

16. Gill PS, Chandraratna P, Meyer PR, Levine AM. Malignant lymphoma: cardiac involvement at initial presentation. (submitted).

17. Burkitt D. A sarcoma involving the jaws in African children. Br J Surg 1958; 46:218–223.

18. MacKintosh FR, Colby TV, Podolsky WJ, et al. Central nervous system involvement in non-Hodgkin's lymphoma: an analysis of 105 cases. Cancer 1982; 49:586–595.

19. Gill PS, Levine AM, Meyer PR, et al. Primary central nervous system lymphoma in homosexual men: clinical, immunologic, and pathologic features. Am J Med 1985; 78:742–748.

20. Sarngodharan MG, Popovic M, Bruch J, Schüpbach J, Gallo RC. Antibodies reactive with human T-lymphotropic retroviruses (HTLV-III) in the serum of patients with AIDS. Science 1984; 224:506–508.

21. Rasheed S, Norman GL, Gill PS, Meyer PR, Cheng L, Levine AM. Virus neutralizing activity, serologic heterogeneity and retrovirus isolation from homosexual men in the Los Angeles area. Virology 1986; 150:1–9.
22. Rasheed S, Norman GL, Gill PS, Meyer PR, Payne BC, Levine AM. Isolation of retrovirus from malignant B-cell lymphoma in homosexual men. (submitted).
23. Henle W, Henle G, Horwitz CA. Epstein-Barr virus specific diagnostic tests in infectious mononucleosis. Human Pathol 1974; 5:551–565.
24. Skarin AT, Canellos GP, Rosenthal DS, et al. Improved prognosis of diffuse histiocytic and undifferentiated lymphoma by use of high dose methotrexate alternating with standard agents (M-BACOD). J Clin Oncol 1983; 1:91–98.
25. Gill PS, Levine AM, Holdorf D, Pinter-Brown L, Krailo M, Rasheed S. High grade AIDS-related lymphomas. Results of prospective multiagent chemotherapy trials. Proc ASCO 1986; 5:5.
26. McKelvey EM, Gottlieb JA, Wilson HE, et al. Hydroxyldaunomycin (adriamycin) combination chemotherapy in malignant lymphoma. Cancer 1976; 38:1484–1493.
27. deClercq E. Suramin: a potent inhibitor of the reverse transcriptase of RNA tumor viruses. Cancer Lett 1979; 8:9–22.
28. Baltimore D. Viral RNA-dependent DNA polymerase. Nature (Lond) 1970; 226:1209–1211.
29. Levine AM, Gill PS, Hawkins J, Formenti S, Aguilar S, Rasheed S. Suramin antiviral therapy in acquired immunodeficiency syndrome (AIDS) and AIDS-related lymphoma: preliminary results. Blood 1985; 66:114a. (Abstract).
30. Montagnier L, Gruest J, Chamaret S, et al. Adaptation of lymphadenopathy associated virus (LAV) to replication in EBV-transformed B lymphoblastoid cell lines. Science 1984; 225:63–66.
31. Carter RL. Infectious mononucleosis: model for self-limiting lymphoproliferation. Lancet 1975; i:846–849.
32. Levitin NL, King NW, Daniel MD, Aldrich WR, Blake BJ, Hunt RD. Experimental transmission of macaque AIDS by means of inoculation of macaque lymphoma tissue. Lancet 1983; ii:599–602.
33. Hunt RD, Blake BJ, Chalifoux LV, Schgal PK, King NW, Letvin NL. Transmission of naturally occurring lymphoma in macaque monkeys. Proc Natl Acad Sci USA 1983; 80:5085–5089.

An Overview of Pediatric AIDS: Approaches to Diagnosis and Outcome Assessment

Wade P. Parks
Gwendolyn B. Scott
University of Miami
School of Medicine
Miami, Florida

Introduction

Complaints of repeated infections, growth failure, diarrhea, and oral candiasis in infants are well known to pediatricians. Even children with documented immunodeficiencies who are seen in tertiary care centers present an extraordinarily long list of differential diagnoses to the subspecialist.[1] Thus, the initial sporadic appearances of infants with these complaints in 1980–1981 were, and continue to be, major diagnostic problems to clinicians. At most centers, cases of pediatric AIDS were initially diagnosed as viral-related immunodeficiency states, usually in association with cytomegalovirus or Epstein-Barr virus. The concurrence of adult cases of AIDS in San Francisco, New York City, and Miami[2-6] and an increasing number of pediatric cases served to clarify the clinical diagnositic situation. As more cases were seen, the recognition of an acquired immunodeficiency syndrome in infants was proposed from four centers.[7-10] Subsequent studies[11] have shown that the majority of cases in the pediatric age range are the result of the perinatal acquisition of HTLV-III/LAV virus from persistently infected mothers. Initial efforts at centers with the majority of cases were to prepare definitions of the clinical disease that would allow more accurate diagnosis and reporting of cases. The early definitions were tailored to fit the adult definitions of AIDS proposed for CDC surveillance purposes. Thus, early definitions emphasized *Pneumocystis carinii* pneumonia (PCP) and Kaposi's sarcoma (KS).[12]

This approach, however, has not proven particularly useful for describing children with either disease or infection, and alternative approaches to diagnosis have been necessary. One approach that has been seriously considered is the use of AIDS-related complex (ARC) for children, analogous to the way it has been employed for adults. This has served to identify children with serious clinical disease who do not meet CDC surveillance definitions for AIDS. However, the types of conditions and clinical problems seen in children are significantly different than those noted in adults. This difference has made the AIDS/ARC separation in children even less clear than it is in adults. Thus, there is still a pressing need for alternative approaches. We have elected to revise again our approach and to define cases as "HTLV-III/LAV infections" associated with seven distinctive clinical syndromes. Classification of HTLV-III/LAV infections into clinical syndromes has allowed a more detailed analysis of the epidemiology and natural history of the various syndromes, and has provided for a more accurate basis of the recognition of sporadic pediatric cases.

This chapter will discuss the issues of clinical and laboratory definitions of pediatric AIDS and, in particular, consider the various syndrome definitions that are currently employed at our center. The epidemiology and natural history of the syndromes will be explored, and particular attention will be paid to a recently described syndrome, lymphocytic interstitial pneumonitis (LIP). This syndrome is analogous to an infection of sheep caused by a lentivirus called progressive pneumonia, or maedi. The virology of pediatric AIDS will be presented, and the utility of children for the study of AIDS virus in this setting will be noted. Finally, future prospects for prevention, chemotherapy, and immunoprophylaxsis of this particularly striking example of an human retrovirus infection will be analyzed.

Clinical Presentation and Diagnosis

The diagnosis of AIDS in an infant requires a high index of suspicion by the clinician to order appropriate laboratory tests and to conduct epidemiological investigations that support the diagnosis of an HTLV-III/LAV infection. This is especially true in isolated or sporadic cases. The problem of diagnosis is particularly compounded when an infant does not have a definitive opportunistic infection or Kaposi's sarcoma that would enable a more conventional diagnosis. As shown in Table 1, the types of clinical findings noted in series of pediatric AIDS patients are extremely common in general pediatrics. What distinguishes the problems listed in Table 1 from those noted in general pediatric populations is their persistence and severity. The definitions of these findings as they apply to pediatric AIDS are presented in a subsequent section, but complaints such as failure to thrive, oral candidiasis, and diarrhea are not unusual in general pediatrics.

In contrast to the generality of many signs in pediatric AIDS, the importance of severe bacterial infection as a presenting sign in infants with HTLV-III/LAV infections has not been adequately appreciated. Bacterial infections with encapsulated pyogenic pathogens such as *Streptococcus pneumoniae* and *Hemophilus influenzae* are particularly common. Bacterial infections not only include septicemia, pneumonia, and chronic otitis media, but also have been frequent causes of meningitis. Further, recurrences of severe bacterial diseases in given patients have been noted. The most common findings in pediatric AIDS are recurrent infections and the presumed secondary failure to thrive.

Given the lack of specificity in clinical findings in a given infant, it is often months before laboratory tests are undertaken that may lead to the diagnosis

TABLE 1 Clinical Findings in 85 Consecutive Infants with HTLV-III/LAV Infection

Clinical finding	%
Failure to thrive	65
Persistent *Candida* infection	70
Generalized lymphadenopathy	74
Diarrhea	
Recurrent	31
Protracted	33
Recurrent bacterial infections:	
Bacteremia	29
Pneumococcus	14
H. influenzae	59
Pneumonia	48
Chronic otitis media	14
Parotitis	

of AIDS. Laboratory findings in infants and children with HTLV-III/LAV infection are shown in Table 2. The most common impressive finding has been that of a polyclonal hypergammaglobulinemia, which presumably results from either increased stimulation of B cells and/or decreased suppression by T-lymphocytes. This finding is usually restricted to the IgG subset, but has also been seen in IgA and IgM, and occasionally patients have hypogammaglobu-linemia as well. Children have higher absolute levels of T-lymphocytes than do adults. Consequently, the criteria for lymphopenia in adults (lymphocyte counts $<500/mm^3$) are rarely observed in children, except in terminal situations. However, because children's normal levels are in the range of $4000/mm^3$, an absolute lymphocyte count below $2000/mm^3$ in a child suggests a relative T-cell lymphopenia. Lymphopenia is often very difficult to interpret without quantification of lymphocyte subsets. When special testing is done, T4$^+$ cells are seen to be selectively depleted relative to T8$^+$ cells. This results in an inverted T-lymphocyte subset ratio. The widely appreciated increased suppressor levels associated with *Herpesvirus* infections also result in inverted ratios.[13,14] In pediatric AIDS, there is a decrease in T4$^+$ cells, which results in low or inverted T4/T8 ratios (<1.0). However, this is not of itself an adequate criteria for diagnosis, but in combination with a polyclonal increase in IgG levels, an inverted T-lymphocyte ratio provides laboratory confirmation of a tentative or presumptive diagnosis of acquired immunodeficiency in a given infant.

More detailed investigations such as lymphocyte responsiveness and spe-

TABLE 2 Laboratory Findings in Infants and Children with HTLV-III/LAV Infections

Hypergammaglobulinemia/hypogammaglobulinemia
Depressed T-helper cells
Reversed lymphocyte subset ratio
Depressed lymphocyte responses to mitogen
Decreased specific antibody responses

Anemia[a]
Leukopenia
Thrombocytopenia
Elevated level of circulating immune complexes
Elevated serum transaminase levels

[a]Items listed in the second group are less specific but commonly observed.

cific antibody responses reveal abnormalities in patients with full-blown AIDS that would not be unexpected in light of the profound effects of the virus on the immune system. Important exclusionary criteria include congenital immunodeficiencies. Thus, pediatric AIDS patients should have *normal* levels of erythrocyte adenosine deaminase and purine nucleoside phosphorylase. Issues of laboratory testing for viral antibodies and viral isolation will be discussed separately.

The combination of selected clinical findings and the described patterns of laboratory results provides the clinician with a presumptive diagnosis of an acquired immunodeficiency disease syndrome in infants. However, the clinical diagnosis of AIDS has proven significantly more difficult in infants than in adults, and this has become a particular problem in attempts to align the criteria for the diagnosis of AIDS in children with the criteria for adults.[15] The types of infectious disease problems faced by children are quite different than those of adults, and consequently the patterns of disease are often different in children than in adults. In a proportion of cases, the same types of infections have been seen in infants that have been noted in adults.[15] The types of opportunistic infections and number of Kaposi's tumors seen in children are shown in Table 3. *Pneumocystis carinii* pneumonia has been noted in 32% of pediatric cases. *Candida* esophagitis is also common, as are disseminated cytomegalovirus (CMV) infections. It should be noted that disseminated CMV infections occurring within the first 6 months of life disqualify a patient for the surveillance definition of pediatric AIDS according to CDC criteria.[12] This presents a special problem in the case of infants with documented HTLV-III/LAV infection and perinatal cytomegalovirus infection. Since perinatally

TABLE 3 Relative Incidence of Opportunistic Infections/Kaposi's Sarcoma in Pediatric AIDS Cases

Infection/Tumor	No.[a]	%
Pneumocystis carinii pneumonia	12	32
Candida esophagitis	8	22
Disseminated cytomegalovirus infection	9	24
Invasive herpes simplex infection	1	1
Cryptosporidiosis	2	3
Kaposi's sarcoma (disseminated)	7	19

[a]Nine patients had more than one opportunistic infection/Kaposi's sarcoma.

acquired HTLV-III and CMV are often concurrent infections in our series, one of the major clinical manifestations of HTLV-III/LAV infection is often CMV-associated disease. The issues of diagnosing Kaposi's sarcoma in children will be discussed in a later section, but cases of disseminated lymphadenopathic Kaposi's, such as we have described,[16] are not diagnosed until autopsy and are of little use in antemortem clinical diagnosis. The location of Kaposi's lesions in the lymph nodes of infants and children also contrasts with the dermatological manifestation of KS in adult patients. In summary, the types of infections that qualify a patient for the CDC surveillance definition of AIDS are noted in children, but other pathological processes that have been divided into specific syndromes are far more common.

The syndrome approach to pediatric HTLV-III/LAV infections appears to describe clinical observations more accurately than attempts to fit observations from children into definitions for adult patients. Table 4 indicates the relative incidence of the major syndromes other than the opportunistic infections in our series of pediatric patients with HTLV-III/LAV infections. The syndrome that will be considered most extensively in this review is the lymphoid interstitial pneumonitis, which has been diagnosed in 41% of all patients and is perhaps a variant of the less common, in children, lymphadenopathic syndrome. Together, these syndromes account for almost half of the observed cases. Syndromes of hepatitis, cardiomyopathy, protein calorie malnutrition

TABLE 4 Relative Incidence of Syndromes Other than Opportunistic Infection/Kaposi's Sarcoma in Pediatric Patients[a]

Syndrome	%
Lymphoid interstitial pneumonitis	41
Encephalopathy	7
Protein calorie malnutrition	8
Hepatitis	10
Lymphadenopathic syndrome	7
Cardiomyopathy	—
Encephalopathy	—

[a]Some children at different times will have more than a single syndrome. The relationship of syndromes with each other is still under evaluation.

(analogous to the thin-man syndrome in adults), and encephalopathy have been noted. These latter syndromes are significantly less common than lymphoid interstitial pneumonitis. Collectively, diagnoses of opportunistic infections and lymphoid interstitial pneumonitis encompass the majority of pediatric AIDS cases. However, because of the exclusion of CMV, less than 50% of observed cases of HTLV-III/LAV infection with severe clinical manifestations qualify for the CDC surveillance definition of AIDS. Adding the lymphocytic interstitial pneumonitis (LIP) to the criteria for pediatric AIDS will increase the number of cases accepted by the CDC. However, as will be noted, infants with LIP have a significantly different natural history than that noted in infants with opportunistic infections.

There is a broad spectrum of disease associated with HTLV-III/LAV in pediatric patients. On one end of the spectrum are children with severe opportunistic infections and a high mortality rate. On the other end of the spectrum are children who are asymptomatic or merely have mild to moderate pulmonary infiltrates associated with the lymphocytic interstitial pneumonitis syndrome. This range of manifestations of HTLV-III/LAV infection in children further complicates the diagnosis by a pediatric specialist or infectious disease subspecialist confronted with an isolated case of AIDS, and probably is a major factor in the apparent under-reporting of pediatric AIDS cases nationwide.

Epidemiology and Natural History

The incidence of AIDS cases diagnosed in children under 13 years of age nationally is less than 2% of the total number of AIDS cases diagnosed.[17] The distribution of these cases according to the likely source of infection reveals that 76% of the cases occur in infants born to HTLV-III/LAV-infected mothers. It is likely that mothers who are infected with HTLV-III/LAV transmit the virus to their infants at some point near parturition. There is one report of postnatal transmission through breast milk.[18] The other major mode of transmission that results in HTLV-III/LAV infection in pediatric patients is through transfusions; thus hemophiliacs and children with other coagulation disorders or children receiving multiple transfusions, including those who are undergoing surgery, premature infants, or those that require blood or blood products for other reasons, are at increased risk. Presumably the ELISA screening test for HTLV-III/LAV has significantly decreased the likelihood of acquiring AIDS by this route. Thus, the perinatal route is currently the major mode of viral transmission.

The incidence of pediatric AIDS cases nationally is difficult to assess because the majority of cases are reported out of very few selected geographic centers, namely New York, Newark, and Miami.[19] This is an unusual situation that is still not adequately explained, and may simply reflect the experience of these centers in the diagnosis of AIDS. It remains surprising that roughly 20 to 25% of the entire national series has been reported by a single hospital in Miami. This raises a question concerning the existence of cases in other hospitals that may be undetected at the present time. On the other hand, reported cases of pediatric AIDS are occurring in the same geographic centers where cases of adult AIDS are at the highest incidence. For example, New York, Miami, and Newark have the highest number of pediatric AIDS cases and also are three of the top four cities nationally in terms of the AIDS incidence per million cases. On a year-by-year basis, an increase in pediatric AIDS cases has been noted each year, with an approximate 50% increase in incidence each year from 1980 to 1986 in our series. Current estimates are that over 30 infants with HTLV-III/LAV infection will be diagnosed in the current year in Miami. With the increased use of serological assays, it is possible that even more children will be diagnosed who have only minor clinical symptoms associated with the virus. If so, these infants will likely remain persistently infected and can be considered as potential reservoirs of the virus.

The natural history of pediatric AIDS has been approached in several ways. Our investigations have utilized a longitudinal evaluation wherein all affected infants and comparison patients and their respective households are examined every 3 months in a special immunology clinic and are also seen at other times if clinical needs dictate. This study design provides the basis for detailed studies of clinical disease and laboratory parameters. As shown in Table 5, the proportion of "AIDS" in a series of 85 HTLV-III/LAV-positive patients exceeds 50% of cases, although only a proportion of children may meet the CDC surveillance definition of AIDS. There are only 3 children who have no significant evidence of clinical disease who are HTLV-III/LAV-infected. These data, however, are biased by virtue of the fact that all pediatric AIDS cases and households discovered to date are those that have presented with clinical

TABLE 5   Clinical Classification and Outcome of 85 Diagnosed Pediatric HTLV-III/LAV Infections

Diagnostic category	No.	%	Mortality %
AIDS	44	52	62
Non-AIDS	37	44	6
Asymptomatic	3	4	0

disease. There may be children and households with viruses of lower virulence where HTLV-III/LAV infection is common, but disease is uncommon.

In our experience (Table 5), the mortality of infants with a diagnosis of AIDS is 62%; the mortality rate in the non-AIDS cases is only 15%. Nevertheless, there is significant clinical disease in the non-AIDS patients, and multiple hospitalizations are common for such patients. Hospitalizations are necessary for clinical manifestations discussed previously. Thus, mortality shows a rough correlation with the diagnostic criteria that are used, and/or the opportunistic infections favored in the diagnosis of AIDS are associated with a higher mortality. A peak in mortality occurs in the first 7 months of life, and then a second peak is noted between 2 and 3 years of age. Infants who have survived beyond 3 years of age generally have an improved prognosis, especially if they have grown. Long-term neurological and developmental outcomes are not yet available, in part because the number of patients is still very small. However, several relatively asymptomatic infants who are over 4 years of age with documented perinatal infection have been now followed longitudinally for several years and are doing well.

Mothers of infants with perinatally acquired HTLV-III/LAV infection are themselves persistently infected and at high risk to develop disease.[11] Mothers are usually members of documented risk groups. Ten percent of mothers in our series were sexual partners of either intravenous (IV) drug abusers or bisexual men. In Miami, approximately 75% of the total number of cases has been observed in mothers who were born in Haiti and have recently come to the United States. More recently, the proportion of mothers who are IV drug abusers or sexual partners of IV drug abusers has grown dramatically.

The risk of perinatal infection from infected women to infants is still somewhat controversial. The data from our center include a study of 20 infants born to infected mothers who had already delivered one infant with AIDS; 13 (or 65%) of the subsequent offspring had clinical evidence of HTLV-III/LAV infection within several months after birth. These represent a biased population in that the women were selected on the basis of already having transmitted the virus perinatally. It is not known what the incidence of infected offspring will be in a study of all HTLV-III/LAV-infected pregnant women. These studies are underway and would suggest that the risk of transmission in all HTLV-III/LAV-infected women may be lower (M. Rogers, personal communication).

The natural history of pediatric AIDS is apparently dependent on the initial clinical presentation. For example, the mortality rate in children with opportunistic infections or Kaposi's sarcoma is very high, as previously mentioned. However, in children with lymphoid interstitial pneumonitis (LIP), the mortality rate is less than 15%. This may reflect a significantly different virus host outcome than is the case in HTLV-III/LAV-infected infants with opportunistic infections. The reasons for these differences are unclear. The natural history of less common syndromes, such as the encephalopathy,[20] protein calorie malnutrition,[21] and hepatitis,[22] include too few cases to make definitive assessments at the present time. It is likely that each syndrome will have a distinctive natural history, and require a larger data base than currently exists.

A syndrome of persistent pulmonary infiltrates or lymphoid interstitial pneumonitis syndrome was reported in the initial series,[9] and was not associated with *Pneumocystis* or cytomegalovirus. A definition is provided in Table 6. The major differential after lung biopsy is distinguishing lymphoid interstitial pneumonitis (LIP) from a desquamitave interstitial pneumonitis.[23] The more common condition is that of LIP, which is characterized by diffuse and local lymphoid hyperplasia in the interstitial spaces. Occasional plasma cells may also be noted. These collections of cells are more common in areas of mild consolidation, and were present uniformly in infants who had significant clinical disease requiring lung biopsy. Infants with LIP present at a later age than those infants with opportunistic infections. The mean age of onset of opportunistic infections was approximately 6 months of age. In contrast, the mean onset of LIP was 14 months. Another major distinguishing characteristic of LIP patients was marked lymphadenopathy; all had hepatosplenomegaly and generalized lymphadenopathy (defined as lymph nodes greater than 2 cm in diameter in two noncontiguous areas). Many infants with LIP develop signs and symptoms of chronic lung disease. Clubbing of the digits has been seen in approximately 25% of affected infants. Six patients have become persistently hypoxemic with a PaO_2 of less than 60 mm Hg. Four have become oxygen-dependent and have required home oxygen therapy. The patients with LIP have elevated IgG levels, ranging from 2400 to 11,000 mg%, with no observed relationship between the level of IgG and the severity of LIP. Although in

TABLE 6   Definitions of Clinical Features of Pulmonary Syndromes Associated with Pediatric AIDS

Interstitial pneumonitis syndrome
Persistent bilateral reticulonodular interstitial infiltrates with or without hilar lymphadenopathy present on chest X-ray for a period of at least 2 months, with no pathogen identified and unresponsive to antibiotic treatment

or

Biopsy-proven lymphoid interstitial pneumonia
Pathogens such as cytomegalovirus, pneumocystis, tuberculosis, etc. may be associated with this pathological entity and are not exclusionary

---

certain instances there is a severe pulmonary sequelae, the mortality is relatively low as compared with that in the opportunistic infection syndrome.

At present, it is unclear why some children develop LIP. It is our impression that LIP may be a reflection of a host immune response. Of particular interest is the relationship between the histopathology and the lesions described in another lentivirus infection of sheep, known as maedi[24] or progressive pneumonia virus.[25] Lentivirus diseases present a model for human lentiviral disease.[26] Together with visna, the neurological and pulmonary manifestations of this family of viruses show surprising similarity. Given the characteristic histopathology and the radiographic appearance of the lung fields in these infants, the diagnosis of LIP in its characteristic form is not difficult, especially in association with an elevated IgG. LIP should call attention to the possible diagnosis of perinatal HTLV-III/LAV infection.

A list of the other clinical definitions is contained in Table 7. The use of these definitions has facilitated classification, and is the basis of ongoing natural history studies of the different syndromes associated with HTLV-III/LAV infection. Two particularly intersting conditions that have not been reported from other centers are the protein calorie malnutrition syndrome and the cardiomyopathy syndrome. These conditions are striking when seen, and pediatricians who may see cases of perinatal HTLV-III infection should be alerted to their existence.

There is an issue concerning the diagnosis of Kaposi's sarcoma in pediatric AIDS. Lesions similar to those noted in pediatric AIDS patients in our series[16] have been reported from Africa[27] in children as diffuse lymphadenopathic KS. However, the degree of proliferation of the endothelial tissue and the invasive criteria for these lesions used by adult pathologists suggest that "Kaposi-like" or Kaposi's-associated lesions is a more appropriate diagnostic term for the lymphadenopathic disease that we have noted. In many patients, lesions can be found only by careful examination of multiple lymph node sections. In patients with extensive lesions and who otherwise have no obvious clinical explanation for poor progress, it is our experience that the lesions are associated with a high mortality in infants. This may reflect the fact that these lesions are usually found only postmortem, although they have also been noted in lymph node biopsies.

Virology

HTLV-III/LAV infection of infants generally derives from maternal infection.[11] Until recently, documentation of the source of the virus had not been possible. By isolation of both maternal and infant viruses, it has now been shown by restriction mapping of the viral isolates that the viruses from the mother and

TABLE 7 Definitions of Clinical Features in Syndromes Associated with Pediatric AIDS

I. **Wasting syndrome**
   A. Failure to thrive: failure to maintain growth at an expected rate predicted by standard growth curves
   B. Diarrhea: (a) Recurrent diarrhea—two or more episodes of diarrhea within a 2 month period, with dehydration requiring hospitalization. Specific pathogens are not usually identified, but the presence of bacterial pathogens is not exclusionary. (b) Protracted diarrhea—daily loose, watery, frequent stools occurring over a 2-week period, with associated weight loss requiring hospitalization and parenteral nutrition. The presence of pathogens, such as *Salmonella* and *Giardia* are exclusionary.
   C. Protein calorie malnutrition: deficit in weight for height. Abnormal anthropometric measurements of mid-arm circumference. Laboratory criteria for diagnosis include low serum albumin (<3.0) with elevated serum cholesterol, and anemia (Hgb <10 gm%). Clinical findings include lethargy, irritability, edema, and hepatomegaly. Hair is frequently coarse and sparse, and dermatitis may be present.

II. **Infection syndrome**: unusually severe infections occurring in an infant without otherwise predisposing factors.
   A. Recurrent pneumonia: two or more episodes of acute pneumonia, documented by consolidation on chest X-rays, usually in different lobes over a 4-month period that responds to antimicrobial therapy with resolution of clinical symptoms and clearing of the chest X-ray.
   B. Recurrent bacterial sepsis: more than one episode of bacterial organisms, particularly *S. pneumoniae* and *H. influenzae,* documented within a 1-year period.
   C. Chronic draining otitis media: otitis media with perforation and repeated acute infections and drainage of purulent fluid at least twice during a 6-month period.
   D. Recurrent herpes stomatitis: typical clinical picture of vesicular lesions on tongue, lips and gingiva, with positive cultures for herpes simplex occurring more than once over a 1-year period.
   E. Persistent infection of the oral mucosa with *Candida* sp.: extensive involvement of the buccal mucosa, tongue, and pharynx with *Candida* infection persisting for greater than 1 month in a child who is not receiving antibiotics. The *Candida* infection is unresponsive to the conventional therapies (i.e. mycostatin or Gentian violet).
   F. Other: Varicella zoster, recurrent.
      Molluscum contagiosum, recurrent.
      Condylomata, recurrent.

TABLE 7 *Continued*

III. **Lymphadenopathy syndrome**
   A. Generalized lymphadenopathy: nontender lymph nodes greater than 1 cm found in two or more *noncontiguous* sites, present for greater than 2 months with no obvious pathogen identified as etiology (i.e., tuberculosis, routine bacterial etiologies). Patients with elevated CMV, *Toxoplasma,* and EBV titers are not excluded since these infections may be associated with HTLV-III/LAV infection.
   B. Hepatomegaly: persistent physical finding of liver span increased for age, with or without liver enzyme abnormalities. Screen for common causes of viral heptatitis A or B are negative.
   C. Splenomegaly: persistent physical finding of a palpable spleen for greater than 2 months, without evidence of hemolysis or sequestration.
   D. Parotitis: nontender enlarged parotid gland present for greater than 1 month, with elevated serum amylase. Acute bacterial infection or obstruction must be ruled out.

IV. **Cardiomyopathy:** persistent cardiac enlargement with findings below in absence of concurrent evidence of enteroviral etiology of infection.
   A. Clinical findings of heart failure: tachypnea, rales (in absence of definite pulmonary process), gallop, murmur (usually of mitral insufficiency), hepatomegaly.
   B. Laboratory findings: (a) chest X-ray—cardiomegaly (>55% cardiothoracic ratio), with or without pulmonary edema. (b) Echocardiogram—LV >2 SD above age and matched normals. Shortening fraction and/or velocity of circumferential shortening >2 SD below normal and/or LV systolic time interval ratio >2 SD above normal, and/or evidence of pericardial effusion.
   C. Electrocardiogram: left ventricular hypertrophy and ST-T wave abnormalities.

V. **Hepatitis syndrome:** hepatomegaly and elevation of liver function tests (>2× upper limits of normal) that persist for at least 2 months in the absence of evidence of other etiologies (hepatitis A or B, EBV, CMV, *Mycobacterium tuberculosis*). Disease may progress with development of jaundice, prolonged PT/PTT, and may be associated with liver failure. Liver biopsy shows noncaseating granulomas.

VI. **Encephalopathy syndromes:** progressive neurological condition usually beginning in the lower extremities, and which may involve the trunk and upper extremities. Associated with loss of developmental milestones and pyramidal tract signs. Diagnosis includes cortical atrophy on CAT scan and normal cerebrospinal fluid values for cells, protein, and glucose. Diagnosis excludes all known causes, such as enteroviral, CMV, rubella, *Herpesvirus,* mumps, CMV, and toxoplasmosis. Other clinical features noted or reported include secondary microcephaly, generalized seizures, withdrawal, truncal ataxia, and loss of academic skills.

child are highly related, thus documenting that the parents are the source of the virus in several cases in our series. (Shaw, Hahn, and Hutto, personal communication). A current problem in the diagnosis of HTLV-III/LAV infection in pediatric AIDS concerns serological testing in the first year of life. Infants acquire high-titered anti-HTLV-III/LAV antibody from their mothers and, to date, no assay for IgM anti-HTLV-III/LAV has been developed. It may be that infants do not respond with a strong IgM response analogous to those responses noted in congenital rubella.[28] Consequently, a virological diagnosis in our laboratory is based on isolation of virus as well as persistent retention of IgG antibody in the infant's serum. Virus isolation from infants is relatively common in pediatric AIDS patients, and several groups have isolated virus in this setting.[29] As already mentioned, infants have higher concentrations of lymphocytes and, consequently, smaller amounts of blood are required to obtain comparable numbers of lymphocytes. The isolation rate of HTLV-III/LAV from infants with documented AIDS and positive serology now approaches 90%.

Isolation of virus from mothers is a different matter. Only approximately 60% of the mothers yielded virus in multiple virus isolation attempts, even though virtually 100% have high levels of antibodies to numerous HTLV-III/LAV polypeptides. The infants develop antibodies both to p24 and to the envelope gene products of HTLV-III/LAV. The time course of the development of these antibodies is currently under study. No evidence has been found that would suggest that either antibody status, virus status, or even neutralizing antibody status correlate prognostically with clinical outcome in infants with infection when age variables are controlled in perinatal infections.

At the present time, virus isolation and serology are used principally as a means of establishing that a given patient is, in fact, HTLV-III/LAV-positive. Infants have been studied over 7 years and have remained persistently positive through that period of time, suggesting that infection with HTLV-III/LAV is likely persistent for life and is not always associated with clinical disease in children. Analysis of sequential isolates from children demonstrates that strains undergo marked genetic variation. The significance of this variation is not clear, but it is remarkable in its frequency and degree. The importance of these changes for clinical outcome and in terms of pathogenesis is not clear at present.

Future Prospects for Prevention, Treatment, and Immunoprophylaxis

A major approach to prevention involves education of groups of women who are at high risk for being infected by the AIDS virus. Such groups have been identified using HTLV-III/LAV antibody tests, and are defined in terms of relative seroprevalence. An appreciation of the cultural complexity of these groups is still evolving. A particular focus of educational effort will be female intravenous drug abusers or sexual partners of high risk males (such as IV drug abusers), the female sexual partners of men with AIDS, ARC, or asymptomatic AIDS virus infection, recent emigrants from Africa or Haiti, and other individuals who are exposed to blood or blood products for any number of disorders or problems. At present, individuals who have antibody are being counselled to avoid pregnancy until further information is available. However, the likelihood of detecting groups with highest seroprevalence depends on screening programs, which unfortunately seldom reach those individuals at greatest risk. Antibody-positive individuals should obviously be counselled regarding blood donations, sexual activity, and the need for frequent physical examinations. Of considerable relevance for educational programs are antibody-negative women who are in high risk groups. These women should be counselled regarding their sexual practices and their selection of sexual partners. It is likely that high risk women, even if seronegative, should be advised against donating blood or organs because of their risk of being infected.

Evidence of the success of intervention programs, such as counselling in any of the risk groups just mentioned, has seldom been presented. For example, there is no evidence that intervention with IV drug abusers in any area related to behavior modification has been effective over time. Nevertheless, educational efforts targeted at women at risk remain the best prospect for avoidance of infection by sexual or IV routes; then, secondarily, there can be prevention of perinatal AIDS. Without successful intervention programs, it is unlikely that a diminution in the number of pediatric AIDS cases will be seen.

In the area of treatment, exciting advances have recently been made. There are a number of drugs, including azidothymidine,[30] ribavirin,[31] and, in the near future, 2,3-dideoxynucleosides,[32] that are being tested for clinical safety and efficacy. These compounds interfere with the replication of the HTLV virus in infected cells, and reduce the likelihood of cells being infected by the AIDS virus. (See chapters by Mitsuya et al., and Yarchoan and Broder.) The consequence of this may be to suppress the spread of infection within the individual and to prevent transmission to contacts. However, many of these currently proposed antiviral drugs may have teratogenic and mutagenic properties associated with their mode of action. Such compounds would not be appropriate for infected pregnant women; however, they may well be useful for the treatment of children with perinatal AIDS. In fact, phase I pediatric studies with azidothymidine will begin soon. Any potential to reduce transmission as well as improve outcome offers children infected with HTLV-III/LAV the greatest prospect for a near-normal life. It is not at all clear what late outcome may be in terms of neurological results, but at the present time, chemotherapy of infected children is the most promising approach. It is likely that combination chemotherapy and perhaps even immunological reconstitution will be essential components of a comprehensive treatment program for children with perinatal AIDS.

It should be noted that these children will also have to undergo intensive educational and counselling designed to decrease the likelihood of their transmitting the virus to infected contacts over the course of their entire life. This will require an enormous effort on the part of the medical profession, the patients themselves, their families, and a support network that, of necessity, will be involved in the comprehensive care of infected children.

Prospects for immunoprophylaxis center around an understanding of both the natural history of the viral infection in individuals (and children particularly), as well as an understanding of the host's immune responses to virus infection. Currently, it would appear that antibodies to the envelope's external glycoprotein, gp120, analogous to most other viral infections, are an important aspect of the immunopathogenesis of HTLV-III/LAV virus infection. High-titered antibody to the gp120 with cross-reactivity with other isolates could be produced by vaccination with purified glycoprotein. Ultimately, such a vaccine is likely to be the product of recombinant DNA technology. This type of killed vaccine would require multiple injections and administration to groups at highest risk. Parenthetically, it should be noticed that the groups at highest risk are also, in many instances, the same people for whom it is most difficult to deliver all other medical services. In fact, this is likely to be the major problem in the delivery of any vaccine to prevent perinatal AIDS virus infection. However, the prospects for developing vaccines with broadly reactive immunogenicity are promising, and this approach may well be of value as in the case of heptatits B, in which perinatally infected infants are immunized at birth *and* given HBV-immune serum globulin. A similar approach ultimately may be feasible for pediatric AIDS. Perhaps the vaccination of sexual contacts in high risk groups will also decrease the development of perinatal AIDS

As our understanding of pediatric AIDS has grown, so too have the prospects for control. This multifaceted disease involves multiple organs and presents in many forms. It is, in fact, these variations that provide both the impetus and the basis of a multifactorial approach to the treatment and prevention of further infections in children.

References

1. Ammann AJ, Hong R. Disorders of the T cell system. In: Stiehm ER, Fulginiti VA, eds. Immunologic disorders in infants and children, 2nd ed. Philadelphia: WB Saunders, 1980:286–348.
2. Masur H, Michelis MA, Greene JB, et al. An outbreak of community acquired *Pneumocystis carinii* pneumonia: initial manifestations of cellular immune dysfunctions. N Engl J Med 1981; 305:1431–1438.

3. Siegal FP, Lopez C, Hammer GS, et al. Severe acquired immunodeficiency in male homosexuals, manifested by chronic perianal ulcerative herpes simplex lesions. N Engl J Med 1981; 305:1439–1444.

4. Gottlieb MS, Schroff R, Schanker HM. *Pneumocystis carinii* pneumonia and mucosal candidiasis in previously healthy homosexual men: evidence of a new acquired cellular immunodeficiency. N Engl J Med 1981; 305:1425–1431.

5. Vieira J, Frank E, Spira TJ, Landesman SH. Acquired immune deficiency in Haitians: opportunistic infections in previously healthy Haitian immigrants. N Engl J Med 1983; 308:125–129.

6. Pitchenik AE, Fischl MA, Dickinson GM, et al. Opportunistic infections and Kaposi's sarcoma among Haitians: evidence of a new acquired immunodeficiency state. Ann Intern Med 1983; 98:277–284.

7. Rubinstein A, Sicklick M, Gupta A, et al. Acquired immunodeficiency with reversed T4/T8 ratios in infants born to promiscuous and drug-addicted mothers. JAMA 1983; 249:2350–2356.

8. Oleske J, Minnefor A, Cooper R Jr, et al. Immune deficiency syndrome in children. JAMA 1983; 249:2345–2349.

9. Scott GB, Buck BE, Leterman JG, et al. Acquired immunodeficiency syndrome in infants. N Engl J Med 1984; 310:76–81.

10. Cowan MJ, Ammann AJ. Acquired immunodeficiency syndrome in infants and children. In: Gallin JI, Fauci AS, eds. Advances in host defense mechanisms. New York: Raven Press, 1985:99–107.

11. Scott GB, Fischl MA, Klimas N, et al. Mothers of infants with the acquired immunodeficiency syndrome: evidence for both symptomatic and asymptomatic carriers. JAMA 1985; 253:363–366.

12. Centers for Disease Control. Update: acquired immunodeficiency syndrome (AIDS)—United States, MMWR 1984; 32(52).

13. Carney WP, Rubin RH, Hoffman RA, et al. Analysis of T lymphocyte subsets in cytomegalovirus mononucleosis. J Immunol 1981; 126:2114–2116.

14. Reinherz EL, O'Brien C, Rosenthal P, et al. The cellular basis for viral-induced immunodeficiency: analysis by monoclonal antibodies. J Immunol 1980; 125:1269–1274.

15. Thomas PA, Jaffe HW, Spira TJ, et al. Unexplained immunodeficiency in children: a surveillance report. JAMA 1984; 252:639–644.

16. Buck BE, Scott GB, Valdes-Dapena M, Parks WP. Kaposi's sarcoma in two infants with acquired immunodeficiency syndrome. J Pediatr 1983; 103:11–13.

17. Centers for Disease Control. Acquired immunodeficiency syndrome (AIDS). Weekly Surveillance Report 1986:Jan. 13.

18. Ziegler JB, Cooper DA, Johnson RO, Gold J. Postnatal transmission of AIDS-associated retrovirus from mother to infant. Lancet 1985; i:896–897.

19. Centers for Disease Control. Update: acquired immunodeficiency syndrome (AIDS)—United States, MMWR 1984; 33(21).

20. Epstein L, Sharer L, Joshi V, et al. Progressive encephalopathy in children with acquired immunodeficiency syndrome. Ann Neurol 1985; 17:488–496.

21. Scott GB, Parks WP, Jonas M. Protein calorie malnutrition as a presenting manifestation of human retrovirus (HTLV-III) infection in infants and children. Pre-

sented at International Conference on Acquired Immunodeficiency Syndrome, Atlanta, Georgia, April 14–17, 1985.

22. Duffy LF, Daum F, Kahn E, et al. Hepatitis in children with acquired immunodeficiency syndrome. Gastroenterology 1986; 90:173–181.

23. Joshi VV, Oleske JM, Minnefor AB, et al. Pathology of suspected acquired immunodeficiency syndrome in children: a study of eight cases. Ped Pathol 1984; 2:71–87.

24. Siguidsson B, Grimsson HM, Palssom H. Maedi, a chronic progressive infection of sheep lungs. J Infect Dis 1952; 90:233–241.

25. Querat G, Barban V, Sauze N, et al. Highly lytic and persistent lentiviruses naturally present in sheep with progressive pneumonia are genetically distinct. J Virol 1984; 52:672–679.

26. Narayan O, Griffin DE, Clements JE. Virus mutation during slow infection: temporal development and characterization of mutants of visna virus recovered from sheep. J Gen Virol 1978; 41:343–352.

27. Safai B, Good RA. Kaposi's sarcoma: a review and recent developments. Clin Bull 1980; 10:62–69.

28. Alford CA, Griffiths PD. Rubella. In: Remington JS, Klein JO, eds. Infectious diseases of the fetus and newborn. Philadelphia: WB Saunders, 1983:69–103.

29. Gallo RC, Salahuddin CZ, Popovic M, et al. Frequent detection and isolation of cytopathic retroviruses (HTLV-III) from patients with AIDS and at risk for AIDS. Science 1984; 224:500–503.

30. Mitsuya H, Weinhold KJ, Furman PA, et al. 3′-Azido-3′-deoxythymidine (BW A509U): an antiviral agent that inhibits the infectivity and cytopathic effect of human T-lymphotrophic virus type III/lymphadenopathy-associated virus *in vitro*. Proc Natl Acad Sci USA 1985; 82:7096–7100.

31. McCormick JB, Getchell JP, Mitchell SW, Hicks DR. Lancet 1984; ii:1367–1369.

32. Mitsuya H, Broder S. Inhibition of the *in vitro* infectivity and cytopathic effect of HTLV-III/LAV by 2′,3′-dideoxynucleosides. Proc Natl Acad Sci USA 1986; 93:1911–1915.

16

HTLV-III/LAV-Related Neurological Disease

Joseph R. Berger
University of Miami
School of Medicine
Miami, Florida

Lionel Resnick
University of Miami
School of Medicine
Miami, Florida
and Mount Sinai Medical Center
Miami Beach, Florida

Background

Human T-cell lymphotropic virus type III/lymphadenopathy-associated virus (HTLV-III/LAV) has been recognized as the cause of the acquired immunodeficiency syndrome (AIDS) and AIDS-related complex (ARC).[1-5] AIDS is currently defined by the Centers for Disease Control as "a reliably diagnosed disease that is at least moderately indicative of an underlying cellular immunodeficiency in a person who has had no known underlying cause of cellular immunodeficiency nor any other cause of reduced resistance reported to be associated with that disease."[6] The immunodeficiency is typically characterized by the presence of an opportunistic infection, such as *Pneumocystis carinii* pneumonia or the development of Kaposi's sarcoma in an individual less than 60 years old. With the availability of serological and virological tests for HTLV-III/LAV, the accepted opportunistic infections have been refined to include individuals with disseminated histoplasmosis, isosporiasis, bronchial and pulmonary candidiasis, non-Hodgkin's lymphoma, histologically confirmed Kaposi's sarcoma in patients over 60 years old, and chronic lymphoid interstitial pneumonia in children less than 13 years of age with positive tests for HTLV-III/LAV.[7] The specificity of the case definition has been increased by excluding as AIDS those individuals with negative results on antibody testing to HTLV-III/LAV with no other positive HTLV-III/LAV test in the absence of a low number of T-helper lymphocytes or low ratio of T-helper to T-suppressor lymphocytes.[7]

AIDS is often preceded by a prodromal illness characterized by fever, malaise, lymphadenopathy, weight loss, and diarrhea referred to as ARC.[8,9] Infection with HTLV-III/LAV, whether subclinical or manifested by ARC or AIDS, is a substantial risk factor for the development of neurological illness. Neurological disease occurring in association with HTLV-III/LAV infection is extraordinarily common. In a preliminary communication, Bredesen and Messing[10] reported that 30% of 175 patients with AIDS or ARC developed neurological symptoms or signs during an average follow-up period of 6 months. The incidence of neurological disease complicating AIDS was 39% in a series by Levy et al.[11] and 41% in a series by Snider et al.[12] In the former study, one-third of the patients were symptomatic with neurological disease at the time of presentation.[11] These investigators believed that their figures were probably an underestimation of the true incidence of neurological disease because unselected autopsy data on the same group of patients revealed evidence of abnormal central nervous system (CNS) pathology in 30 of 41.[11] This incidence of neuropathological abnormalities in AIDS patients is quite similar to that reported by Nielsen et al.,[13] in which 31 of 40 patients had CNS disease. In another study, three of every four patients with AIDS developed a neurological complication, and, though it was felt that these complications typically developed late in the course of the illness,[14] that has not been our experience. Berger et al.[15] detected neurological illness in 83 (63%) of 132 with AIDS evaluated over a 52-month period at Jackson Memorial Hospital, Miami, Florida. In 26 (20%) patients, neurological disease heralded the onset of AIDS. This incidence of neurological disease as the harbinger of the immunodeficiency state complicating HTLV-III/LAV is higher than the 10% reported in other series.[10,12] Furthermore, the neurological complications of HTLV-III/LAV may appear before the development of any associated immunological abnormalities.[16]

The spectrum of neurological disease complicating HTLV-III/LAV is quite broad (Table 1). These illnesses can be divided into those that result from direct involvement of the nervous system by HTLV-III/LAV and those that result as a consequence of immunosuppression. The latter include a variety of infectious complications, brain hemorrhage secondary to immune thrombocytopenia, embolic stroke secondary to marantic endocarditis, and neoplasm (either primary or metastatic). The neoplastic complications may have an etiology related to infection. For example, preliminary evidence links brain lymphoma, peculiarly common to AIDS patients, with Epstein-Barr virus infection.[17]

There is, as yet, no recognized characteristics of patients with HTLV-III/LAV that predict the subsequent development of neurological illness or its nature. The risk groups for AIDS (homosexual men, recent Haitian immigrants, parenteral drug abusers, and hemophiliacs) appear to be distributed in their appropriate proportions in AIDS patients with neurological disease. However, the nature of the neurological disease may vary among each of the risk groups. For instance, Haitian patients appear to have a greater predilection for toxoplasma encephalitis.[18] The risk factors of HTLV-III/LAV-related neurological disease remain undefined. The high degree of neurotropism exhibited by the virus conceivably places all HTLV-III/LAV-infected individuals at risk for its development.

HTLV-III/LAV Neurotropism

In 1984, a new human retrovirus was isolated and subsequently demonstrated to be the etiological agent of AIDS and ARC. The virus has been referred to as human T-lymphotropic virus type III (HTLV-III) because it was the third type of human T-lymphotropic virus to be discovered. Despite its propensity to infect lymphocytes, its nucleic acid sequence is distinct from that of HTLV-I and HTLV-II.[19] It has also been referred to as lymphadenopathy-associated virus (LAV) because AIDS is often preceded by lymphadenopathy. A major contribution to the pathological consequences of infection by HTLV-III/LAV results from the infection of helper/inducer (OKT4/leu 3a$^+$) lymphocytes and probably of other cell types exerting a direct cytopathic effect and/or indirect effect on cells involved in cellular and humoral immunity.[20] While many of the neurological consequences of HTLV-III/LAV infection are the result of infectious processes resulting from the immunodeficient state, it appears that some of the neurological complications are the direct result of HTLV-III/LAV because it is not only lymphotropic, but also neurotropic. Evidence that supports HTLV-III/LAV neurotropism includes isolation of the HTLV-III/LAV from cerebrospinal fluid (CSF) and neural tissues,[16,21] detection of HTLV-III/LAV DNA and RNA in the brain, and intrablood-brain barrier synthesis of HTLV-III/LAV-specific IgG.[24]

HTLV-III/LAV has been recovered from patents presenting with acute and chronic meningitis, meningoencephalitis, dementia, myelopathy, and peripheral neuropathy.[16] Furthermore, HTLV-III/LAV has been isolated from CSF, brain, spinal cord, and peripheral nerves of patients with AIDS-related neurological dysfunction.[16] The presence of the virus in the brain of patients with

TABLE 1 Neurological Complications of AIDS

Infectious complications
A. Encephalitis
   1. Viral
      a. HTLV-III/LAV
      b. Cytomegalovirus
      c. Herpes simplex I
      d. Herpes simplex II
      e. Herpes zoster
      f. Adenovirus*
      g. Undetermined
   2. Bacterial
      a. *Treponema pallidum*
   3. Parasitic
      a. *Toxoplasmosis gondii*
      b. *Taenia solium* (cysticercosis)
B. Meningitis
   1. Viral
      a. HTLV-III/LAV
      b. Undetermined
   2. Bacterial
      a. *Mycobacterium tuberculosis*
      b. *Mycobacterium avium-intracellulare*
      c. *E. coli*
      d. *Treponema pallidum*
      e. Polymicrobial bacterial infection
   3. Fungal
      a. *Cryptococcus neoformans*
      b. *Aspergillus fumigatus*
      c. *Histoplasma capsulatum*
      d. *Coccidioides immitis*
C. Brain abscess
   1. Bacterial
      a. *Mycobacterium tuberculosis*
      b. *Mycobacterium avium-intracellulare*
      c. Polymicrobial bacterial infection
      d. Others
   2. Fungal
      a. *Cryptococcus neoformans*
      b. *Candida albicans*
      c. Others
   3. Parasitic
      a. *Toxoplasmosis gondii*
      b. *Taenia solium* (cysticercosis)
D. Myelopathy
   1. Viral
      a. HTLV-III/LAV vacuolar myelopathy

TABLE 1 *Continued*

        b. Cytomegalovirus*
        c. Herpes simplex II
        d. Herpes zoster
        e. Epstein-Barr virus (?)
        f. Others
    2. Bacterial
        a. Syphilitic meningomyelitis
    3. Compressive secondary to epidural abscess
  E. Neuropathy
    1. Viral
        a. HTLV-III/LAV*
        b. Cytomegalovirus*
        c. Herpes simplex*
        d. Herpes zoster (post herpetic neuralgia)
  F. Myositis
        Etiology unknown
  G. Progressive multifocal luekoencephalopathy
      (secondary to papovavirus)

Neoplastic

A. Primary tumors
    1. Brain lymphoma
B. Metastatic disease (including carcinomatous meningitis and compressive myelopathy)
    1. Non-Hodgkin's lymphoma
    2. Hodgkin's lymphoma
    3. Kaposi's sarcoma
    4. Plasmacytoma[a]

Metabolic disorders

A. Drug side effect
B. Electrolyte abnormality
C. Vitamin deficiency
    1. Folate
    2. Vitamin B-12
    3. Vitamin E*

Vascular complications

A. Hemorrhage secondary to immune thrombocytopenia
    1. Subarachnoid hemorrhage
    2. Intracerebral hemorrage
B. Embolic stroke secondary to marantic endocarditis
C. Parainfectious cerebral arteritis*
D. Vascular compromise secondary to *Aspergillus fumigatus*

*Possible association.

AIDS is strongly supported by the ability to transfer HTLV-III/LAV infection to chimpanzees by inoculation of brain tissue from patients with AIDS.[21]

Brains from 15 patients with AIDS encephalopathy were examined by Southern blot analysis and in situ hybridization, and revealed the presence of HTLV-III/LAV DNA in five patients and viral-specific RNA in four patients.[23] Utilizing Southern blot analysis for the detection of HTLV-III/LAV DNA, the brain had a higher percentage of positive samples than peripheral blood, lymph node, bone marrow, and spleen of patients with AIDS and ARC.[19]

Additionally, patients with neurological manifestations associated with AIDS or ARC have antibodies directed against HTLV-III/LAV in the CSF.[24] Unique oligoclonal IgG bands have been detected in the CSF, and quantitations of the intrablood-brain barrier IgG synthesis rate reveal both an elevated total IgG synthesis and HTLV-III/LAV-specific IgG synthesis. In eight of nine patients, a higher percentage of HTLV-III/LAV-specific IgG was found in the CSF compared with the serum, suggesting that HTLV-III/LAV infection of neurological tissue is not uncommon (Table 2).

The tropism for the nervous system by HTLV-III/LAV is not without precedent. Certain strains of the murine leukemia virus, also a retrovirus, induce neurological disease in wild mice.[25] The latter develop a chronic progressive paralytic disorder following infection. Additionally, a primary retroviral encephalitis has been observed in macaque monkeys inoculated with simian T-cell lymphotropic virus, a retrovirus that has growth, morphologic, and antigenic properties indicating that it is related to HTLV-III/LAV.[26] HTLV-III/LAV also has morphological and genetic similarities to visna, a lentivirus that causes chronic degenerative neurologic disease of sheep.[27] Like HTLV-III/LAV, visna infects the brain and lymphocytes, has cytopathic effects, and persists in cells in substantial amounts as unintegrated viral DNA.[28,29] The presence of unintegrated DNA in the brain represents a replicative intermediate stage in the life cycle of HTLV-III/LAV, suggesting its active replication in the brain.[23]

Unlike the relatively noninflammatory brain lesions described in AIDS encephalopathy, visna virus infection is associated with an intense mononuclear inflammatory response.[30] The apparent absence of an inflammatory response in the brains of AIDS patients may be the result of the profound cellular immunodeficiency, a feature not present in sheep infected with visna virus.[30]

Acute Neurological Disease Related to HTLV-III/LAV
Primary Infection

An acute illness clinically similar to infectious mononucleosis or influenza may accompany primary HTLV-III/LAV infection.[31-33] typically, the illness occurs

TABLE 2 Intrablood-Brain Barrier: Total and HTLV-III Specific IgG Synthesis

Patient number	Cerebrospinal fluid†				Serum‡				Intrablood-brain barrier IgG synthesis[a]		Cerebrospinal fluid/serum Specific HTLV-III IgG[b]	Oligoclonal IgG bands[c]	Intrablood-brain barrier albumin formation[d] (mg/day)
	Total		HTLV-III-specific IgG		Total		HTLV-III-specific IgG		Total (mg/day)	Specific for HTLV-III (%)			
	IgG (mg/dl)	Albumin (mg/dl)	mg/dl	% of total IgG	IgG (mg/dl)	Albumin (mg/dl)	mg/dl	% of total IgG					
1	22.8	41.0	0.61	2.7	2291	5688	57.0	2.5	69	3	+	12	82
2	27.2	34.6	0.21	0.8	3739	3276	13.8	0.4	36	2	+	3	102
3	21.0	73.6	0.18	0.9	2412	4784	11.3	0.5	15	3	+	2	264
4	12.4	42.4	0.02	0.2	2432	4482	4.8	0.2	2	0	?	0	96
5	6.4	19.4	0.02	0.4	3015	4121	4.1	0.1	−11	0	+	0	8
6	20.9	21.9	0.58	2.8	2613	2349	10.3	0.4	41	6	+	ND	58
7	20.9	17.5	0.42	2.0	2549	2618	1.5	0.2	57	4	+	ND	31
8	7.8	28.8	0.20	2.5	1614	4500	9.4	0.6	10	8	+	ND	46
9	3.4	13.3	0.10	2.8	1153	2917	7.0	0.6	1	0	+	ND	3

†Normal cerebrospinal fluid IgG (mg-dl): 0.9–8.2; normal cerebrospinal fluid albumin (mg/dl): 5.5–34.3.

‡Normal serum IgG (mg/dl): 900–1800. Normal serum albumin (mg/dl): 3600–5600.

[a]IgG synthesis (mg/day) = $\left[\left(IgG_{CSF} - \dfrac{IgG\ serum}{369}\right) - \left(ALB_{CSF} - \dfrac{ALB\ serum}{230}\right) \times \left(\dfrac{IgG\ serum}{ALB\ serum}\right) \times (0.43)\right] \times 5$. Normal intrablood-brain barrier IgG synthesis is < 3 mg/day.

[b]HTLV-III-specific IgG, $\dfrac{CSF}{serum}$ ratio > 1 is scored (+). ? indicates the inability to make a definitive assessment.

[c]Oligoclonal IgG bands = IgG bands found exclusively or more intense in cerebrospinal fluid compared with the autologous serum.

[d]Albumin formation (mg/day) equals: $\left(ALB_{CSF} - \dfrac{ALB_{Serum}}{230}\right) \times 5$. Normal intrablood-brain barrier albumin formation is < 80 mg/day.

Source: Adapted from Ref. 24.

suddenly after an estimated incubation of 3 to 6 weeks,[33] but the incubation period may be shorter.[32] The sources of the infection in the patients studied have included needlestick in a nurse,[31] shared needles among drug abusers,[33] and exposure via homosexual relationships.[32,33] In two studies, [32,34] seroconversion was the means employed to identify acute HTLV-III/LAV infection, whereas in another study,[33] virus isolation was combined with seroconversion. The characteristics of the acute illness include fever with sweats and rigors, arthralgias, and myalgias.[32-34] Patients may also complain of anorexia, nausea, sore throat, abdominal cramps, and diarrhea.[32] Physical examination may reveal fever, generalized lymphadenopathy, pharyngeal injection, splenomegaly, splenic tenderness, maculopapular rash, and urticaria.[32,33,35] Laboratory studies may reveal thrombocytopenia, lymphopenia, and inversion of the T4 to T8 ratio.[32] Seroconversion occurs 8 to 12 weeks after presumed exposure.[33]

The nervous system is also affected during acute HTLV-III/LAV infection. An aseptic meningitis was appreciated in two of three patients in one study.[33] Headache, meningismus, and photophobia are characteristic symptoms and may occur when other features of the illness appear to be resolving. Generalized seizures and encephalopathy[34] may be observed, as well as a chronic meningitis with a course longer than 2 weeks. Despite neurological symptomatology, the CSF may remain normal. However, CSF examination often reveals a mononuclear pleocytosis and mildly elevated protein (<100 mg%). HTLV-III/LAV may be isolated from the CSF,[16] and intrablood-brain barrier synthesis of antibody to HTLV-III/LAV may be detected.[24]

HTLV-III/LAV Encephalopathy

A "subacute viral encephalitis" is probably the most common neurological complication of AIDS.[12] Kaminsky et al.[36] identified it in 8 of 52 patients with AIDS. In a series from Cornell/Memorial Sloan-Kettering of 50 AIDS patients with neurological disease, it was observed in 18 (36%).[12] In larger series from the University of California-San Francisco, "subacute encephalitis" was seen in 35 of 156 AIDS patients with neurological disease.[11] In a prospective study,[37] cognitive dysfunction was eventually observed in over 50% of 180 AIDS patients evaluated neurologically over a 3-year period. The clinical recognition of this disease is undoubtedly an underestimate of its true incidence because its features are frequently ascribed to metabolic derangement or marked debilitation. The latter, however, is usually insufficient to cause the neurological disability detected.[12]

Typically, the onset of the encephalopathy is insidious and its progression is over months.[38] On occasion, its course is more rapid. Problems with mentation are characteristic, and include memory impairment and difficulty with problem-solving. Bradyphrenia, a slowness in thinking, may be detected early, but cognitive function may be normal at this stage of the illness.[39] The patient becomes withdrawn, and business and social interactions become infrequent. The affect may appear blunted. Complaints of easy fatiguability, malaise, and loss of sexual drive are common.[13] Personality changes, which are often early manifestations of the illness, include severe depression, marked anxiety, and paranoid psychosis.[40] The dementia that is displayed, at least early in the clinical course, has many of the features of "subcortical dementia" akin to that observed in patients with Parkinson's disease and Huntington's chorea. The hallmarks of this dementia include slow performance, mildly impaired memory, impaired higher level reasoning, and associated affective disorders.[41]

The patient may complain of headache,[11,12] diffuse weakness,[39] or painful dysesthesia of distal extremities.[12] The latter accompanies the peripheral neuropathy that often complicates this disorder.[12] Seizures are also observed.[11,12,39] Seizures occurred in two of 18 patients in one study.[12] Many patients appear to have a low threshold for the development of CNS side effects secondary to medications. Parkinsonism and dystonia as a consequence of an exquisite sensitivity to neuroleptics, such as chlorpromazine, and metoclopromide, are noted quite frequently in these patients.[42] When the entity is fully developed, the physical examination typically reveals psychomotor retardation. The speech is slow and monotonous, and word-finding difficulties may be apparent. In very advanced states, mutism may supervene. Hemianopsia has been reported complicating this illness,[11] but is decidedly rare. Visual problems are usually the result of coexistent retinitis, either due to cytomegalovirus (CMV), toxoplasmosis, or other complications. Eye movements are preserved, but diminished blink rates may be noted. A loss of facial expression, sialorrhea, diminished ability to make rapid tongue movements, dysarthria, and seborrheic dermatitis mimic features of Parkinson's disease. A generalized motor weakness to confrontation muscle strength testing is not unusual.[39] The patient often is unable to arise from a squat or simply from bed as a result. Debilitation from overwhelming illness may be responsible for the latter, and we and others[12] have observed a myopathy occurring concomitantly in an occasional patient. Distal lower extremity weakness resulting from involvement of the peripheral nerves is seen on occasion;[12] however, in most instances, the weakness appears to be the result of corticospinal tract involvement. Focal motor and sensory signs have also been reported,[11,13] but have been unusual in our experience and should raise suspicion about a coexistent focal process. Paratonic rigidity, characterized by stiffening of the limbs in response to contact and a resistance to passive changes in position and posture with the strength of the antagonists increasing as the examiner uses increasing force to change the position of the limb[43] may be detected.[12] The latter may be a feature of pyramidal or extrapyramidal disease.[43] Tremulousness is common. The tremors are best seen when the patient sustains a posture such as holding the arms and fingers outstretched. On occasion, the tremors may increase with action and, even more rarely, occur during rest. Myoclonus has also been reported.[12,44] In one series,[12] myoclonus was observed in five of 18 patients. The muscle stretch reflexes are normal or hyperactive with the exception of the ankle jerks, which are not infrequently depressed or absent as a result of concomitant peripheral neuropathy.[12] Hoffman's and Babinski's signs, indicative of corticospinal tract dysfunction, may be detected. Frontal release signs, such as snout, root, grasp, and nuchocephalic, are observed frequently, but are not invariable.[11] A prominent palmomental reflex, twitching of the mentalis muscle of the chin on stroking the ipsilateral thenar eminence, is commonly observed. Sensory examination may reveal components of a distal sensory neuropathy. The gait is often hesitant and uncertain. Rarely, a spastic-ataxic gait or paraparesis may be observed,[23] possibly the result of HTLV-III/LAV-related vacuolar myelopathy.[45]

Diagnositic studies are most helpful in ruling out other neurological disorders that may complicate AIDS, including fungal and tuberculous meningitis, toxoplasmosis, progressive multifocal leukoencephalopathy, and brain lymphoma. Computed tomography (CT) of the brain may be normal, but more often demonstrates cerebral atrophy characterized by sulcal widening and ventricular dilatation.[11-13,36] Illnesses that result in focal CT abnormalities may coexist.

Magnetic resonance imaging (MRI) is a new technique that has not yet been adequately studied in this disorder. In a limited series of patients with HTLV-III/LAV encephalopathy, MRI proved helpful in detecting coexistent brain disorders, such as progressive multifocal leukoencephalopathy, not detected by CT. Levy et al.[11] described one AIDS patient with a clinical picture of dementia, abulia, left hemiparesis and frontal release signs, and neuropathological findings at autopsy that strongly suggested "subacute encephalitis," who had an unremarkable CT of the brain, but an MRI that demonstrated bifrontal increases in T2 relaxation time consistent with edema and inflammation. The experience at the University of Miami School of Medicine with MRI in "subacute encephalitis" has been somewhat limited to date, but in most instances, it adds little more than the CT scan of the brain.

The CSF examination generally reveals a normal opening pressure. The most common CSF abnormality is an increased protein, typically on the order of 50 to 100 mg%.[11,12,39] Other CSF abnormalities that may be observed include a mild mononuclear pleocytosis and a mildly decreased glucose.[11,12,39] HTLV-III/LAV may be cultured from the CSF.[22] Levy et al.[22] demonstrated its presence in 14 of 15 CSF samples in AIDS patients with neurological disease, but with one exception, these patients had low titers of antibody to HTLV-

III/LAV in the CSF. Cultures for other viruses are typically negative.[12] How-ever, Levy et al.[22] reported two patients positive for CMV on culture and three that were positive for herpes simplex I (one of their patients was positive for both viruses). Microbiological studies for bacteria, fungi, and parasites are negative unless other illnesses coexist.

The electroencephalogram may be normal or display diffuse slowing. En-zensberger et al.[46] found slow alpha rhythm in 50% of 26 male homosexuals with AIDS in the absence of neurological disease. Five of 13 patients with this rhythm disturbance subsequently developed an acute or subacute encephalitis, most often attributed to toxoplasmosis and the other eight patients developed a chronic encephalitis believed to be due to HTLV-III/LAV.[46] Snider et al.[12] detected diffuse slowing of the electroencephalogram in all but one patient with subacute encephalitis. Occasionally, paroxysmal features may be noted, particularly in those patients with seizures as a feature of their illness.

Gross neuropathological studies[13] of the brains of patients with HTLV-III/LAV encephalopathy reveal cortical atrophy with sulcal widening and ven-tricular dilatation. Meningeal fibrosis may be seen.[13] The myelin may exhbit diffuse pallor. Microscopic examination frequently, though not invariably, reveals abnormality. The cerebrum, cerebellum, brainstem, and spinal cord may all be involved,[13] but the hypothalamus and brainstem are frequently the areas that seem to be most severely affected.[11] Nielsen et al.[13] divided the changes into those affecting the gray matter and those affecting the white matter. In the gray matter, multiple microglial nodules (Fig. 1) composed of oval to rod-shaped mononuclear cells with scant cytoplasm are noted. They are frequently located in the subpial region or adjacent to small vessels.[13] In one series, eight of 19 brains demonstrated large cells with single intranuclear basophilic inclusions and multiple small cytoplasmic basophilic inclusions.[13] Some of these cells were astrocytes. Astrocytic scars and diffuse astrocytosis are observed in end-stage disease.[13] Perivascular or parenchymal lymphocytic infiltrates are notably absent.[13]

The white matter pathology is characterized by a smaller number of micro-glial nodules and areas of paravascular demyelination. Lipid-laden macro-phages associated with microglial cells, multinucleate cells, and reactive astro-cytes are seen.[13] Evidence of coexistent CMV infection may be detected patho-logically. Two of eight brains in one series[13] and three of four brains in another[36] revealed CMV inclusions on histopathological study; Nielsen et al.[13] demonstrated electron microscopic findings compatible with CMV in one patient. Despite these findings, CMV could not be cultured directly from the brain.[13] Similarly, "owl eye" inclusions have been noted in areas of brain and spinal cord demyelination in other studies.[47] Diffuse astrocytosis was seen in the white matter of all the brains in Nielsen study, and eight of 19 showed

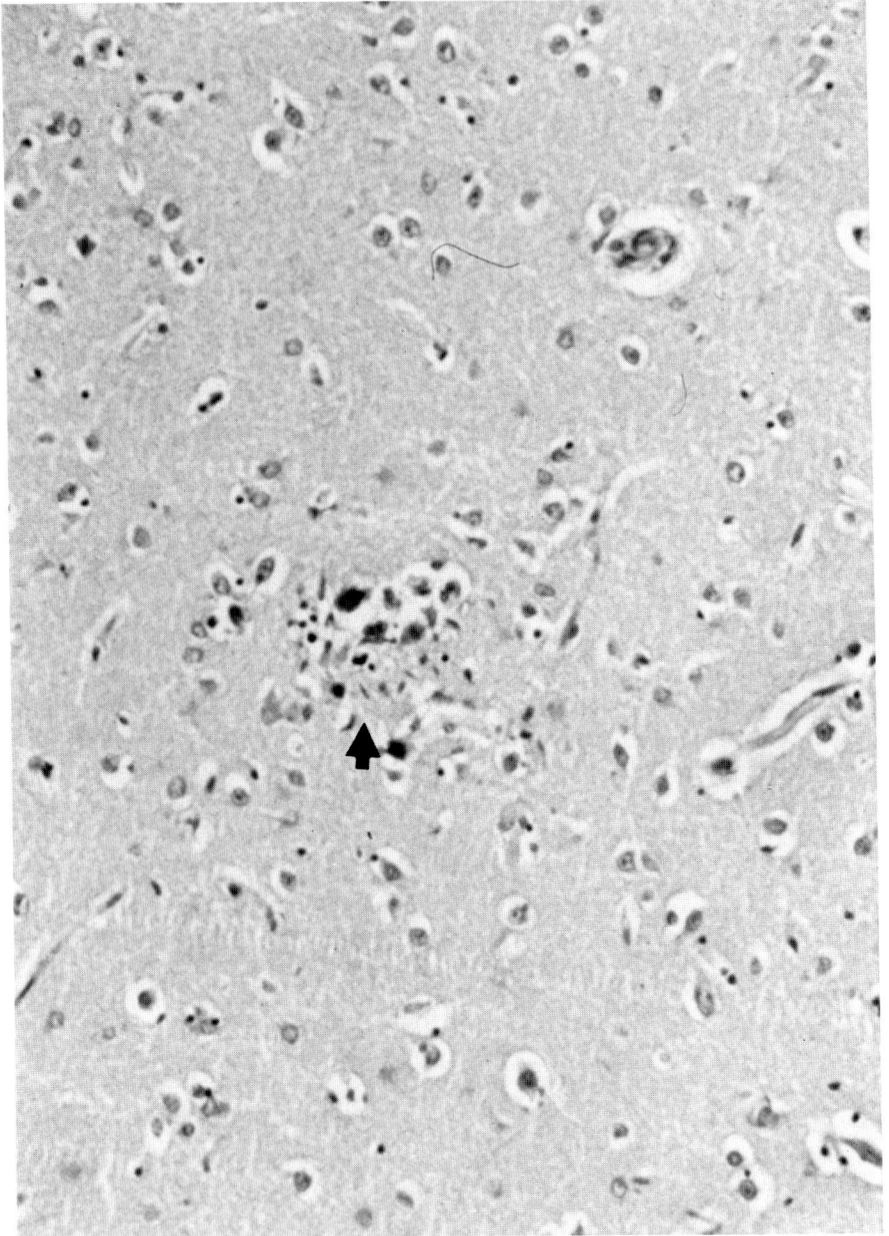

FIGURE 1   Microglial nodule in HTLV-III/LAV encephalopathy.

vacuolization of the centrum semiovale. In 20%, the white matter or the gray matter appears to be predominantly involved to the relative exclusion of the other.[13]

We and others[45] have observed AIDS patients with an unexplained progressive dementia characteristic of HTLV-III/LAV encephalopathy occurring in the absence of any neuropathological findings. Though HTLV-III/LAV has been isolated from the CSF and brains of patients with dementia,[16,22] as well as from patients without neurological disease,[22] it is uncertain whether all had neuropathological findings.

A progressive encephalopathy clinically similar to that described in adults has been observed in children as well.[23,48,49] The disorder is characterized by a loss of intellectual and motor milestones.[23,48,49] Weakness with pyramidal tract signs is observed,[48,49] though hypotonia has also been noted.[49] Seizures, myoclonus, and cortical blindness have been described.[48] Secondary microcephaly may develop.[48,49] CT of the brain typically reveals cortical atrophy and ventricular dilatation and, on occasion, calcification of the basal ganglia.[49] In addition to generalized slowing on the electroencephalogram, abnormalities may also be detected in brainstem auditory- and visual-evoked potentials.[49] Neuropathological findings in children with HTLV-III/LAV encephalopathy are similar to those of adults. The abnormalities include gross cortical atrophy, nonspecific white matter changes, microglial nodules, intranuclear inclusions, and corticospinal tract degeneration.[48,49]

HTLV-III/LAV Myelopathy

A unique degenerative condition of the spinal cord is commonly seen in association with HTLV-III/LAV infection.[12,45,50,51] Petito et al.[45] observed it at autopsy in 20 of 89 consecutively studied patients with AIDS. HTLV-III/LAV is the suggested pathogen since the retrovirus has been cultured from the cerebrospinal fluid and spinal cords of patients with AIDS-related myelopathy.[16] Furthermore, the myelopathy appears to be clinically and pathologically distinguishable from other viral myelitides, such as herpes simplex,[52,53] that also occur in association with HTLV-III/LAV infection.

Leg weakness and incontinence are the most common symptoms.[45] The gait is impaired. Frequently, these complaints are attributed to general debilitation, and the true nature of the process remains undiagnosed until autopsy examination of the spinal cord. Examination typically reveals spastic paraparesis. Ataxia may be noted as well, though neither spasticity nor ataxia need be present. Monoparesis and quadriparesis are occasionally observed. Hyperflexia and extensor plantar responses (Babinski signs) may be detected in the absence of weakness. Occasionally, muscle stretch reflexes may be absent, presumably as a result of coexistent peripheral neuropathy. In our experience, paresthesia and discomfort in the legs are not uncommon. Sensory examination often reveals that vibratory and position sense are affected to a greater degree than pinprick, temperature, or light touch. Significant impairment of the latter modalities is suggestive of concomitant peripheral neuropathy. Bladder and bowel disturbances are common. In one study,[45] incontinence was observed in 60% of the patients with myelopathy.

Petito et al.[45] correlated the frequency with which symptoms were observed with neuropathological severity. Patients with AIDS-related spinal cord pathology were classified into three groups based on the severity of the illness as quantified neuropathologically. All those with severe involvement exhibited clinical features of spinal cord disease, whereas only five of seven with moderate changes and two of eight with mild changes did.

Encephalopathy and peripheral neuropathy are frequently superimposed on the myelopathy. Progressive dementia was noted in 14 of 20 patients in one study.[45] Symptoms were characteristic of HTLV-III/LAV encephalopathy and included lethargy, psychomotor retardation, impaired concentration, and memory loss.

The value of diagnostic studies in this condition is to rule out other possible etiologies. Myelography is negative. The value of MRI of the spinal cord in this condition remains uncertain.

With the exception of patients with severe myelopathy, the spinal cord and subdural and epidural spaces are normal to gross examination.[45] Histologically, loss of myelin and spongy degeneration are noted.[45,51] The lateral columns are affected to a greater extent than posterior columns, and the spinal cord is least involved anteriorly (Fig. 2).[45] The vacuolization of spinal white matter occurs in association with lipid-laden macrophages, and is most extensive in middle and lower thoracic regions. The spinal pathology may be asymmetric and is not confined to particular tracts,[45] though Goldstick et al.[51] described involvement of the posterior columns increasing in intensity with rostral progression, whereas pyramidal tract involvement increased caudally. Vacuolization appears to result from intramyelin swelling. Axons are preserved except in areas of severe vacuolization. Similar white matter vacuolization may be detected elsewhere in the CNS. Microglial nodules may be noted in the spinal gray matter,[45,51] and five of 20 patients had central chromatolysis of anterior horn motor cells.[45] Inflammation and intranuclear viral inclusions are not observed, and immunohistochemical studies are negative for virus.[45]

HTLV-III/LAV-Related Peripheral Neuropathy

All forms of peripheral neuropathy have been reported to occur in association with AIDS. Peripheral neuropathy may herald the onset of AIDS, as we[54] and

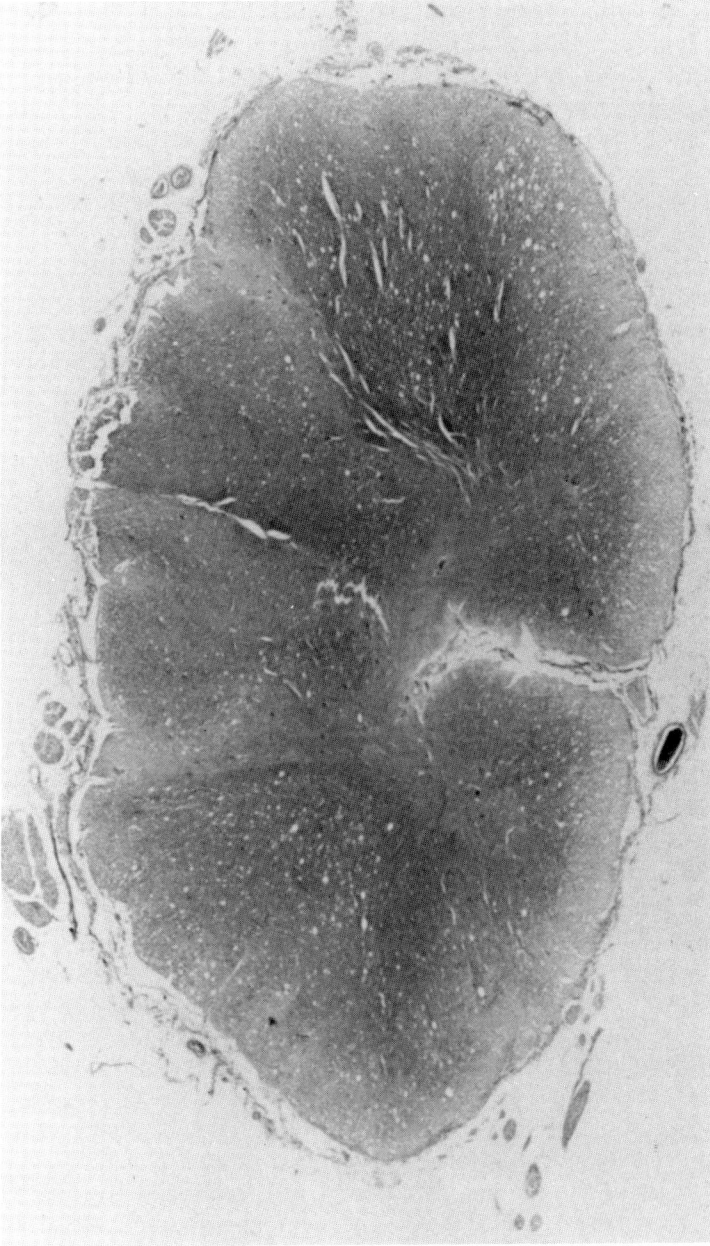

FIGURE 2 HTLV-III/LAV-related myelopathy in an AIDS patient. Specimen stained with luxol fast blue and hematoxylin and eosin. Demyelination and vacuolization are present throughout the white matter.

others[10] have reported. Occasionally, the peripheral neuropathy is ascribable to specific etiologies, such as alcohol, diabetes mellitus, nutritional deficiencies, and drug side effects. The causation may, in fact, be multifactorial. That HTLV-III/LAV is the pathogen responsible for peripheral neuropathy in some cases is suggested by the frequent association of AIDS and peripheral neuropathy, the absence of known etiologies in the majority of instances, the well-recognized neurotropism of HTLV-III/LAV,[16,21] and recovery of HTLV-III/LAV from the peripheral nerve.[16]

Among 25 patients with ARC or AIDS with peripheral neuropathy examined at Jackson Memorial Hospital, Miami, Florida, a mixed sensorimotor neuropathy was most common, but relatively pure sensory and pure motor peripheral neuropathies were also observed. The former typically presents with painful dysesthesia in the distal lower extremities. In one study, seven of eight patients with peripheral neuropathy experienced painful dysesthesia.[12] The onset and progression of the disorder are typically slow and gradual. Diminished sensory perception for vibration in the toes is appreciated early. Decreased pinprick sensation in a symmetric "stocking" distribution is also noted. Temperature and, to some degrees, light touch perception may be similarly impaired. Position sense may be affected later, resulting in or contributing to an ataxic gait. Weakness generally starts in the distal lower extremities. At first, the patient may find it difficult to walk on heels or toes. Muscle atrophy may also be observed. Muscle stretch reflexes are depressed or absent in the lower extremities. Sensory abnormalities are detected more often and are present to a greater degree than motor abnormalities,[12] except in instances of inflammatory neuropathy. Motor involvement that is greater than sensory involvement, asymmetric sensory findings, and cranial nerve dysfunction are all suggestive of the presence of an inflammatory neuropathy, a form of peripheral neuropathy that has also been recognized to complicate HTLV-III/LAV infection.[55]

Electromyography and nerve conduction studies confirm the presence of a mixed sensorimotor neuropathy, with either features of demyelination[12] or axonal degeneration[55] predominating. Electromyographic evidence of denervation may be minimal.[12] Although CSF examination may be normal, an elevated protein, borderline glucose, and mild mononuclear pleocytosis may be observed. Elevated CSF IgG and IgG/albumin index have been reported.[55] Nerve biopsy has, on occasion, demonstrated epineural and endoneural perivascular inflammation with axonal degeneration or demyelination.[55] Concomitant *Herpesvirus* infection was observed in five of eight patients with peripheral neuropathy described in one study,[12] though viral serological studies revealed no consistent relationship to the peripheral neuropathy.[12]

Treatment has been largely unsatisfactory. In one study of inflammatory peripheral neuropathy,[55] steroids proved to be unhelpful in four patients, though plasmaphereisis-lymphapheresis appeared to be beneficial in one patient. The dysesthetic component of the neuropathy may respond to carbamazepine or diphenylhydantoin therapy.

Guillain-Barré syndrome may also complicate HTLV-III/LAV infection. Though the disorder has been reported in association with other viruses, such as Epstein-Barr virus and cytomegalovirus,[56-58] a direct relation to HTLV-III/LAV is possible for reasons previously stated. We have observed six cases occurring in association with HTLV-III/LAV infection over a 3 year period. The illness conforms to the criteria established for the diagnosis of Guillain-Barré syndrome.[59] Although sensory symptoms are absent to minimal, vague discomfort in the extremities and paresthesias were noted in some patients. The onset and progression of Guillain-Barré syndrome complicating HTLV-III/LAV infection are generally more abrupt and rapidly progressive than that of the mixed sensorimotor neuropathy. Nerve conduction studies typically demonstrate slowed velocity indicative of a demyelinating neuropathy. CSF examination reveals the characteristic albuminocytological dissociation, though mononuclear pleocytosis may occur as well. Increased CSF IgG and oligoclonal bands may be detected. A gradual improvement in strength has been the rule in our experience.

Diagnosis and Treatment of HTLV-III/LAV-Related Disease

The diagnosis of HTLV-III/LAV-related neurological disease is essentially a diagnosis of exclusion. A strong attempt should be made to rule out potentially treatable neurological disorders. Because neurological disease may be the presenting manifestation of HTLV-III/LAV,[10,54] a high index of suspicion should be maintained, particularly in patients at high risk for AIDS and in patients presenting with unusual neurological disease.

With respect to HTLV-III/LAV encephalopathy, the clinical picture may be mimicked by metabolic derangements, other infectious illnesses, and CNS neoplasm. Each of these entities is seen in increased frequency in patients with AIDS. Laboratory studies should routinely include the following: serum electrolytes, calcium, glucose, blood urea nitrogen, liver function tests, VDRL, and FTA. Toxicology screens may be warranted in certain circumstances. Radiographic imaging of the brain is mandated in patients suspected of having HTLV-III/LAV encephalopathy, primarily to rule out other pathology. If available, MRI should be the initial study performed because it is more sensitive than CT in detecting brain pathology in AIDS.[60] MRI is especially useful in detecting lesions of the white matter and small lesions surrounded by edema.[60] Because of the disadvantages of MRI in characterizing the nature of lesions, 1 hour-delayed, double-dose contrast CT of the brain is recommended when the MRI is abnormal or when the study is unavailable.[60,61] Focal pathology as indicated by CT scan or MRI is unexpected in HTLV-III/LAV encephalitis unless other forms of brain pathology coexist. Strong consideration should be given to biopsy of focal pathology[62-64] demonstrated by CT scan in patients with ARC or AIDS because of the diversity of abnormalities observed, the presence of potentially treatable disease, and the difficulty in diagnosing these conditions by noninvasive means. Lumbar puncture is mandated when meningitis is suspected. The opening and closing pressures should be recorded. Studies of the CSF should include not only protein, glucose, and cell count, but also culture and sensitivity for bacteria and mycobacteria, fungal cultures, cryptococcal antigen assays, VDRL, cytology, and immunoelectrophoresis. Though not diagnostic of the nature of the underlying pathology, an electroencephalogram is recommended in patients with seizures or in instances where uncertainty exists as to whether abnormal behavior is the result of organic or psychiatric disease.

In patients with HTLV-III/LAV myelopathy, vitamin B-12 deficiency and syphilitic meningomyelitis should be considered in the differential diagnosis, and B-12 levels and VDRL and FTA should be obtained. CSF examination is also warranted. The clinical picture is seldom suggestive of a compressive myelopathy resulting from an extradural or intradural mass lesion or cervical spondylosis, though bacterial and fungal abscesses, neoplasm (particularly lymphoma), and hemorrhage associated with thrombocytopenia may result in myelopathy in patients with AIDS. For the former reason, myelography may not be necessary in many of these patients. If, however, there remains any question as to the nature of the spinal cord pathology, myelography may be indicated. Metrizamide meylography followed by CT of the spine at the level of the suspected pathology is undertaken. Delayed scans may prove helpful in detecting intrameduallary lesions. MRI of the spine and spinal cord may prove exceptionally useful and, in many instances, obviate the need for myelography.

The approach to the patient with a symmetric peripheral neuropathy should include attempts to exclude metabolic and toxic etiologies such as alcohol, diabetes mellitus, vitamin deficiency, and drug or toxin exposure. The history is helpful, but laboratory studies should include glucose tolerance test, thyroid function tests, vitamin B-12 and folate levels, and serum protein electrophoresis. If the peripheral neuropathy is asymmetric, it is more likely to be the result of inflammatory neuropathy or, less often, a complication of nerve root involvement by meningeal carcinomatosis. Lumbar puncture with assay of IgG levels and cytology is indicated. Nerve biopsy may be very helpful in establishing the presence of an inflammatory neuropathy. Regardless of the nature of the neuropathy, nerve conduction studies and electromyography are warranted to better elucidate its nature (i.e., demyelinating or axonal degeneration). Also, unsuspected sensory or motor involvement can often be detected with electrophysiological studies. Patients with inflammatory peripheral neuropathies may respond to steroids or plasmapheresis.

Unfortunately, no specific therapy exists for HTLV-III/LAV-related neurological disease. It is important to withdraw potentially offending medications from the patient with HTLV-III/LAV encephalopathy and address the metabolic parameters that may be complicating the neurological dysfunction. The treatment of coexistent systemic infections may also improve mentation. To date, there are insufficient data on experimental therapies, such as interferon, ribavirin, or HPA-23, to routinely recommend them in this setting.

The finding of large quantities of HTLV-III/LAV in the CNS tissues of patients with AIDS is important in the quest to define the biological behavior of the virus. It will be important to determine which type of cell is infected with HTLV-III/LAV and how the virus affects these cells in vitro and in vivo. Could the multiple tissue tropism of HTLV-III/LAV be the result of antigenic similarities in cell surface receptors? Therapeutic strategies for the patient with HTLV-III/LAV infection with require serious consideration of not only the incorporation of its genetic material into the host genome and the altered host immunity resulting from infection, but also the virus' presence in the central nervous system sanctuary. Effective antiviral therapy must be able to penetrate the blood-brain barrier.

References

1. Gallo RC, Salahuddin SZ, Popvic M, Shearer GM, Kaplan M, Haynes BF, Paker TJ, Redfield R, Oleske J, Safai B, White G, Foster P, Markham PD. Science 1984; 224:500.
2. Popovic M, Sarngadharan MG, Read E, Gallo RC. Science 1984; 224:497.
3. Broder S, Gallo RC. N Engl J Med 1984; 311:1291.
4. Safai B, Sarngadharan MG, Groopman JE, Arnett K, Popovic M, Sliski A, Schupbach J, Gallo RC. Lancet 1984; i:1438.
5. Gallo RC, Wong-Staal, F. Ann Intern Med 1985; 103:679.
6. Centers for Disease Control. MMWR 1982; 31:507.
8. Miller B, Stansfield SK, Zack MM, Curran JW, Kaplan JE, Schonberger LB, Falk H, Spira TJ, Mildvan D. JAMA 1984; 25:242.
9. Mitsuya H, Guo HG, Megson M, Trainor C, Reitz MS, Broder S. Science 1984; 223:1293.
10. Bredesen DE, Messing R. Ann Neurol 1983; 14:141. Abstract.
11. Levy RM, Bredesen DE, Rosenblum ML. J Neurosurg 1985; 62:475.
12. Snider WD, Simpson DM, Nielsen S, Gold JWM, Metroka CE, Posner JB. Ann Neurol 1983; 14:403.
13. Nielsen SL, Petito CK, Urmacher CD, Posner JB. Am J Clin Pathol 1984; 82:678.
14. Grapen P. JAMA 1982; 248:2941.

15. Berger JR, Moskowitz L, Fischl M, Kelley RE. South Med J (in press).
16. Ho DD, Rota TR, Schooley RT, Kaplan JC, Allan JD, Groopman JE, Resnick L, Felsenstein D, Andrews CA, Hirsch MS. N Engl J Med 1985; 313:1493–1497.
17. Hochberg FH, Miller G, Schooley RT, Hirsch MS, Feorino P, Henle W. N Engl J Med 1983; 309:745.
18. Sher JH. Lancet 1983; i:1225. Letter.
19. Shaw GM, Hahn BH, Arya SK, Groopman JE, Gallo RC, Wong-Staal F. Science 1984; 226:1165.
20. Klatzmann D, Barre-Sinoussi F, Nugeyre MT, Dauguet C, Vilmer E, Griscelli C, Brun-Vezinet F, Rouzioux C, Gluckman JC, Chermann JC, Montagnier L. Science 1984; 225:59.
21. Gajdusek, Amyx HL, Gibbs CJ, Asher DM, Rodgers-Johnson P, Epstein LG, Sarin PS, Gallo RC, Maluish A, Arthur MO, Montagnier L, Mildvan D. Lancet 1985; i:55.
22. Levy JA, Shimabukuro J, Hollander H, Mills J, Kaminsky L. Lancet 1985; ii:586.
23. Shaw GM, Harper ME, Hahn BH, Epstein LG, Gajdusek DC, Price RW, Navia BA, Petito CK, O'Hara CJ, Groopman JE, Cho ES, Oleske JM, Wong-Staal F, Gallo RC. Science 1985; 227:177.
24. Resnick L, Di Marzo-Veronese F, Schupbach J, Tourtellotte WW, Ho DD, Muller F, Shapshak P, Vogt M, Groopman JE, Markham PD, Gallo RC. N Engl J Med 1985; 313:1498.
25. Gardner MB. Curr Topics Microbiol Immunol 1978; 79:215.
26. Letvin NL, Daniel MD, Seghal PK, Desrosiers RC, Hunt RD, Walson LM, Mackey JJ, Schmidt DK, Chalifoux LV, King NW. Science 1985; 230:71.
27. Gonda MA, Wong-Staal F, Gallo RC, Clements JE, Narayan O, Gilden RV, Science 1985; 227:173.
28. Clements JE, D'Antonio N, Narayan O. Virology 1980; 102:46.
29. Clements JE, Narayan O. Virology 1981; 113:412.
30. Petursson G, Nathanson N, Georgsson G, Panitch H, Palsson PA. Lab Invest 1976; 35:402.
31. Editorial. Lancet 1984; ii:1376.
32. Cooper DA, Gold J, Maclean PM, Donovan B, Finlayson R, Barnes TG, Michelmore HM, Brooke P, Penny R. Lancet 1985; i:537.
33. Ho DD, Sarngadharan MG, Resnick L, Di Marzo-Veronese F, Rota TR, Hirsch M. Ann Intern Med 1985; 103:880.
34. Carne CA, Tedder RS, Smith A, Sutherland S, Elkington SG, Daly HM, Preston FE, Groshe S. Lancet 1985; ii:1206.
35. Tucker J, Ludlam CA, Craig A, Philp I, Steel CM, Tedder RS, Cheingsong-Popov K, Macnicol MF, McClelland DBL, Boulton FE. Lancet 1985; i:585.
36. Kaminsky DL, Mathur U, Yancovitz S, Croxson TS, Yang WC, Mildvan D. Interscience Conf. Antimcrob. Agents. Chemother 1983; 23:197. Abstract.
37. Tross JC, Holland S, Wetzler S. In: International Conference on the Acquired Immunodeficiency Syndrome (AIDS). 1985. Abstract.
38. Holland JC, Tross S. Ann Intern Med 1985; 103:760.
39. Britton CB, Miller JR, Neuro Clin 1984; 2:315.
40. Britton CB, Marquardt D, Koppel B, Garvey G, Miller JR. Ann Neurol 1985; 12:80. Abstract.

41. Albert ML, Feldman RG, Willis AL. J Neurol Neurosurg Psych 1974; 37:121.
42. Hollander H, Golden J, Mendelson T, Cortland D. 1985; 2:186.
43. DeJong RN. In: The neurologic examination, IV ed. Hagerstown, Maryland: Harper & Row, 1979.
44. Jordan BD, Navia BA, Petito C, Cho ES, Price RW. Front Radiol Ther Oncol 1985; 19:82.
45. Petito CK, Navia BA, Cho ES, Jordan BD, George DC, Price RW. N Engl J Med 1985; 312:874.
46. Enzensberger W, Fischer PA, Helm EB, Stille W. Lancet 1985; i:1047.
47. Moskowitz LB, Gregorios JB, Hensley GT, Berger JR. Arch Pathol Lab Med 1984; 108:873.
48. Epstein LG, Sharer LR, Joshi VV, Fojas MM, Koenigsberger MR, Oleske JM. Ann Neurol 1985; 17:488.
49. Belman AL, Ultmann MH, Horoupian D, Novick B, Spiro AJ, Rubinstein A, Kurtzberg D, Cone-Wesson B. Ann Neurol 1985; 18:560.
50. Goldstick L, Mandybur TI, Means E. J Neuropathol Exp Neurol 1984; 43:294.
51. Goldstick L, Mandybur TI, Bode R. Neurology 1985; 35:103.
52. Tucker T, Dix R, Katzen C, Divis RL, Schmidley JW. Ann Neurol 1985; 18:74.
53. Britton CB, Mesa-Tejada R, Fenoglio CM, Hays AP, Garvey GG, Miller JR. Neurology 1985; 35: 1071.
54. Berger JR, Moskowitz L, Fischl M, Kelley RE, Neurology (Suppl 1) 1984; 34:134. Abstract.
55. Lipkin I, Parry G, Kiprov D, Abrams D. Neurology 1985; 35:1479.
56. Kabins S, Keller R, Nariqi S, Peitchel R. Arch Intern Med 1976; 136:933.
57. Klenola E, Weckman N, Hattia K, Kaariainen L. Acta Med Scand 1967; 181:603.
58. Leonard JC, Tobin JOH. Q J Med 1971; 159:435.
59. Asbury AK. Ann Neurol (Suppl) 1981; 9:1.
60. Post MJD, Sheldon JJ, Hensley GT, Soila K, Tobias J, Chan JC, Quencer RM, Moskowitz LB. Radiology 1986; 158:141.
61. Post MJD, Kursunoglu SJ, Hensley GT, Chan JC, Moskowitz LB, Hoffman TA. AJNR 1985; 6:743.
62. Levy RM, Pons VG, Rosenblum ML. J Neurosurg 1984; 61:9.
63. Snow RB, Lavyne MH, Neurosurgery 1985; 16:148.
64. Moskowitz LB, Hensley GT, Chan JC, Conley FK, Post MJD, Gonzalez-Arias SM. Arch Pathol Lab Med 1984; 108:368.

Dermatological (Non-Kaposi's Sarcoma) Manifestations Associated with HTLV-III/LAV Infection

Lionel Resnick
Jay S. Herbst
Mount Sinai Medical Center
Miami Beach, Florida

The most commonly known cutaneous manifestation of the acquired immunodeficiency syndrome (AIDS), Kaposi's sarcoma, was recognized in the earliest descriptions of the syndrome.[1,2] The rarity of Kaposi's sarcoma in the affected populations made this dermatological manifestation a conspicuous part of the syndrome. We are now aware that AIDS is one clinical manifestation of the spectrum of human T-cell lymphotropic virus type III (HTLV-III)/lymphadenopathy-associated virus (LAV) infection. The majority of patients with HTLV-III/LAV infection are clinically asymptomatic. Patients who present with signs and symptoms associated with HTLV-III/LAV infection have been clinically defined as having primary HTLV-III/LAV infection, AIDS-related complex (ARC), or AIDS.[3,4] Patients with HTLV-III/LAV infection develop a defect of cellular immunity characterized by depletion of T-helper cells, defects in delayed hypersensitivity, and the occurrence of multiple

TABLE 1   Dermatological
Manifestations (Non-Kaposi's
Sarcoma) Associated with
HTLV-III/LAV Infection

Infections
  Viruses
    Herpesvirus
      Herpes simplex
      Varicella zoster
    Pox virus
      Molluscum contagiosum
    Papilloma virus
      Verruca vulgaris
      Condyloma acuminatum
  Fungi
    Candida albicans (thrush)
    Cryptococcus neoformans
    Histoplasma capsulatum
  Protozoan
    Amebiasis
      Acanthamoeba castellani
  Bacteria and mycobacteria
    Staphylococcus
    Mycobacterium intracellulare
    Mycobacterium tuberculosis
Malignancies
  Lymphomas
    Hodgkin's lymphoma
    Non-Hodgkin's lymphoma
    Burkitt's lymphoma
  Carcinomas
    Squamous cell carcinoma
    Cloacogenic carcinoma
Miscellaneous
  Drug eruptions
    Sulfonamides
    Suramin
  Primary HTLV-III/LAV infection
  Seborrheic dermatitis
  Oral "hairy" leukoplakia
  Granuloma annulare-like eruption

opportunistic infections and malignancies. Recent clinical observations[5] suggest that patients infected with HTLV-III/LAV have an increased incidence of skin eruptions. The skin, as a window of internal disease, can develop lesions that may suggest to the physician that a patient has been exposed to HTLV-III/LAV infection. Dermatological manifestations associated with HTLV-III/LAV infection can be classified into three general categories (Table 1): infections, malignancies, and miscellaneous cutaneous eruptions.

Mucocutaneous Infections

Common and uncommon cutaneous infections can occur in clinically unusual forms in patients with HTLV-III/LAV infection. Mucocutaneous infections can be caused by viruses, fungi, protozoa, bacteria, and mycobacteria, all resulting from impaired host immunity. A decreased number of Ia-positive Langerhan's cells in the skin of patients with HTLV-III/LAV infection suggests that they may have a defect in the antigen-presenting function of the cellular immune system at the level of the skin, which predisposes to infections by multiple organisms.[6] These infections are extremely difficult to treat and have a high recurrence rate.

Viruses

Herpesviruses: Herpes simplex virus (HSV) type I and type II infections have occurred as localized and disseminated infections. Many patients have atypical, severe, and often persistent oral and genital herpetic infections. Patients with recurring herpes simplex virus infections of the genital area have a prolonged healing time, accompanied by deep ulcerations with persistent shedding of virus. HSV can frequently be cultured from the skin lesions. Severe, chronic, ulcerative HSV infection involving the perianal region is a frequent type of herpetic disease seen in homosexual men (Fig. 1).[7] These patients present with perianal pain associated with exudative ulcerations, which persist for months unless aggressively treated with acyclovir. The rectal mucosa may also become involved, giving rise to herpetic proctitis.[8] Patients present with anorectal pain, discharge, tenesmus, hematochezia, and anogenital eruptions. Difficulty in urinating with urinary retention and sacral parasthesias may also occur.

The occurrence of a *Varicella* infection in young children exposed to HTLV-III/LAV can be life-threatening, with extensive cutaneous and internal manifestations (Fig. 2).

The clinical appearance of zoster, an ulcerative vesicobullous eruption that usually occurs in a dermatomal distribution, can present in either a localized

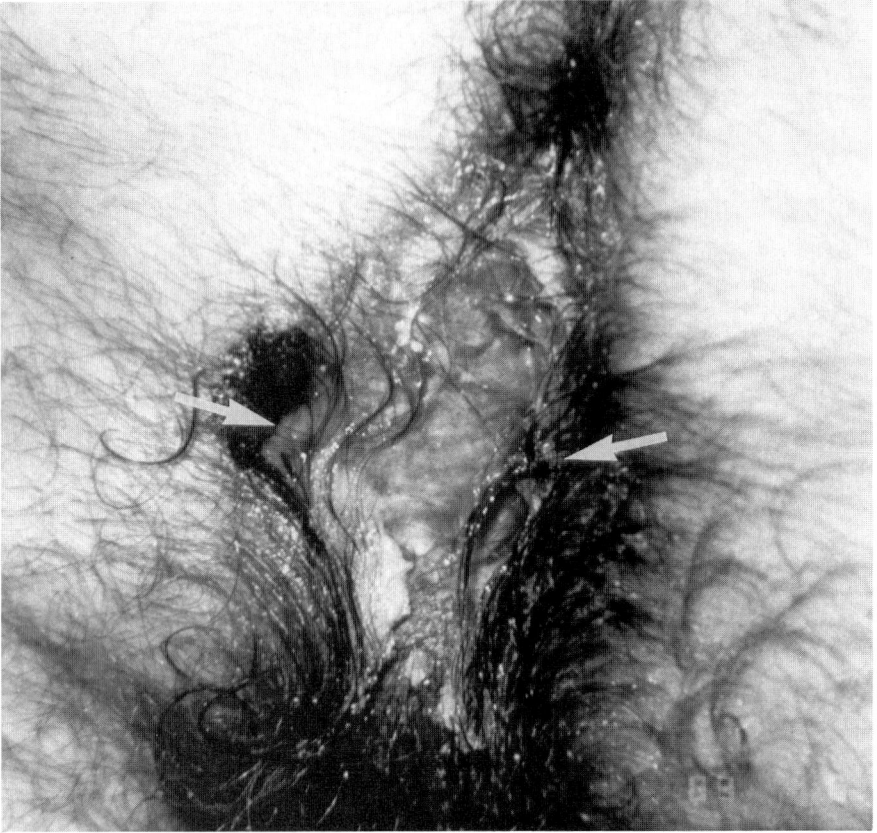

FIGURE 1   Ulcerative perianal herpes simplex.

or disseminated form (Fig. 3).[9] Zoster with dissemination can be associated with encephalitis, pneumonitis, and hepatitis, and is often fatal. Aggressive therapy with acyclovir may be life-saving.

Pox virus: Molluscum contagiosum is a pox virus infection most commonly seen in young children. Molluscum contagiosum may also occur in adolescents, especially in the genital region, where it is transmitted by sexual contact. Typically, infections consist of fewer than 20 lesions that resolve spontaneously over 3 to 12 months. Disseminated, persistent, umbilicated papules (more than 100) due to molluscum contagiosum have occurred in patients infected with HTLV-III/LAV infection (Fig. 4).[10]

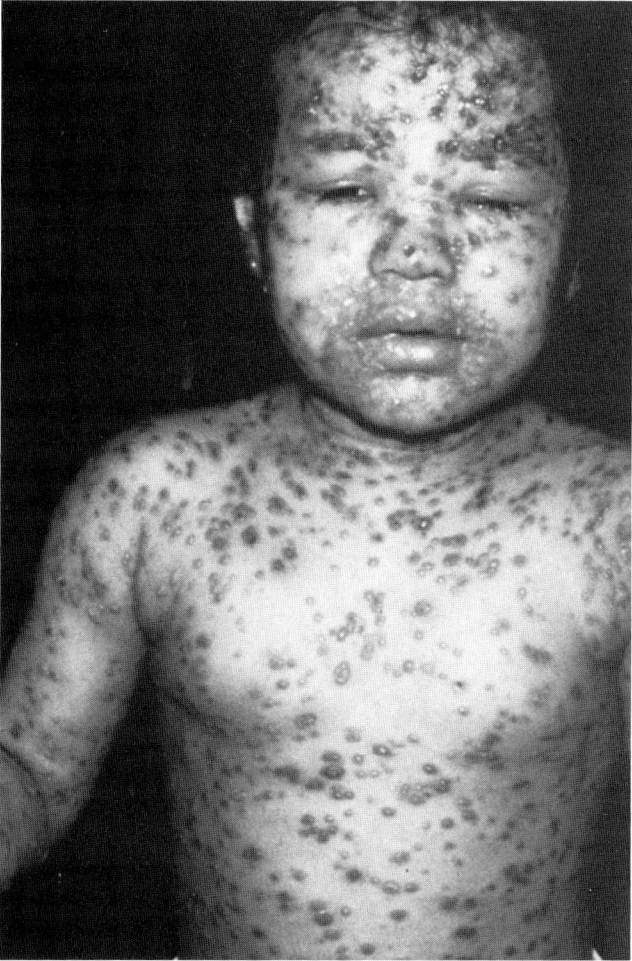

FIGURE 2   Disseminated hemorrhagic *Varicella* (chicken pox).

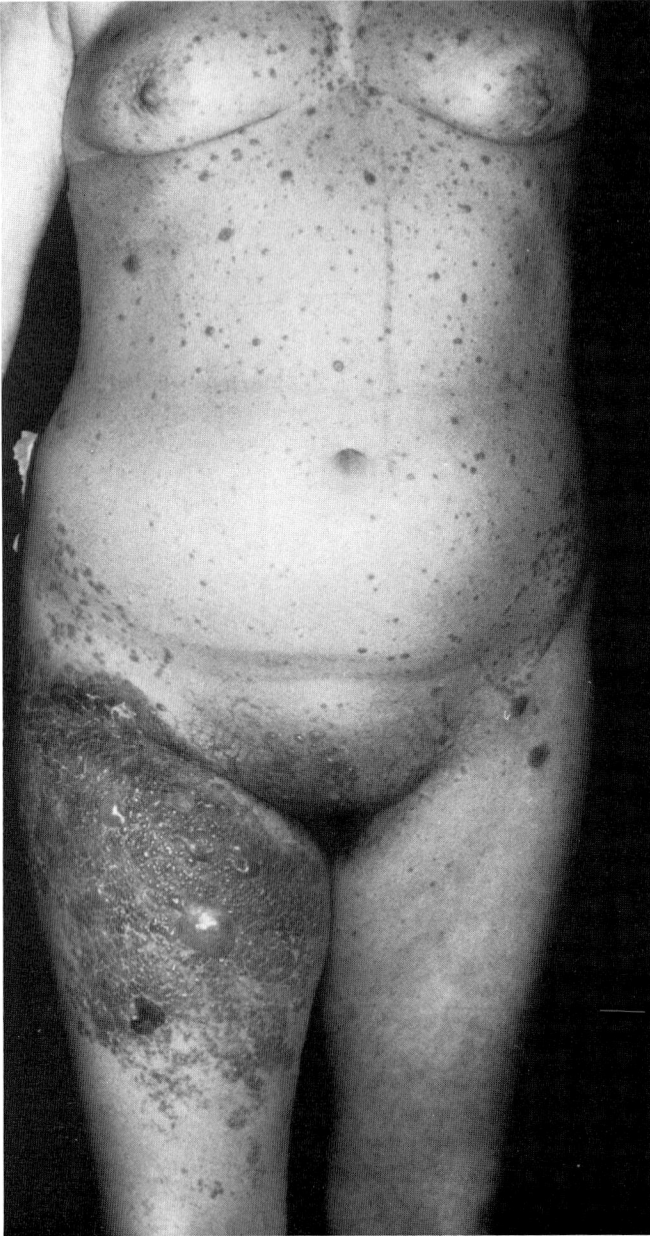

FIGURE 3   Disseminated herpes zoster.

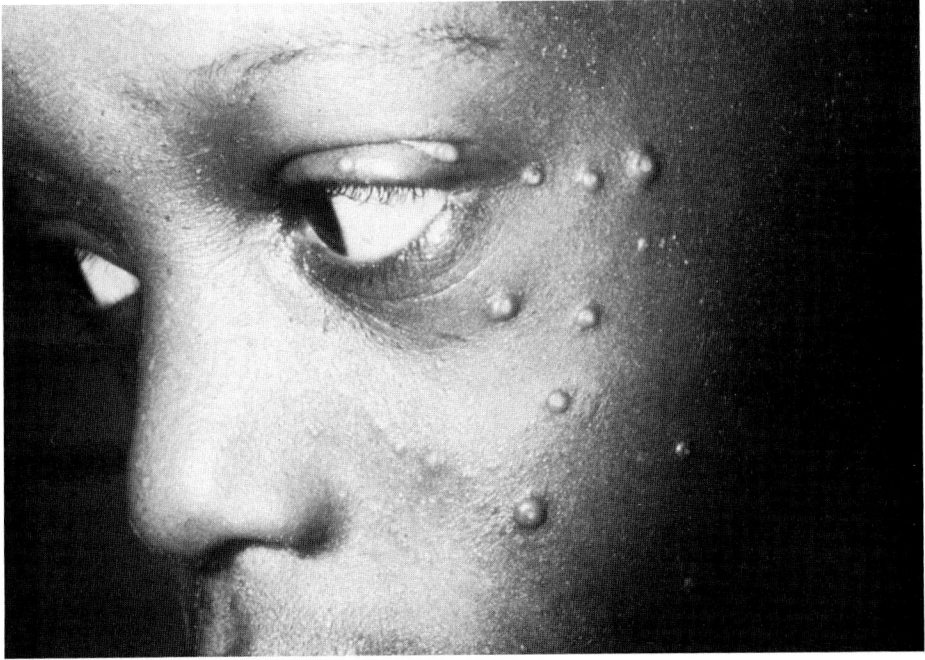

FIGURE 4   Molluscum contagiosum; umbilicated papules on the face.

Papilloma virus: Multiple filiform or flat warts (verucca vulgaris) usually involving the beard area, have been described in homosexual men with HTLV-III/LAV infection.[5] Genital warts (condyloma acuminata) are common, especially of the anorectal area in homosexuals.[11] The presence of genital warts in a child can sometimes provide a clue of child abuse (Fig. 5).

Fungi

Yeast: Oral candidiasis (thrush) is now being commonly recognized as a possible indicator of immune deficiency. The presence of unexplained oral candidiasis predicts the development of serious opportunistic infections and the development of AIDS.[12] Grayish-white membranous plaques with a moist, reddish base usually involve the buccal mucosa and the tongue (Fig. 6). The lesions are treated with nystatin and ketaconazole, but recurrences are frequent when treatment is discontinued. Candidal intertrigo, commonly involving the inguinal region, is often severe and tends to spread to the adjacent skin

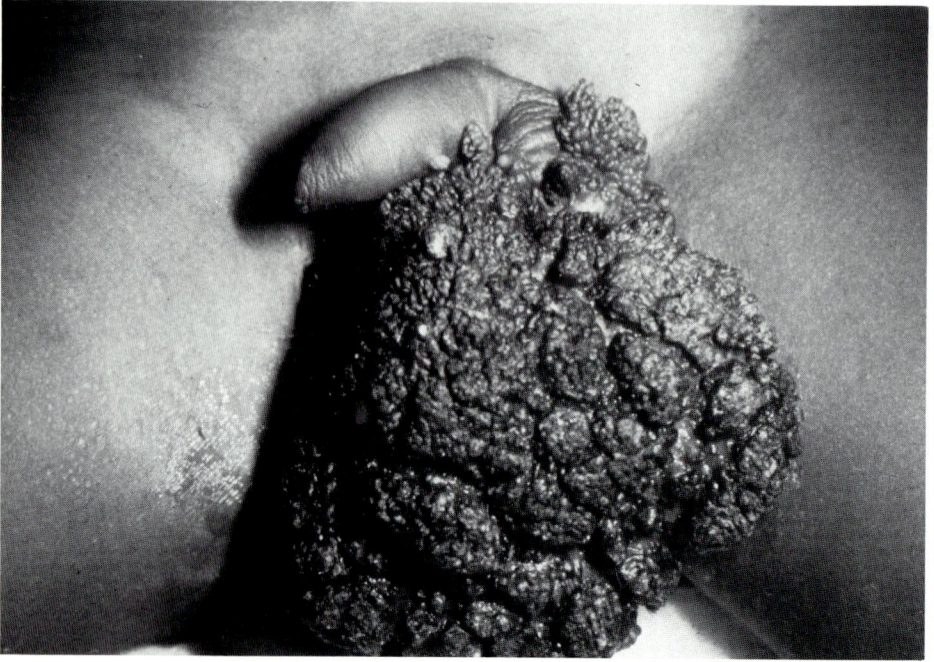

FIGURE 5   Scrotal condyloma acuminata.

of the perineum and gluteal folds. It requires aggressive prolonged therapy for control.

Fungal infections: Disseminated cryptococcus or histoplasmosis infections can present with skin manifestations such as cellulitis, ulcers, vasculitis, vesicles, papules, plaques, and purpura.[13,14] Histological study and culture of skin specimens are essential for diagnosis.

Protozoa: A rare form of cutaneous amebiasis presenting with multiple papules has been reported.[15] Histological sections of a biopsy specimen of a papule revealed amoebic trophozoites of *Acanthamoeba.*

Bacteria and mycobacteria: Multiple skin abscesses or furunculosis occur with staphylococcus, the most frequently cultured organism.[5] Extensive impetigo, occasionally a severe form of bullous impetigo, frequently involves the intertriginous areas and can become disseminated if not treated aggressively with systemic antibodies.

Mycobacterial (*Mycobacterium avium-intracellulare* and tuberculosis) infection can present with skin manifestations.[15] Patients clinically exhibit multiple papules or enlarged lymph nodes with draining sinuses.

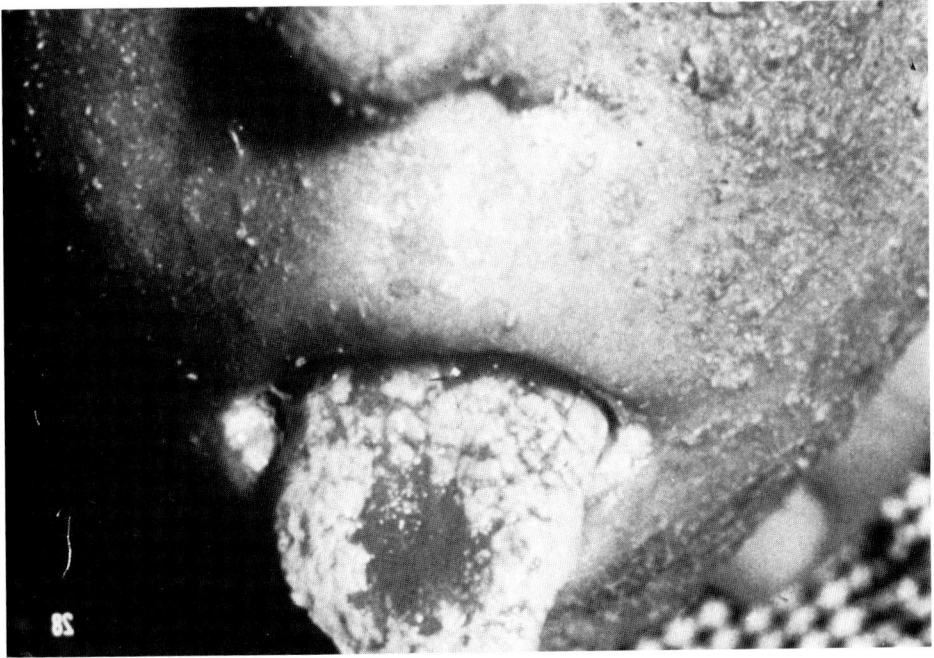

FIGURE 6   Oral candidiasis (thrush) involving the buccal mucosa and tongue.

Patients with HTLV-III/LAV infection should be closely monitored for the development of serious opportunistic infections. The recognition of one or more of these atypical infections in high risk individuals alerts the physician to monitor patients with prodromal signs of immunological deficiency, who may subsequently develop the more typical signs and symptoms of HTLV-III/LAV infection. Although these mucocutaneous infections are seldom life-threatening, their unusual clinical manifestations, prolonged course, and slow response to therapy often make their diagnosis and management difficult.

Malignancies

Lymphomas

An increased incidence of aggressive Hodgkin's and non-Hodgkin's lymphomas occurs in patients with HTLV-III/LAV infection.[16,17] Patients usually present initially with generalized lymphadenopathy, but may also have skin nodules. Epstein-Barr virus (EBV) can produce fatal lymphoproliferative diseases and, occasionally, Burkitt's lymphoma.[18] These lymphomas have been found to contain the EBV genome.[19] The normal immune response produces EBV-specific antibodies and, in conjunction with T-cell-mediated events, prevents the uncontrolled proliferation of cells triggered by EBV infection. Patients with immunological defects appear to be predisposed to the development of EBV-associated tumors. (See chapter by Levine et al.)

Carcinomas

Cutaneous squamous cell and cloacogenic anorectal carcinomas occur with greater than expected frequency.[20,21] Mucocutaneous squamous cell carcinomas have occurred after renal transplantation and in patients receiving immunosuppressive drugs.[22,23] A possible etiological role for herpes viruses and papilloma viruses in the development of squamous cell carcinomas has been postulated.[24]

Cloacogenic carcinoma of the anorectum arises from the transitional zone mucosa. The transitional zone mucosa lies between the proximal rectal columnar mucosa and the squamous mucosa of the anal canal; it is derived from the cloacogenic membrane in the fetus. Cloacogenic carcinoma is normally seen more commonly in women, but now occurs in male homosexuals engaged in long-standing receptive anal intercourse.[21] In view of the common embryological origin of the transitional zone and the uterine cervix, a potential etiological relationship between receptive anal intercourse and the development of cloacogenic carcinoma has been suggested. Just as cervical carcinoma has been linked to early sexual intercourse with multiple partners, cloacogenic carcinoma may have similar risk factors.

It is possible that many of the malignancies seen in patients with HTLV-III/LAV infection are related to potential oncogenic viruses that are able to proliferate in the absence of immune surveillance, thereby giving rise to the malignant state.

Miscellaneous

Drug Eruptions

Cutaneous drug eruptions are frequently seen in patients receiving sulfonamide medications during therapy for *Pneumocystis carinii* pneumonia or toxoplasmosis.[25] Trimethoprim-sulfamethoxazole and pentamadine are utilized for therapy of *Pneumocystis* pneumonia. In contrast to the relatively low frequency of side effects in non-AIDS patients, a much higher incidence of adverse reactions occurs in AIDS patients treated with trimethoprim-sulfamethoxazole.[26] Skin eruptions usually occur between the 8th and 12th days of treatment. Diffuse maculopapular eruptions are most common, but erythema multiforme and urticarial eruptions also occur (Fig. 7). These reactions

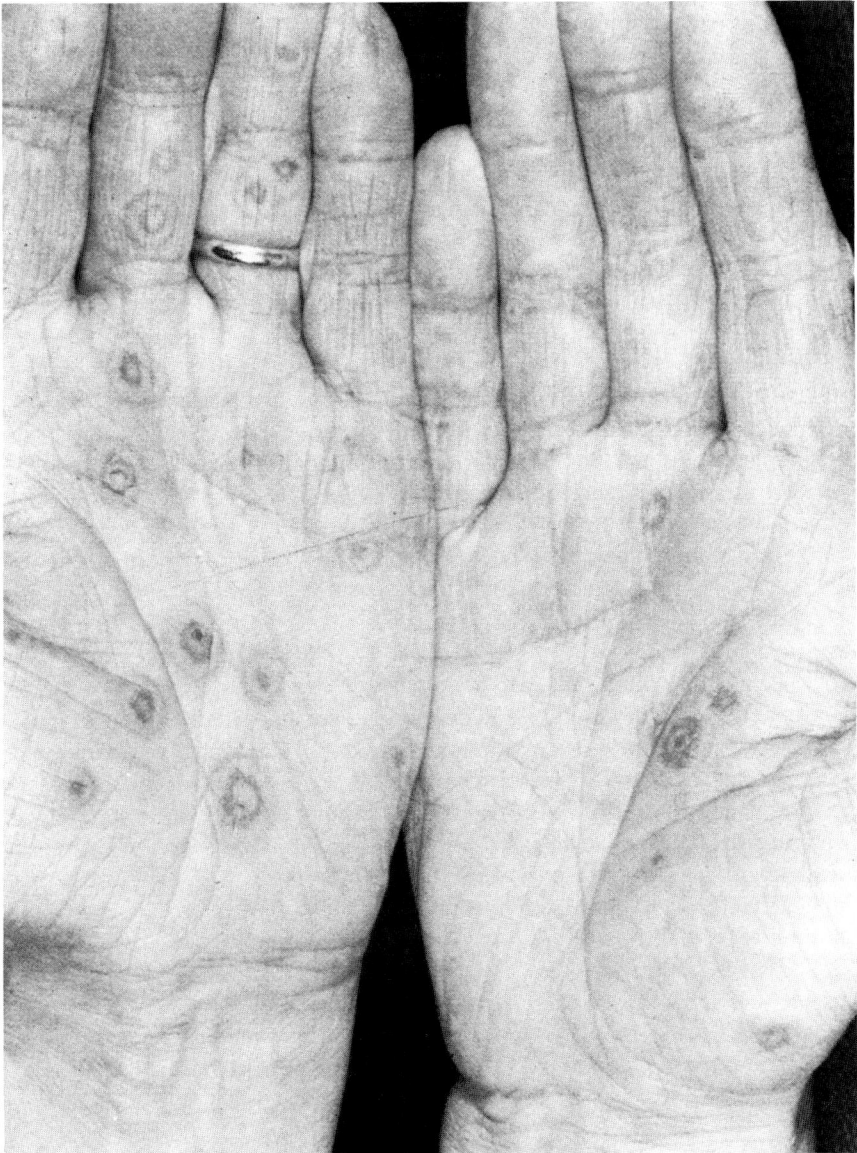

FIGURE 7 Erythema multiforme (target lesions) involving the hands; secondary to sulfonamides.

usually require discontinuation of the drug. With pentamadine or Fansidar (pyrimethamine sulfadoxine) therapy, no increased incidence of adverse reactions has been reported.[27,28] Adverse cutaneous reactions due to the sulfonamides are thought to be immunologically mediated. The reactions have a rapid onset and return immediately after readministration of the drug. Caution and close follow-up are, therefore, warranted when sulfonamides are given to patients with HTLV-III/LAV infection.

Suramin, an inhibitor of HTLV-III/LAV replication, has caused self-limiting photoeruptions associated with burning sensations.[29]

Primary HTLV-III/LAV Infection

A febrile illness of sudden onset associated with anorexia, nausea, myalgia, arthralgia, headache, diarrhea, lymphadenopathy, acute encephalopathy, meningitis, seizures, maculopapular skin eruptions, and urticaria has been described in patients acutely infected with HTLV-III/LAV (Fig. 8).[3,30,31] The illness lasts approximately 2 weeks and is temporally related to seroconversion to HTLV-III/LAV. The early recognition of this syndrome may permit effective therapy before immunological abnormalities have occurred.

Seborrheic Dermatitis

Seborrheic dermatitis is a chronic dermatological disorder of unknown etiology. Patients usually present with greasy-yellowish scales on an erythematous base on the scalp, eyebrows, nasolabial folds, ears, and infraorbital areas. It may also affect the axillae, chest, and groin. In contrast to the usual mild appearance of seborrheic dermatitis, patients with HTLV-III/LAV infection tend to have thicker, greasier scales, giving the appearance of more severe disease. Seborrheic dermatitis in a butterfly pattern on the face is a striking finding (Fig. 9).[32] Numerous organisms have been implicated in the etiology of seborrheic dermatitis, such as *Pityrosporum*, aerobic cocci, and *Corynebacterium acnes*. The population of microorganisms in the areas involved with seborrheic dermatitis is denser than in other parts of the body. The eruption may be related to uninhibited fungal or bacterial growth.

Oral Hairy Leukoplakia

A new form of oral leukoplakia, principally on the lateral borders of the tongue, occurs in patients with HTLV-III/LAV disease.[33,34] Most patients present with white areas on the tongue and, occasionally, of the buccal mucosa (Fig. 10). The areas are slightly raised, a few millimeters in height, poorly demarcated, and

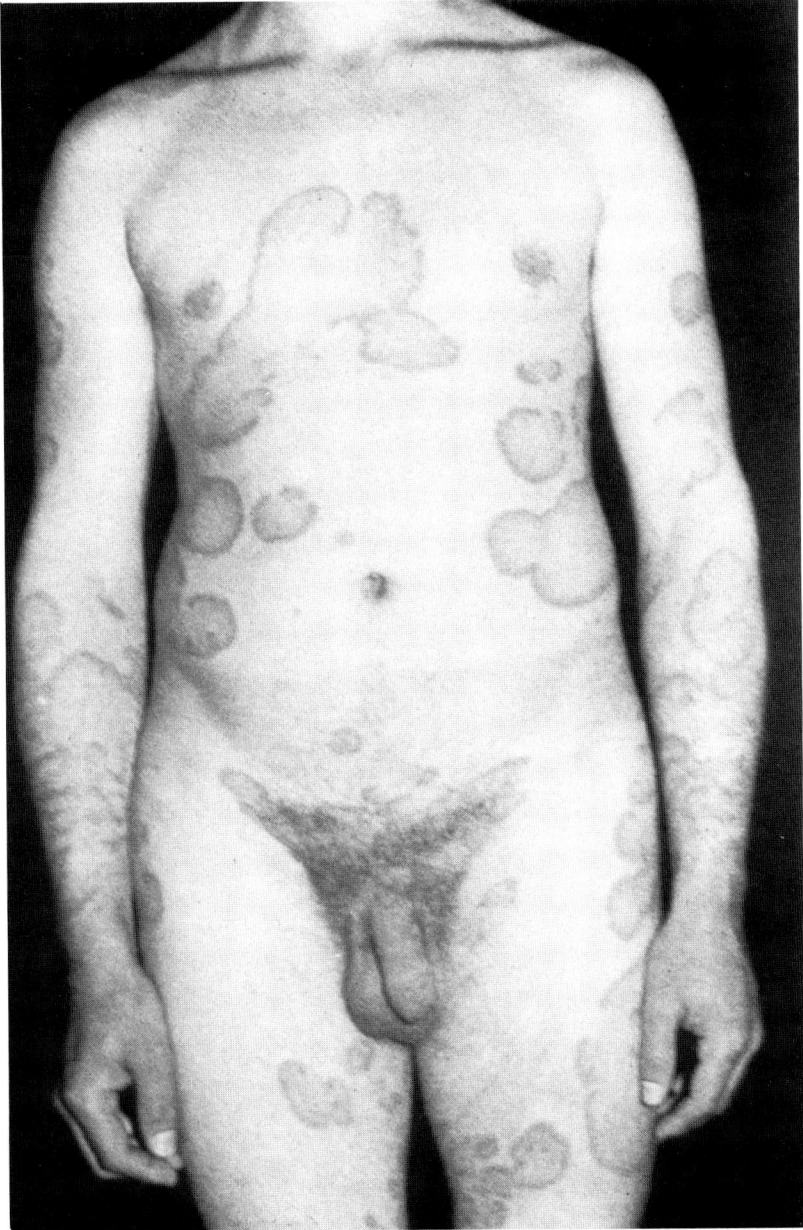

FIGURE 8 Urticarial eruption of primary HTLV-III/LAV infection.

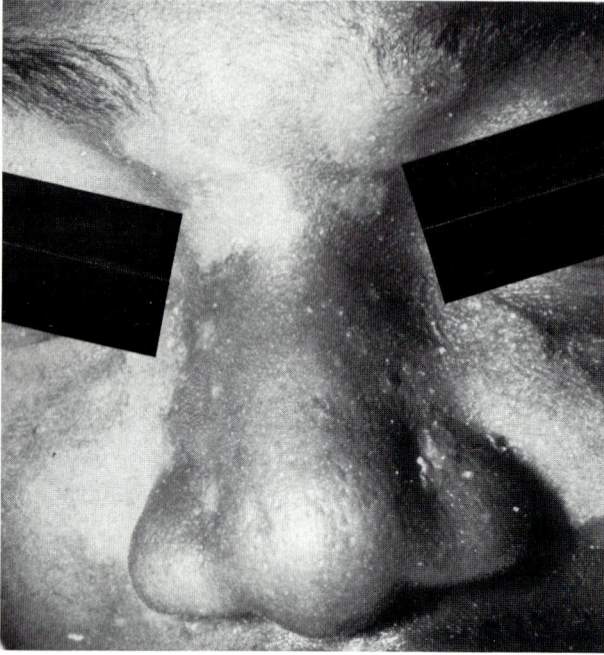

FIGURE 9   Seborrheic dermatitis; butterfly pattern on the face.

have a hairy surface. The histopathology is consistent, distinctive, and unlike that of any previously defined oral white lesion, but does, however, resemble that of warts. Oral hairy leukoplakia has been identified almost exclusively in male homosexuals with HTLV-III/LAV infection. Ninety-nine percent of serum specimens studied revealed the presence of HTLV-III/LAV antibodies. Twenty-five percent of patients with oral hairy leukoplakia went on to develop AIDS over a 3-year period. Laboratory studies utilizing electron microscopy and immunocytochemistry have revealed papilloma virus core antigen in the involved tissue in the majority of patients tested. Herpes-type viral particles have also been seen by electron microscopy, and immunofluorescence studies have revealed a high incidence of intense nuclear-staining of epithelial cells for the viral antigen of Epstein-Barr virus. During DNA hybridization utilizing EBV molecular probes, Southern blots demonstrated EBV DNA in all specimens. The evidence suggests that Epstein-Barr virus is actively replicating within the epithelial cells of oral hairy leukoplakia tissue.

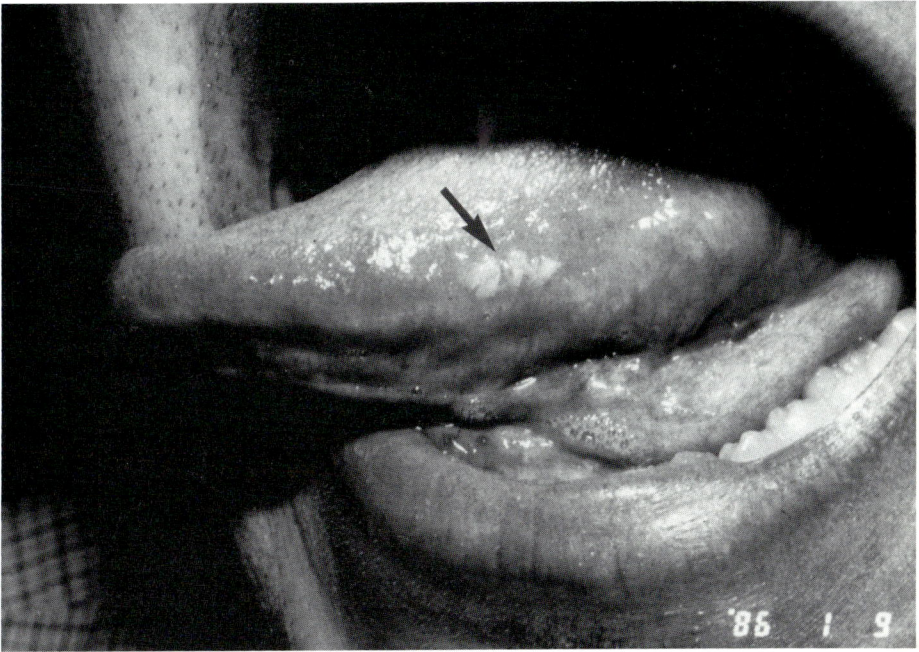

FIGURE 10 Oral "hairy" leukoplakia of the tongue.

Granuloma Annulare-like Eruption

Patients with HTLV-III/LAV infection have presented with multiple-grouped papules on the trunk and neck that mimic granuloma annulare.[35] Biopsy specimens of these papules reveal a histological picture indistinguishable from granuloma annulare. A number of such patients have now been described.

Summary

Clearly, thorough dermatological assessments at regular intervals are an important part of the management of patients with HTLV-III/LAV disease. When present in patients at high risk for HTLV-III/LAV infection (homosexual men, intravenous drug addicts, hemophiliacs), these dermatological disorders should alert the clinician to the possible diagnosis of an HTLV-III/LAV-associated disorder.

Acknowledgments

We wish to thank Phillip Frost, M.D. for helpful discussions and critical review of the manuscript. We are indebted to Neal Penneys, M.D. for providing valuable clinical photographs. We also thank Donna Herbst and Maggi Mackle for technical assistance. This chapter was supported in part by the Key Pharmaceutical Medical Research and Education Foundation, Inc.

References

1. Freidman-Kien AE, Laubenstein LJ, Rubinstein P, Buimovici-Klein E, Marmor M, Stahl R, Spigland I, Kim KS, Zolla-Pazner S. Disseminated Kaposi's sarcoma in homosexual men. Ann Intern Med 1982; 96:693–700.

2. Centers for Disease Control. Kaposi's sarcoma and pneumocystis pneumonia among homosexual men—New York City and California. MMWR 1981; 30:305–308.

3. Ho DD, Sarngadharan MG, Resnick L, DiMarzo-Veronese F, Rota TR, Hirsch MS. Primary human T-lymphotropic virus type III (HTLV-III) infection. Ann Intern Med 1985; 103:880–883.

4. Fauci AS, Masur H, Gelman EP, Markham PD, Hahn BH, Lane CH. The acquired immunodeficiency syndrome: an update. Ann Intern Med 1985; 102:800–813.

5. Hatcher VA. Mucocutaneous infections in acquired immunodeficiency syndrome. In: Friedman-Kien AE, Laubenstein LJ, eds. AIDS: the epidemic of Kaposi's sarcoma and opportunistic infections. New York: Masson Publishing 1984; 245–251.

6. Belsito DV, Sanchez MR, Baer RL, Valentine F, Thorbecke GJ. Reduced Langerhans cell Ia antigen and ATPase activity in patients with the acquired immunodeficiency syndrome. N Engl J Med 1984; 310:1279–1282.

7. Siegal FP, Lopez C, Hammer GS, Brown AE, Kornfeld SJ, Gold J, Hassett J, Hirschman SZ, Cunningham-Rundles C, Adelsberg BR, Parham DM, Siegal M, Cunningham-Rundles S, Armstrong D. Severe acquired immunodeficiency in male homosexuals manifested by chronic perianal ulcerative herpes simplex lesions. N Engl J Med 1981; 305:1439–1444.

8. Goodell SE, Quinn TC, Mkrtichian E, Schuffler MD, Holms KK, Corey L. Herpes simplex virus proctitis in homosexual men. N Engl J MEd 1983; 308:868–871.

9. Cone PA, Schiffman MA. Herpes zoster and the acquired immunodeficiency syndrome. Ann Intern Med 1984; 100:462.

10. Lombardo PC. Molluscum contagiosum and the acquired immunodeficiency syndrome. Arch Dermatol 1985; 121:834–835.

11. Webster SB. Dermatologic diseases of the sexual revolution. Primary Care 1983; 10:429–441.

12. Klein RS, Harris CA, Small CB, Moll B, Lessor M, Friedland GH. Oral candidiasis in high-risk patients as the initial manifestation of the acquired immunodeficiency syndrome. N Engl J Med 1984; 311:354–358.

13. Rook A, Woods B. Cutaneous cryptococcosis. Br J Dermatol 1962; 74:43–49.

14. Studdard J, Sneed WF, Taylor MR, Campbell GD. Cutaneous histoplasmosis. Am Rev Respir Dis 1976; 113:689–693.
15. Penneys NS, Hicks B. Unusual cutaneous lesions associated with acquired immunodeficiency syndrome. J Am Acad Dermatol 1985; 13:845–852.
16. Schoeppel SL, Hoppe RT, Dorfman RF, Horning SJ, Collier AC, Chew TG, Weis LM. Hodgkin's disease in homosexual men with generalized lymphadenopathy. Ann Intern Med 1985; 102:68–70.
17. Levine A, Parkash SG, Meyer PR, Burkes RL, Ross R, Dworsky RD, Krailo M, Parker JW, Lukes RJ Rasheed S. Retrovirus and malignant lymphoma in homosexual men. JAMA 1985; 254:1921–1925.
18. Ziegler JL, Drew WL, Miner RC, Mintz L, Rosenbaum E, Gershow J, Shillitoe E, Beckstead J, Casavant C, Yamamoto K. Outbreak of Burkitt's-like lymphoma in homosexual men. Lancet 1982; ii:631–633.
19. Purtillo DT. Immune deficiency predisposing to Epstein-Barr virus-induced lymphoproliferative diseases: the x-linked lymphoproliferative syndrome as a model. Adv Cancer Res 1981; 34:279–312.
20. Sonnabend J, Witkin SS, Purtillo DT. Acquired immunodeficiency syndrome, opportunistic infections, and malignancies in male homosexuals: a hypothesis of etiologic factors in pathogenesis. JAMA 1983; 249:2370–2374.
21. Cooper HS, Patchefsy AS, Marks G. Cloacogenic carcinoma of the anorectum in homosexual men. An observation of four cases. Dis Col Rect 1979: 22:557–558.
22. Maize JC. Skin cancer in immunosuppressed patients. JAMA 1977; 237:1857–1858.
23. Marshall V. Premalignant and malignant skin tumors in immunosuppressed patients. Transplantation 1974; 17:272–275.
24. Purtillo DT. Viruses, tumors and immune deficiency. Lancet 1982; i:684.
25. Jick H. Adverse reactions to trimethoprim-sulfamethoxazole in hospitalized patients. Rev Inf Dis 1982; 4:426–428.
26. Jaffe HS, Abrams DJ, Ammann AJ, Lewis BJ, Golden JA. Complications of cotrimoxazole in treatment of AIDS-associated pneumocystis carinii pneumonia in homosexual men. Lancet 1983; ii:1109–1111.
27. Gordon FM, Simon GL, Wofsy CB, Mills J. Adverse reactions to trimethoprim-sulfamethoxazole in patients with acquired immunodeficiency syndrome. Ann Intern Med 1984; 100:495–499.
28. Gottlieb MS, Young LS. Adverse reactions to pyrimethamine-sulfadoxine in context of AIDS. Lancet 1985; i:1389.
29. Broder S, Yarchoan R, Collins JM, Lane HC, Markham PD, Klecker RW, Redfield RR, Mitsuya H, Hoth DF, Gelman E, Groopman JE, Resnick L, Gallo RC, Myers CE, Fauci AS. Effects of suramin on HTLV-III/LAV infection presenting as Kaposi's sarcoma or AIDS-related complex: clinical pharmacology and suppression of virus replication in vivo. Lancet 1985; ii:627–630.
30. Cooper DA, Gold J, Maclean P, Donovan B, Finlayson R, Barnes TG, Michelmore HM, Brooke P, Penny R. Acute AIDS retrovirus infection. Lancet 1985; i:537–540.
31. Carne CA, Tedder RS, Smith A, Sutherland S, Elkington SG, Daly HM, Preston FE, Craske J. Acute encephalopathy coincident with seroconversion for anti-HTLV-III. Lancet 1985; ii:1206–1208.

32. Eisenstat BA, Wormser GP. Seborrheic dermatitis and butterfly rash in AIDS. N Engl J Med 1984; 311:189.

33. Greenspan D, Greenspan JS, Conant M, Peterson V, Silverman S, DeSouza Y. Oral "hairy" leukoplakia in male homosexuals: evidence of association with both papilloma virus and a herpes-group virus. Lancet 1984; ii:831–834.

34. Greenspan JS, Greenspan D, Lennette ET, Abrams DI, Conant MA, Peterson V, Freese UK. Replication of Epstein-Barr virus within the epithelial cells of oral "hairy" leukoplakia, and AIDS-associated lesion. N Engl J Med 1985; 313:1564–1571.

35. James WD, Redfield RR, Lupton GP, Meltzer MS, Berger TG, Rodman OG, Markham PD, Sarngadharan MG, Salahuddin SZ, Gallo RC. A papular eruption associated with human T-cell lymphotropic virus type III disease. J Am Acad Dermatol 1985; 13:563–566.

18

Rapid in Vitro Systems for Assessing Activity of Agents Against HTLV-III/LAV

Hiroaki Mitsuya
Makoto Matsukura
Samuel Broder
Clinical Oncology Program
National Cancer Institute
National Institutes of Health
Bethesda, Maryland

The discovery of human T-lymphotropic virus type III (HTLV-III)/lymph-adenopathy-associated virus (LAV) has intensified two practical lines of research that might potentially lead to control of the acquired immunodeficiency syndrome (AIDS) and a set of related diseases: (1) the development of a vaccine to protect persons who are not already infected with HTLV-III/LAV or who are in a very early stage of infection, and (2) the study of agents active against HTLV-III/LAV that may have therapeutic effect in persons who are already infected.

In this chapter, we discuss our in vitro screening system for agents active against HTLV-III/LAV; provide a review of some important nucleoside analogues—particularly those in the 2',3'-dideoxynucleoside family;[1,2] outline additive or synergistic interactions between certain agents; and discuss our general perspective for antiretroviral drug screening and its clinical application in the setting of HTLV-III/LAV infection.

Development of Screening System for Agents Active Against HTLV-III/LAV

In the long term, it may be possible to design antiretroviral agents to treat patients with AIDS based on a molecular analysis of HTLV-III/LAV (particularly analysis of genes such as *pol* and *tat*-III; see the accompanying chapter by Yarchoan and Broder). However, the search for immediate agents active against HTLV-III/LAV relies upon the development of techniques that permit a substantial number of compounds to be screened rapidly in tissue culture for antiviral activity. In the spring of 1984, after a new pathogenic retrovirus (HTLV-III/LAV) was proven to be the causative agent of AIDS and large quantities of purified virus became available,[3-6] we started to develop an anti-HTLV-III/LAV drug screening system in the Clinical Oncology Program of the National Cancer Institute.

We have now utilized a variety of approaches in the screening of drugs for potential usefulness in HTLV-III/LAV-related diseases (Table 1). In the initial step of screening we perform the HTLV-III/LAV cytopathic effect inhibition assay, in which an immortalized T-cell line (ATH8) (vide infra) that is profoundly sensitive to the cytopathic effect of HTLV-III/LAV, as well as normal cloned helper-inducer T-cell lines, are used as target T cells.[1,2] Purified HTLV-III$_B$ is used in the first stage of our drug screening as a source of infectious virions. HTLV-III$_B$ was derived from a pool of American patients with AIDS and is used as a representative of HTLV-III/LAV in the United States.[5] The HTLV-III/LAV cytopathic effect inhibition assay is discussed in detail in the following section. Other in vitro screening has involved five additional steps.

TABLE 1   Strategy for in Vitro Anti-HTLV-III/LAV Drug Screening

---

1. Protection of antigen-specific helper-inducer T cells against the cytopathic effect of HTLV-III$_B$ (a representative of HTLV-III/LAV in the United States) using normal and immortalized target T cells.
2. Protection of target T cells against the cytopathic effect of different HTLV-III/LAV strains as an additional control for the HTLV-III/LAV-isolate variability.
3. Inhibition of the viral p24 *gag* protein expression in H9 cells, following exposure to HTLV-III/LAV.
4. Detection of HTLV-III/LAV DNA (using Southern blot hybridization) and RNA (using Northern blot hybridization) in susceptible T cells exposed to the virus in the presence and absence of the drug.
5. Inhibitory effect of the drug on viral reverse transcriptase production and release by peripheral blood mononuclear cells exposed to the virus.
6. Effects of the drug on immune reactivities of normal T cells in vitro.

---

1. Assessment of the protective effect of drugs against the cytopathic effect of different HTLV-III/LAV isolates as an additional control for HTLV-III/LAV isolate variability. For example, we test the effects of given compounds against HTLV-III/RF-II, which was derived from a Haitian patient with AIDS. This is the most divergent HTLV-III/LAV isolate at this writing, and differs by about 20% in the amino acid and nucleotide sequence of *env* gene from several isolates, including HTLV-III$_B$.[7]

2. Determination of the inhibitory effect of drugs on viral p24 *gag* protein expression in H9 cells—a line developed by Popovic and co-workers[5] that is partially resistant to the cytopathic effect of HTLV-III/LAV—following exposure to the virus by indirect immunofluorescence assay using murine monoclonal antibody.[8] H9 cells are relatively resistant to the cytopathic effect of HTLV-III/LAV, and one can use the p24 *gag* protein expression following exposure to HTLV-III/LAV as an index of viral infectivity and replication in vitro. It is then possible to assess antiviral effect of the compounds by quantitating the HTLV-III/LAV p24 *gag* protein expression in H9 cells that were exposed to the virus but cultured with drugs.

3. Determination of the inhibitory effect on viral DNA synthesis (using Southern blot hybridization) and viral RNA expression (using Northern blot hybridization) in susceptible T cells exposed to the virus in the presence of drugs.

4. Determination of the inhibitory effect of drugs on production and release of reverse transcriptase (RT) into culture medium by normal peripheral blood mononuclear cells or cultured cells exposed to the virus.

5. Finally, assessment of the effects of drugs on immune reactivities of normal T cells in vitro. In this assay, we use normal cloned helper-inducer T cells to monitor the effect of putative drugs on antigen-induced proliferative response and/or helper activity on immunoglobulin production by B cells. We also use normal peripheral blood mononuclear cells to monitor the effect of compounds on lectin-induced (polyclonal) activation of normal T cells.

Generation of an HTLV-III/LAV Cytopathic Effect-Sensitive T-Cell Clone (ATH8)

The hallmark feature of HTLV-III/LAV infection is a progressive depletion of T4$^+$ helper-inducer T cells. It has been shown that immunodeficiency states in patients with HTLV-III/LAV infection are largely paralleled by depletion of peripheral T4$^+$ helper-inducer T cells and/or decreased ratios of helper-inducer T cells to T8$^+$ suppressor/cytotoxic T cells.[9,10] Therefore, we thought at least the initial steps in the drug screening for anti-HTLV-III/LAV activity should include a system to assess the inhibitory effect of drugs on the cytopathic effect of HTLV-III/LAV. We generated an immortalized helper-inducer T-cell clone (ATH8) from a normal volunteer by cloning a normal tetanus-toxoid specific T-cell line in the presence of human T-cell lymphotropic virus type I (HTLV-I) as described previously.[11] ATH8 was selected for this study on the basis of its rapid growth [in the presence of interleukin-2 (IL-2)] and readily apparent sensitivity to the cytopathic effect of the virus. Clone ATH8 bears several distinct copies of HTLV-I in its genome when assessed by Southern blot hybridization using a radiolabelled HTLV-I probe, but, nevertheless, it does not produce detectable amounts of HTLV-I *gag* proteins (H. Mitsuya, M. Reitz, and S. Broder, unpublished data). Detailed methods for generation of helper-inducer T-cell clones and the HTLV-III/LAV cytopathic effect inhibition assay are provided in the Appendix to this chapter. When ATH8 cells are cultured in a test tube, these cells form a pellet at the bottom of the tube and the pellet size reflects the number of viable target T cells (Fig. 1). Under these conditions, the cytopathic effect is amenable to direct visual inspection. When exposed to HTLV-III/LAV, in the absence of protective drugs, the virus exerts a profound cytopathic effect on the target T cells by day 4 in culture, and by day 10, >98% of cells are killed by the virus and the pellet of ATH8 cells is essentially destroyed. The killing of target T cells can be monitored quantitatively as a function of starting dose of virus particles.[2] When ATH8 cells were used in a 7-day assay, 5 virus particles per cell (10^6 virions added to 2×10^5 target cells in a tube) represent the minimum detectable cytopathic dose of virus. (There is some variability from batch to batch, so standardization of each viral preparation is necessary.) When a nontoxic and potentially effective antiviral agent is added in culture at the beginning of the assay, target ATH8 cells are protected against the cytopathic effect of the virus, and can continue to grow, forming a visible cell pellet comparable to that of virus-unexposed ATH8 cells. These observations can be substantiated and quantitated by counting the number of viable cells with a dye exclusion method. For example, as shown in Figure 1, ATH8 cells are almost completely killed by the virus by day 7 of culture following exposure to the virus (top right). However, the addition of 40 μM 2′,3′-dideoxyadenosine (ddAdo) or 2 μM 2′,3′-dideoxycytidine (ddCyd) exhibited complete protection of ATH8 cells against the HTLV-III/LAV cytopathic effect and enabled ATH8 cells to survive and grow (middle right and bottom right) comparably to the virus-unexposed and drug-exposed control cells (top left). It should be noted that the pellet sizes of ATH8 cells exposed only to the drug (middle left and bottom left) were comparable to that of the virus-unexposed and drug-unexposed cells (top left). The HTLV-III/LAV cytopathic effect inhibition

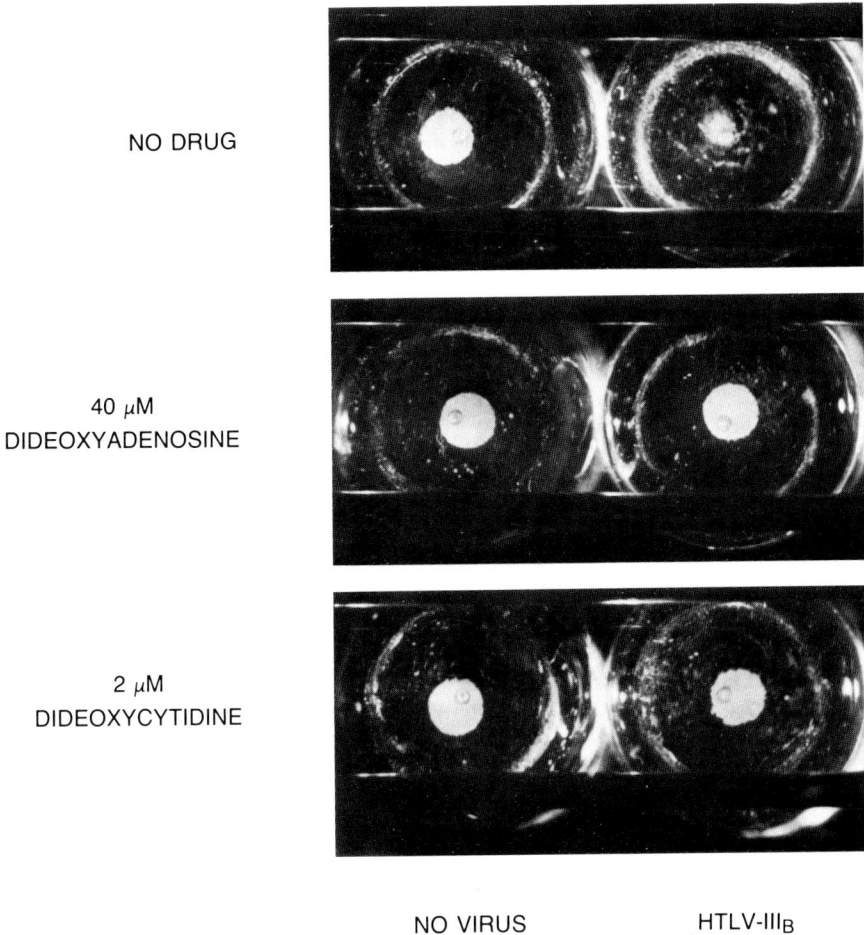

NO DRUG

40 μM
DIDEOXYADENOSINE

2 μM
DIDEOXYCYTIDINE

NO VIRUS   HTLV-III$_B$

FIGURE 1 Cytopathic effect of HTLV-III/LAV on clone ATH8 and protection by 2′,3′-dideoxyadenosine and 2′,3′-dideoxycytidine. ATH8 cells (2 × 10^5) were exposed to HTLV-III$_B$ (3000 virus particles per cell) and cultured in test tubes in the presence or absence of dideoxynucleosides. By day 7 of culture ATH8 cells were almost completely killed by the virus. The cytopathic effect can be seen as a small disrupted pellet which contains debris of cells (top right). In the presence of 2′,3′-dideoxyadenosine or 2′,3′-dideoxycytidine, ATH8 cells were completely protected and continued to grow, which can be seen as large cell pellets (middle right, bottom right) comparable to that of HTLV-III$_B$-unexposed and drug-unexposed ATH8 population (top left). ATH8 cells exposed to only drug (middle left, bottom left) formed large pellets comparable to that of the control virus-unexposed and drug-unexposed cells. (top left).

assay, thus, permits the simultaneous assessment of potential antiviral activity and toxicity of selective compounds.

The traditional in vitro screening systems involve the use of H9 cells. The H9 system requires an immunofluorescence assay or reverse transcriptase assay to monitor the antiviral effects of a putative drug. Harada and co-workers[12] have also observed that HTLV-I-infected cell lines (MT2 and MT4) are sensitive to the cytopathic effect of HTLV-III/LAV, and they developed a plaque-forming assay. The immunofluorescent assay, reverse transcriptase assay, and plaque-forming assay may require some special skills and special equipment. In contrast, the ATH8 test tube system is rapid, is highly sensitive, and is not labor-intensive. It is readily adaptable for mass screening (e.g., in microtiter plates). Moreover, special training would not be necessary on the part of the operator of the test. Thus, in our laboratory development of the HTLV-III/LAV cytopathic effect inhibition assay using clone ATH8 expedited the process of drug screening.

Anti-HTLV-III/LAV Activities of 2′,3′-Dideoxynucleosides

To date, we have screened more than 250 different compounds, including some 120 nucleoside derivatives, for anti-HTLV-III/LAV activity. The structures of many of the nucleoside analogues discussed in this chapter are provided in Figure 2. Recently, we have found that essentially every purine and pyrimidine nucleoside with a 2′,3′-dideoxyribose moiety can block the infectivity and cytopathic effect of HTLV-III/LAV in vitro.[2] Figure 3 illustrates the protective ability of 2′,3′-dideoxynucleosides on the survival and growth of ATH8 cells exposed to HTLV-III/LAV. In this experiment, in the absence of drugs, HTLV-III$_B$ (in the form of cell-free virions) exerted a substantial cytopathic effect and ATH8 cells were almost totally killed by the virus by day 7 of culture (the very left solid columns). In contrast, concentrations >10 μM of 2′,3′-dideoxyadenosine (ddAdo), 2′,3′-dideoxyguanosine (ddGuo), and 2′,3′-dideoxyinosine (ddIno), as well as concentrations >0.5 μM of 2′,3′-dideoxycytidine (ddCyd), completely protected virus-exposed ATH8 cells and enabled them to survive and grow comparably to the drug-treated by HTLV-III$_B$-unexposed control ATH population (open columns). It should be noted that these compounds exhibited a strong antiviral effect at concentrations that were 10 to 20 times lower than those that inhibited growth of the virus-unexposed control ATH8 population. 2′,3′-Dideoxythymidine (ddThd) required relatively high concentrations to exert a protective effect, and, unlike the other comparable dideoxynucleosides tested, its capacity to nullify the cytopathic effect of the virus was lost on day 10 of culture (data not shown). It

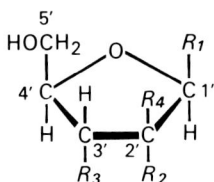

Compound	R_1	R_2	R_3	R_4
2'-deoxyadenosine	adenine	H	OH	H
2',3'-dideoxyadenosine	adenine	H	H	H
3'-azido-2',3'-dideoxyadenosine	adenine	H	N_3	H
3'-amino-2',3'-dideoxyadenosine	adenine	H	NH_2	H
3'-azido-3'-deoxyadenine arabinoside	adenine	H	N_3	OH
2'3'-didehydro-2',3'-dideoxy-adenosine *	adenine	-	-	H
C-2',3'-dideoxyadenosine	adenine	H	H	H
2'-deoxyguanosine	guanine	H	OH	H
2',3'-dideoxyguanosine	guanine	H	H	H
C-2',3'-dideoxyguanosine	guanine	H	H	H
2'-deoxyinosine	hypoxanthine	H	OH	H
2',3'-dideoxyinosine	hypoxanthine	H	H	H
2'-deoxycytidine	cytosine	H	OH	H
2',3'-dideoxycytidine	cytosine	H	H	H
3'-azido-2',3'-dideoxycytidine	cytosine	H	N_3	H
3'-amino-2',3'-dideoxycytidine	cytosine	H	NH_2	H
2'-deoxythymidine	thymine	H	OH	H
2',3'-dideoxythymidine	thymine	H	H	H
3'-fluoro-2',3'-dideoxythymidine	thymine	H	F	H
3'-azido-2',3'-dideoxythymidine	thymine	H	N_3	H
C-2',3'-dideoxythymidine	thymine	H	H	H
C-3'-azido-2',3'-dideoxythymidine	thymine	H	N_3	H

FIGURE 2 Structures of nucleosides tested. The primed numbers (top) refer to positions in the sugar moiety of nucleosides. C denotes that the nucleoside has a sugar moiety of the molecule in a carbocyclic configuration where the oxygen at the apex of the pentagon is replaced with a carbon. *2',3'-didehydro-2',3'-dideoxyadenosine has a double bond between the 2'- and 3'-carbons in the sugar moiety.

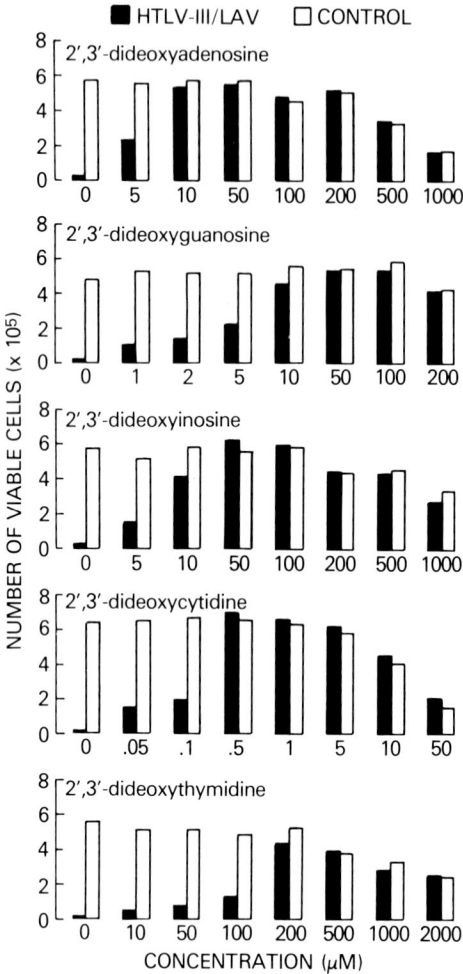

FIGURE 3   Inhibition of cytopathic effect of HTLV-III/LAV by 2′,3′-dideoxynucleo-sides against ATH8 cells. ATH8 cells (2 × 10⁵) were pre-exposed to polybrene, exposed to HTLV-III_B (2000 virus particles per cell) and cultured in test tubes (solid columns) in the presence or absence of various concentrations of 2′,3′-dideoxyadeno-sine, -inosine, -guanosine, -cytidine, or -thymidine. Control cells (open columns) were similarly treated, but were not exposed to the virus. On day 5, total viable cells were counted. (From Ref. 2, by permission of the Proceedings Office of the National Academy of Sciences, U.S.A.)

is worth stressing that it is likely that thymidine kinase (TK) does not act on this analogue of thymidine because comparable amounts of ddThd are converted to ddThd monophosphate in both TK$^+$ and TK$^-$ mouse L cells.[13]

The protective effects of 2',3'-dideoxynucleosides were confirmed in normal cloned helper-inducer T cells (TM3) cocultured with irradiated HTLV-III$_B$-producing H9 cells (H9/HTLV-III$_B$). (H9/HTLV-III$_B$ cells serve as a source of infectious virions, and theoretically both cell-free and cell-associated virus transmission can occur.) When cultured in the absence of drugs, by day 14, H9/HTLV-III$_B$ cells exerted a substantial cytopathic effect on the TM3 population, resulting in a profound decrease in the number of total viable TM3 cells as compared to the virus-unexposed TM3 population. However, 100 μM ddAdo, 100 μM ddIno, and 2 μM ddCyd clearly blocked the cytopathic effect of HTLV-III$_B$.[2]

Furthermore, the anti-HTLV-III/LAV activity of dideoxynucleosides was confirmed by their inhibitory effect on the expression of HTLV-III/LAV p24 *gag* protein in H9 cells (Fig. 4). Following exposure to HTLV-III$_B$ in the form of cell-free virions, by day 10 of culture, 65 to 74% H9 cells were infected and expressed p24 *gag* protein. Ten μM ddAdo, ddGuo, and ddIno, as well as 1 μM ddCyd, however, again exerted potent inhibitory effect on viral infectivity and replication and no H9 cells became detectably positive for *gag* protein throughout the study. As in the cytopathic effect assay, ddThd required relatively higher concentrations to mediate an antiviral effect, and this compound allowed a resumption of viral replication by day 10 of culture (bottom of Fig. 4).

In order to determine whether the 2',3'-dideoxyribose moiety was necessary for the anti-HTLV-III/LAV activity, we explored the capacity of five closely related adenosine congeners [2',3'-dideoxyadenosine, 2'-deoxyadenosine, 3'-deoxyadenosine (also called cordycepin), adenine arabinoside (ara-A), and 2',3',5'-trideoxyadenosine] to block the cytopathic effect of HTLV-III/LAV.[2] These congeners differ only in their sugar moieties. 2',3'-Dideoxyadenosine completely protected the target ATH8 cells against the lysis by HTLV-III$_B$. Neither 2'-deoxyadenosine, 3'-deoxyadenosine, nor ara-A was effective. 2',3',5'-Trideoxyadenosine also failed to protect the cells. These results indicate that at least among closely related adenosine congeners tested, only adenosine with a 2',3'-dideoxyribose moiety has an anti-HTLV-III/LAV activity. It is worth noting that 2',3'-dideoxynucleosides and related compounds such as 3'-azido-3'-deoxythymidine (see the following section) are not new chemicals and in several cases pioneering studies were initiated in the 1960s and 1970s, before human retroviruses were proven to exist. In particular, Robins, Horwitz, Cohen, Prusoff, and others[14-21] have made contributions in studying these nucleosides.

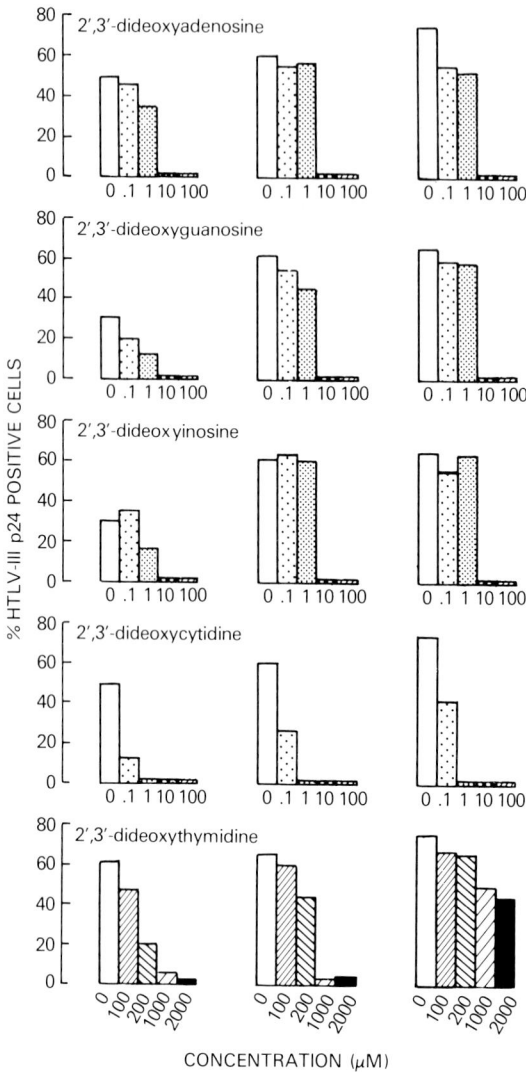

FIGURE 4 Inhibition of the infectivity and replication of HTLV-III/LAV in H9 cells by 2′,3′-dideoxynucleosides for 4 hr and then to polybrene, pelleted, and exposed to HTLV-III$_B$ (3000 virus particles per cell). Cells were resuspended in fresh complete medium and cultured in test tubes. The cells were continuously exposed to 2′,3′-dideoxynucleosides. On days 8 (left), 9 (middle), and 10 (right) in culture, the percentage of the target H9 cells expressing p24 *gag* protein of HTLV-III/LAV was determined by indirect immunofluorescence assay using a murine monoclonal antibody (M26; Ref. 8). (From Ref. 2, by permission of the Proceedings Office of the National Academy of Sciences, U.S.A.)

Inhibition of HTLV-III/LAV DNA Synthesis and RNA Expression in T Cells Exposed to the Virus

In cells infected with HTLV-III/LAV, the virus can be detected as unintegrated and integrated viral DNA as well as viral mRNA.[22,23] It has been shown that Southern and Northern blot hybridization techniques are potentially useful in determiantion of the relative amounts of viral DNA and RNA of the virus-harboring cells and tissues.[23] These molecular techniques enable us to detect HTLV-III/LAV even when the virus is residing in the latent form.

We have asked if viral DNA and mRNA can be detected in susceptible T cells (ATH8) when exposed to the virus but protected by putative drugs. In a typical experiment, ATH8 cells are exposed to the cell-free virions at a multiplicity of 1000 viral particles per cell and cultured in the presence or absence of selective drugs. High molecular weight DNA is extracted at various times and assayed for its content of viral DNA using a radiolabelled HTLV-III/LAV probe. In the absence of protective agents under our culture conditions, viral DNA is first detected by day 2, and a substantial amount of viral DNA is detected on the following day. In contrast, in DNA from ATH8 cells that have been completely protected by effective drugs, neither unintegrated nor integrated DNA is detected. We also ask whether viral mRNA is expressed in target T cells exposed to the virus and cultured with or without protective agents. Figure 5 shows that ddAdo and ddCyd completely inhibited the HTLV-III/LAV mRNA expression in ATH8 cells exposed to the virus. In this experiment, ATH8 cells were exposed to HTLV-III$_B$ (1000 virions per cell), and RNA was extracted from ATH8 cells on days 1, 2, 3, and 8 of culture. Extracted RNA was then assayed for the content of viral mRNA by Northern blot hybridization using a radiolabelled HTLV-III/LAV antisense RNA probe. In the absence of dideoxynucleosides, viral mRNA was detectable on day 2 and was present at a greater level on day 3. The band at 9.3 kb in the blot represents HTLV-III/LAV genomic RNA, that at 4.3 kb represents *env* RNA, and the 2 kb band represents the *tat*-III and 3'*orf* RNA species. In contrast, when cultured in the presence of 50 μM ddAdo or 2 μM ddCyd, viral RNA could not be detected throughout the study. When these cultures were maintained for extensive periods of time in the presence of drugs, we did not detect any viral RNA expression in the cells throughout the 30-day interval of culture (H. Mitsuya, R. Jarrett, M. Matsukura, and S. Broder, unpublished data).

This assay system allows us to assess the capacity of drugs to inhibit HTLV-III/LAV DNA synthesis and mRNA expression in T cells exposed to the virus, and also perhaps allows us to assess the mechanism of the antiviral effects. Our working conclusion is that the dideoxynucleosides can inhibit HTLV-III/LAV at the point of cytoplasmic reverse transcription (vide infra).

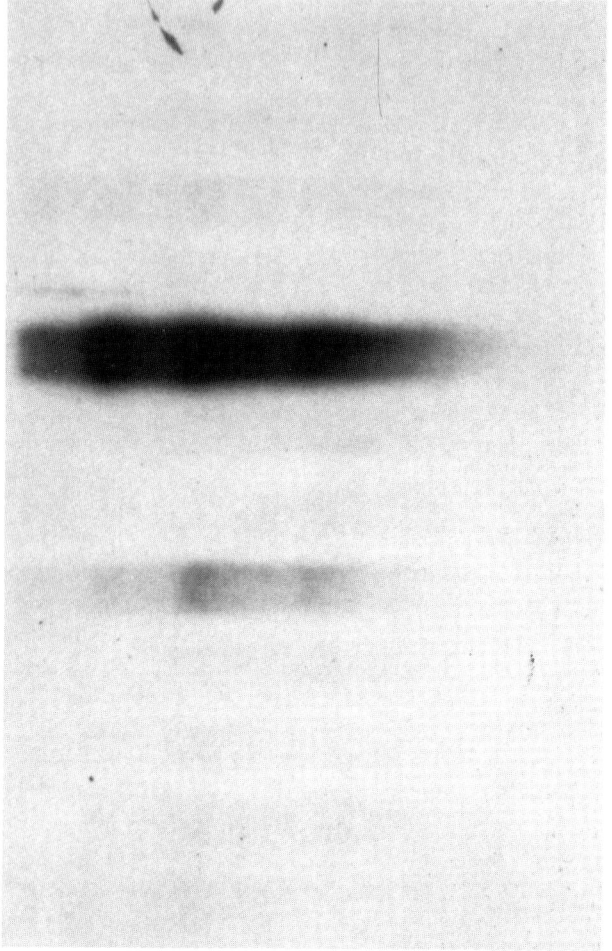

FIGURE 5 Lack of HTLV-III/LAV mRNA expression in ATH8 cells exposed to the virus but protected by 2′,3′-dideoxyadenosine or 2′,3′-dideoxycytidine. 2×10^7 ATH8 cells were treated with polybrene, exposed to HTLV-III$_B$ (1000 virus particles per cell), resuspended, and cultured in the presence or absence of 50 μM 2′,3′-dideoxyadenosine or 2 μM 2′,3′-dideoxycytidine in culture flasks. On days 1, 2, 3, and 8 following exposure to the virus, total RNA was extracted and subjected to Northern blot hybridization using radiolabelled HTLV-III/LAV antisense RNA. The 9.3 kb segment represents HTLV-III/LAV genomic RNA; the 4.3 kb band *env* RNA; and the 2 kb *tat*-III and 3′*orf* RNA species. Control denotes total RNA from ATH8 cells that were not exposed to the virus.

Mechanism(s) of Antiretroviral Activity of 2',3'-Dideoxynucleosides

Figure 6 shows the probable mechanism by which 2',3'-dideoxynucleosides suppress HTLV-III/LAV replication in vitro. When the 3'-carbon of the deoxyribose is modified by certain substitutions, it is not possible to form normal 5' → 3' phosphodiester linkages which are necessary for DNA elongation in the replication of virus from an RNA form to a DNA form. We have shown that 2',3'-dideoxycytidine is converted to a triphosphate by cellular enzymes,[24] and the triphosphate product is utilized by HTLV-III/LAV DNA polymerase [or reverse transcriptase (RT)] and inhibits DNA synthesis mediated by purified HTLV-III/LAV RT (H. Mitsuya, F. Veronese, M. Sarngadharan, and S. Broder, unpublished data). Certain dideoxynucleosides as a triphosphate form can thus act as DNA chain terminators in viral DNA synthesis, although this need not be the only mechanism for antiretroviral activity. It has been shown that the 5'-triphosphate products of ddAdo, ddGuo, ddCyd, and ddThd can rather easily inhibit mammalian DNA polymerases beta, gamma, as well as viral reverse transcriptase of animal retroviruses, but not mammalian DNA polymerase alpha;[13] and a similar observation has been made by us with HTLV-III/LAV (H. Mitsuya, Z. Spigelman, F. Veronese, R. McCaffrey, M. Sarngadharan, and S. Broder, unpublished observations). DNA polymerase alpha is assumed to be the key DNA synthetic enzyme for DNA replication during cell growth, and it also has a role in DNA repair.[13,25-29] These four dideoxynucleosides have rather negligible short-term effects on the growth of cultured mammalian cells.[13] Indeed, at concentrations that suppressed the replication of the virus, virtually all dideoxynucleosides we tested failed to affect the growth and function of normal T cells except at very high doses.[2]

We believe 2',3'-dideoxynucleosides can potentially have an effect against virtually any retrovirus. Recently we have learned that two dideoxynucleosides, ddCyd and 3'-azido-3'-deoxythymidine (an azido derivtive of ddThd), block the infectivity of HTLV-I against normal helper-inducer T cells (S. Matsushita, H. Mitsuya, M. Reitz, and S. Broder, unpublished data). We have also observed that 2',3'-dideoxynucleosides can block the replication of animal lentiviruses (which are believed to be closely related to HTLV-III/LAV in their characteristics and nucleotide sequences),[30,31] such as caprine arthritis-encephalitis virus and equine infectious anemia virus, as well as the focus formation induced by a transforming murine type C retrovirus, Kirsten murine sarcoma virus (J. Dahlberg, H. Mitsuya, S. Broder, and S. Aaronson, unpublished data). These properties, taken together, suggest that at least some dideoxynucleosides are attractive candidates for further development for treatment of human retrovirus-related diseases and may also have important potential in veterinary medicine.

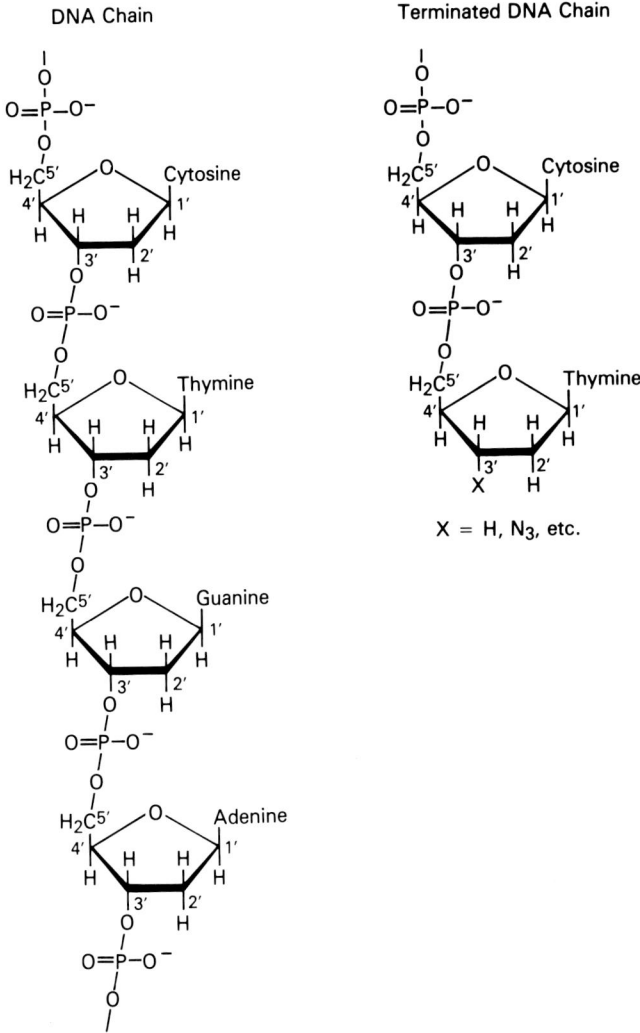

FIGURE 6 Possible mechanism of activity against HTLV-III/LAV of 2′,3′-dideoxy-nucleosides and its derivatives as triphosphate products. When the 3′-carbon of the deoxyribose is modified by certain substitutions (shown by X in right panel), it is not possible to form normal 5′ → 3′ phosphodiester linkages that are necessary for DNA elongation in the replication of the virus from an RNA form to a DNA form. 2′,3′-dideoxynucleosides enter cells, are converted to a triphosphate form by cellular enzymes, are utilized by reverse transcriptase, and act as DNA-chain terminators in the viral DNA synthesis.

TABLE 2 In Vitro Anti-HTLV-III/LAV Activity of Various Nucleosides[a]

Compound	Concentrations (μM)	Protective effect (%)[b]	Cytotoxicity (%)[c]
Adenosine analogues			
2′,3′-dideoxyadenosine	5, 50, 100	25, 99, 101	0, 0, 0
2′,3′-didehydro-2′,3′-dideoxy- adenosine	5, 50, 100	22, 57, 0	5, 47, 99
3′-azido-2′,3′-dideoxyadenosine	5, 10, 100	91, 125, 18	0, 0, 65
3′-amino-2′,3′-dideoxyadenosine	5, 50, 100	4, 11, 3	0, 54, 79
3′-azido-3′-deoxyadenine- arabinoside	5,10	37,30	0,15
C-2′,3′,-dideoxyadenosine[d]	5, 50, 100	12, 20, 26	12, 67, 73
2′-deoxyadenosine	5, 50, 100	5, 4, 4,	0, 1, 16
Guanosine analogues			
2′,3′-dideoxyguanosine	5, 50, 100	85, 104, 80	5, 8, 23
C-2′,4FT-dideoxyguanosine[d]	5, 50, 100	13, 21, 29	2, 25, 56
2′-deoxyguanosine	5, 50, 100	0, 0, 0	0, 55, 71
Inosine analogues			
2′,3′-dideoxyinosine	5, 50, 100	12, 110, 112	0, 0, 0
2′-deoxyinosine	5, 50, 100	0, 0, 0	0, 0, 38
Cytidine analogues			
2′,3′-dideoxycytidine	0.1, 1, 10	12, 119, 96	0, 0, 4
3′-azido-2′,3′-dideoxycytidine	0.2, 2, 20	2, 6, 17	0, 4, 23
3′-amino-2′,3′-dideoxycytidine	0.2, 2, 20	0, 0, 4	27, 70, 82
2′-deoxycytidine	0.1, 1, 10	0, 0, 0	0, 0, 20
Thymidine analogues			
2′,3′-dideoxythymidine	50, 200, 1,000	9, 76, 46	9, 7, 41
3′-azido-2′,3′-dideoxythymidine	1, 5, 50	78, 98, 47	3, 11, 50
3′-fluoro-2′,3′-dideoxythymidine	1, 5, 50	23, 40, 22	41, 65, 77
C-2′,3′-dideoxythymidine[d]	5, 200, 1,000	9, 4, 0	0, 18, 48
C-3′-azido-2′,3′-dideoxy- thymidine[d]	1, 7, 30	0, 5, 0	10, 0, 3
2′-deoxythymidine	50, 200, 1,000	3, 0, 0	4, 42, 86

[a]The HTLV-III/LAV cytopathic effect inhibition assay was performed as described in the Appendix to this chapter. Briefly ATH8 cells (2×10^5) were pre-exposed to polybrene, exposed to HTLV-III$_B$ (3,000 virus particles/cell), and cultured in test tubes in the presence or absence of various concentrations of nucleosides. Control cells were similarly treated, but were not exposed to the virus. On day 7, viable cells were counted. Left,

Anti-HTLV-III/LAV Activities of Other 2',3'-Dideoxynucleoside Analogues

We then tested the capacity of a variety of nucleoside derivatives with a 2',3'-dideoxy- configuration to inhibit the replication of the virus using the HTLV-III/LAV cytopathic inhibition assay. The summary of antiviral activity and cytotoxicity of the nucleoside derivatives tested are provided in Table 2. First we tested 2',3'-didehydro-2',3'-dideoxyadenosine (a compound with a double-bond between the 2'- and 3'-carbons of the sugar) because Atkinson et al.[32] have shown that 2',3'-didehydro-2',3'-dideoxythymidine triphosphate is also active as a DNA-chain terminator. 2',3'-Didehydro-2',3'-dideoxyadenosine was moderately protective against the virus; however, this agent was also toxic and the protective effect was lost on day 10 of culture (Table 2; H. Mitsuya and S. Broder, unpublished data). Perhaps this is because certain didehydro-dideoxy derivatives are much less stable than the dideoxy derivatives, as Sanger and his colleagues[33] described.

3'-Azido-3'-deoxythymidine (AZT or BW A509U) is one of the 2',3'-dideoxynucleoside derivatives in which the 3'-hydroxyl (-OH) group is replaced by an azido (-N3) group (see Fig. 2).[15,19,21] We have shown that AZT is effective in vitro in protecting normal helper-inducer T cells against the

---

middle, and right numbers in the column for concentrations correspond to left, middle, and right numbers in other columns respectively. 3'-Azido-2',3'-dideoxycytidine, 3'-amino-2',3'-dideoxycytidine, 2',3'-didehydro-2',3'-dideoxyadenosine, and 3'-fluoro-2',3'-dideoxythymidine were provided by the Developmental Therapeutics Program, Division of Cancer Treatment, National Cancer Institute.

[b]The percentage of protective effect of nucleoside on the survival and growth of ATH8 cells exposed to the virus was determined by the following forumula: 100 × [(number of total viable cells exposed to HTLV-III/LAV and cultured in the presence of the nucleoside) − (number of total viable cells exposed to HTLV-III/LAV and cultured in the absence of the nucleoside)]/[(number of total viable cells cultured alone) − (number of total viable cells exposed to HTLV-III/LAV and cultured in the absence of the nucleoside)]. By this formula, when the number of viable cells exposed to the virus and drug is the same as the number of viable cells cultured alone, 100% is given. For example, the protective effect and toxicity (vide infra) brought about by 1000 μM 2',3'-dideoxyadenosine (see the top, very right two columns in Fig. 3, which show protective effect and toxicity simultaneously) are expressed as 25% and 70%, respectively. Calculated percentages equal to or less than zero are expressed as 0%.

[c]The percentage of cytotoxicity of nucleoside on the growth of ATH8 cells was determined by the following formula: 100 × [1 − (number of total viable cells cultured in the presence of the nucleoside)/(number of total viable cells cultured alone)]. Calculated percentages equal to or less than zero are expressed as 0%.

[d]C denotes that the nucleoside has a sugar moiety of the molecule in a carbocyclic configuration where the heterocyclic oxygen is replaced with a carbon.

cytopathic effect of HTLV-III$_B$, inhibiting the replication of a genetically divergent isolate of HTLV-III/LAV (RF-II), inhibiting HTLV-III/LAV p 24 *gag* protein expression in H9 cells, and suppressing the production of reverse transcriptase in normal peripheral blood lymphocytes exposed to the virus. Based in part on these in vitro data, a Phase I trial of AZT in patients with AIDS and AIDS-related complex (ARC) was initiated at the National Cancer Institute and Duke University Medical Center in collaboration with Wellcome Research Laboratories.[34] AZT is discussed in further detail in the accompanying chapter by Yarchoan and Broder.

In contrast to AZT, 3'-azido-2',3'-dideoxyadenosine and 3'-azido-2',3'-dideoxycytidine were much less effective against the virus and more cytotoxic than their parental dideoxynucleosides (Fig. 7 and Table 2). 3'-Fluoro-2',3'-dideoxythymidine was also effective against the virus but more cytotoxic than AZT. 3'-Azido-3'-deoxyadenine arabinoside was only partially active against the virus (Table 2). We found that with a 3'-NH$_2$ modification ddAdo and ddCyd became almost completely inert against the virus and became more cytotoxic at the range of concentrations used. (Fig. 7).

Carbocyclic analogues of certain nucleosides (analogues in which the heterocyclic oxygen has been replaced with a carbon in the sugar ring) have been reported to be highly active against certain viruses such as types 1 and 2 herpes simplex virus and vaccinia virus, while the corresponding nucleosides without a carbocyclic structure are not active or modestly active.[35,36] In our assay, however, all carbocyclic dideoxynucleoside derivatives tested (kind gifts from Dr. Y. F. Shealy) exerted much less of a protective effect and greater cytotoxicity at the concentrations used when compared to the parent dideoxynucleosides (Table 2). These data suggest that the heterocyclic oxygen of the sugar moiety (see Fig. 2) plays an essential role for 2',3'-dideoxynucleosides to act as anti-HTLV-III agents.

To date, we have tested some 65 nucleosides that do not have the 2',3'-dideoxy configuration. These nucleosides showed no activity against HTLV-III/LAV. Although the magnitude of the antiviral activity of 2',3'-dideoxynucleoside derivatives varies from one nucleoside to another as described above, our data appear to support the current hypothesis that the 2',3'-dideoxy configuration in the sugar moiety of the nucleoside is closely associated with observed activity against HTLV-III/LAV in vitro.

In Vitro Antiviral Effect of Combinations of Putative Drugs

The use of a combination of drugs may theoretically allow simultaneous interference with multiple steps of the HTLV-III/LAV's life cycle, may lessen

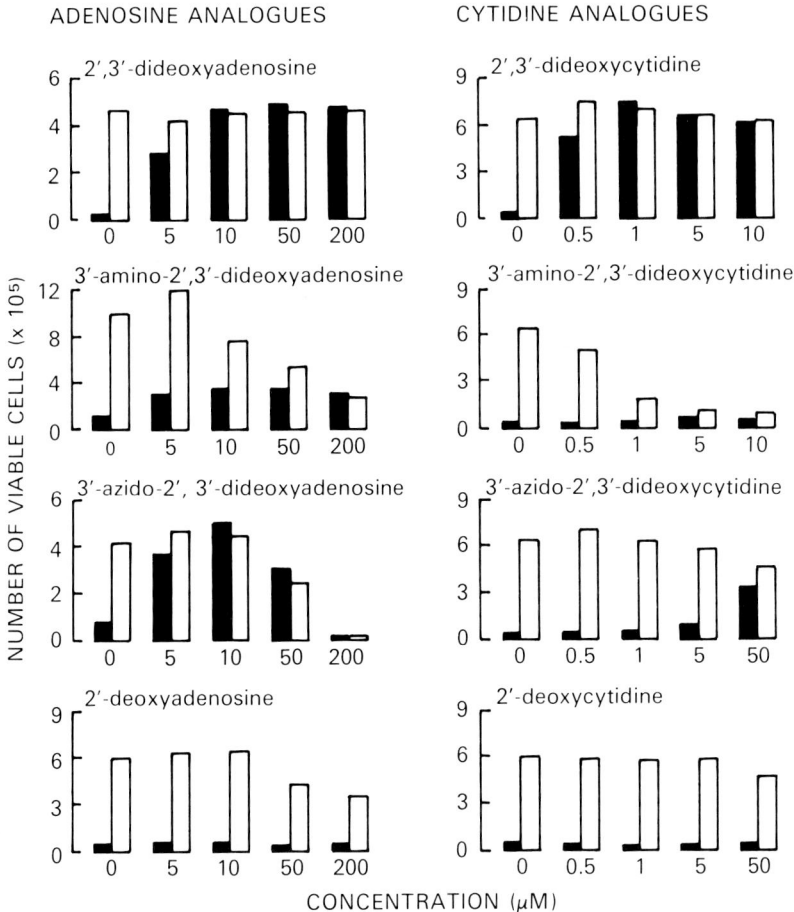

FIGURE 7 Antiviral effect of adenosine and cytidine congeners. ATH8 cells (2×10^5) were exposed to HTLV-III$_B$ (2000 virus particles per cell) and were cultured in test tubes (solid columns) in the presence or absence of various concentrations of nucleosides. Control cells (open columns) were similarly treated, but were not exposed to the virus. On day 5, total viable cells were counted.

the chance of development of viral resistance by mutation, and might forestall certain kinds of toxicity.

For example, we tested the antiviral activity of a combination of suramin (which is the first compound reported to have anti-HTLV-III/LAV activity in vitro)[37,38] and AZT (or BW A509U) in the HTLV-III/LAV cytopathic effect inhibition assay (Fig. 8A). When ATH8 cells were exposed to the virus, in the

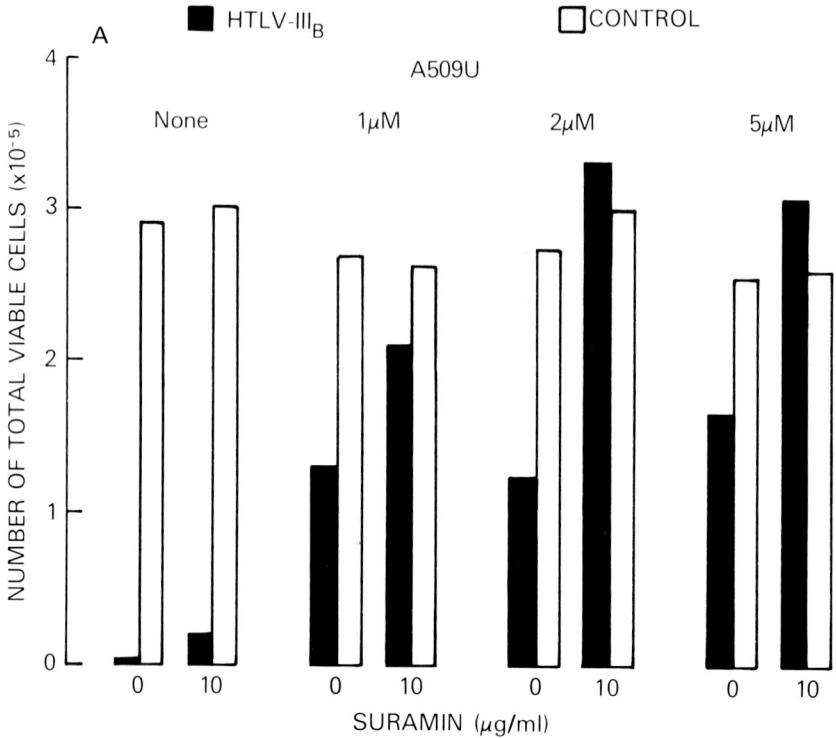

FIGURE 8 HTLV-III/LAV cytopathic effect inhibition by combination of putative drugs. ATH8 cells (2 × 10⁵) were exposed to HTLV-III_B (2000 virus particles per cell) and were cultured in test tubes (solid columns) in the presence or absence of compounds. Control cells (open columns) were similarly treated, but were not exposed to the virus. On day 5, total viable cells were counted. Panel A shows a synergistic antiviral effect of suramin and 3'-azido-3'-deoxythymidine (A509U). Panel B shows a synergistic antiviral effect of acyclovir (ACV) and 3'-azido-3'-deoxythymidine (AZT). Panel C shows at least an additive antiviral effect of 2',3'-dideoxyadenosine (ddAdo) and 2',3'-dideoxycytidine (ddCyd).

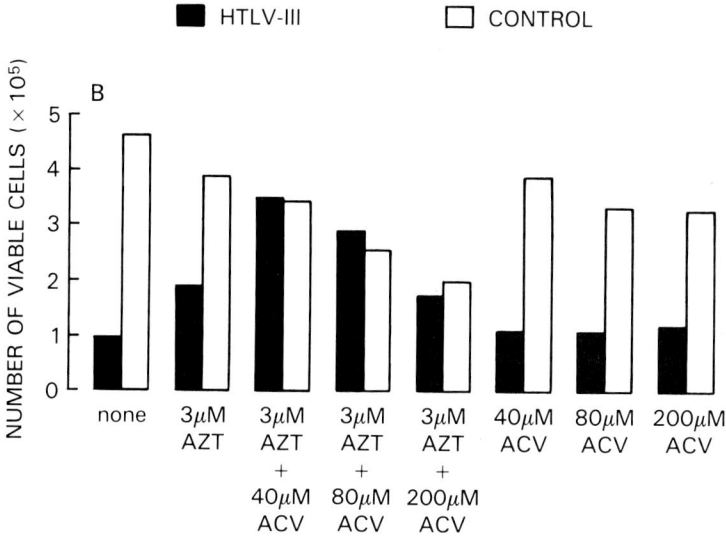

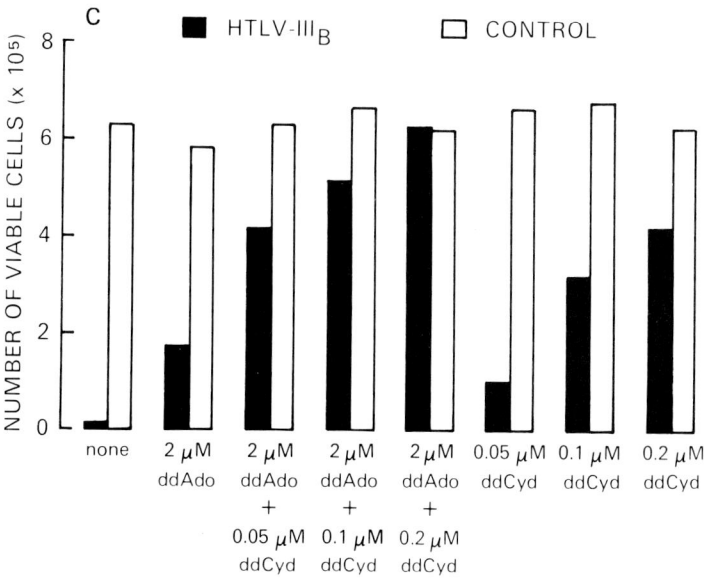

absence of protective agent most ATH8 cells were killed by day 5 in culture. Suramin alone (10 µg/ml) gave only a marginal protective effect. One µM AZT alone also gave a partial protective effect on ATH8 cells. However, a combination of 10 µg/ml suramin plus 1 to 5 µM AZT exerted a more than additive effect on the virus-exposed ATH8 cells without damaging their survival and growth. While suramin does not appear to have a role as a single agent in the treatment of HTLV-III/LAV-related diseases,[39] it is possible that suramin might have a role when combined with other antivirals.

We also have tested whether a combination of AZT and acyclovir could show an additive or synergistic effect on the replication of the virus (Fig. 8B). In our system, at all concentrations used, acyclovir alone did not show any protective effect on ATH8 cells against the virus. Three µM AZT showed a partial protective effect on ATH8 cells when exposed to a very potent preparation of virus. Interestingly, a combination of 3 µM AZT and 40 µM acyclovir apparently exhibited a synergistic effect against the virus. However, it was noted that >80 µM acyclovir with a 3 µM AZT also gave at least an additive cytotoxic effect on the growth of the target T cells. We do not yet have an explanation for the observed synergistic antiviral effect of acyclovir when combined with AZT. Investigation of the mechanism is underway.

We have learned that cell lines exposed to high doses of AZT show decreased levels of thymidine triphosphate in vitro (J. Balzarini, D. Cooney, D. Johns, and S. Broder, unpublished data). It is likely that a pyrimidine starvation results in late drug toxicity in patients. Indeed, in some patients receiving high doses of AZT, megaloblastic and other toxic changes in the bone marrow have been observed. Therefore, if a combination of drugs allows a lesser amount of each drug to be given to reduce drug toxicity, it may permit long-term administration without unacceptable side effects.

We have seen at least an additive antiviral activity without damaging viability and growth of target T cells using a set of two of 2′,3′-dideoxy-nucleosides. We asked whether the combination of a 2′,3′-dideoxypurine and a 2′,3′-dideoxypyrimidine derivative could give additive or synergistic antiviral effects. As shown in Figure 8C, 2 µM ddAdo gave a partial protective effect on ATH8 cells exposed to the virus, while 0.05 µM ddCyd exerted only a marginal protective effect. However, with the combinations of 2 µM ddAdo and 0.05 µM ddCyd, a substantial antiviral effect was observed. The combination of 2 µM ddAdo and 0.2 µM ddCyd completely protected the target T cells without any inhibition of cell growth.

We are also exploring the capacity of thymidine to potentiate the antiviral activity of 2′,3′-dideoxycytidine. When thymidine is converted to a nucleotide (triphosphate product) in a cell, it can allosterically enhance the activity of 2′-deoxycytidine kinase, thereby increasing the anabolism of dideoxycytidine to an active form; at the same time there is an allosteric inhibition of ribonucleotide reductase and this can ultimately reduce the pool of competing 2'-deoxycytidine-5'-triphosphate (vide infra). Thus, the combination of thymidine and 2',3'-dideoxycytidine, at least in vitro, provides an example of potent synergy against HTLV-III/LAV based on an understanding of specific metabolic pathways in a cell (S. Balzarini, D. Cooney, D. Johns, and S. Broder, unpublished data).

Taken together, these results suggest that at least under certain conditions a combination of agents would very likely be useful for treatment of HTLV-III/LAV-related diseases. This area seems to be a fruitful field for future research.

Reversal of 2',3'-Dideoxynucleoside Protection Against the HTLV-III/LAV Cytopathic Effect by 2'-Deoxynucleosides

When nucleoside derivatives are used as therapeutic agents, it is perhaps not surprising that their effect is reversed by the addition of exogenous normal nucleosides. For example, the antitumor activity of cytosine arabinoside (ara-C) can be reversed by 2'-deoxycytidine in vitro[40] and in vivo.[41] We have also shown that the in vitro anti-HTLV-III/LAV activity of AZT could be reversed by the addition of exogenous thymidine.[1]

We then asked whether normal substrates could reverse the anti-HTLV-III/LAV activity of putative nucleoside drugs by acting as competitive agents in vitro. For example, we have tested whether 2'-deoxynucleosides reversed the antiviral effect of ddCyd or ddAdo (Fig. 9). When ATH8 cells were exposed to HTLV-III$_B$ but partially protected by 0.3 μM ddCyd, the addition of an equal amount of 2'-deoxycytidine resulted in a substantial loss of antiviral activity (Fig. 9A). The addition of 1 and 10 μM 2'-deoxycytidine nullified the antiviral effect of 0.3 μM ddCyd. In other words, the normal substrate "rescued" the virus. The protective effects of ddThd and ddGuo were also reversed by the addition of 2'-deoxythymidine and 2'-deoxyguanosine respectively (data not shown). In contrast, the antiviral effect brought about by 2 μM ddAdo (a suboptimal concentration) was not reversed by the addition of even up to 50 μM 2'-deoxyadenosine (Fig. 9B). No reversal of ddAdo could be seen when up to 20-fold higher concentrations of either 2'-deoxyinosine, -guanosine, -cytidine, or -thymidine were added to the culture (M. Matsukura, H. Mitsuya, and S. Broder, unpublished data). We do not yet know the mechanism of failure to reverse the antiviral effect of ddAdo at this writing. Such investigation is currently under way.

These data might conceivably be useful to predict the in vivo effectiveness of antiviral nucleoside derivatives since host cells produce or salvage their own

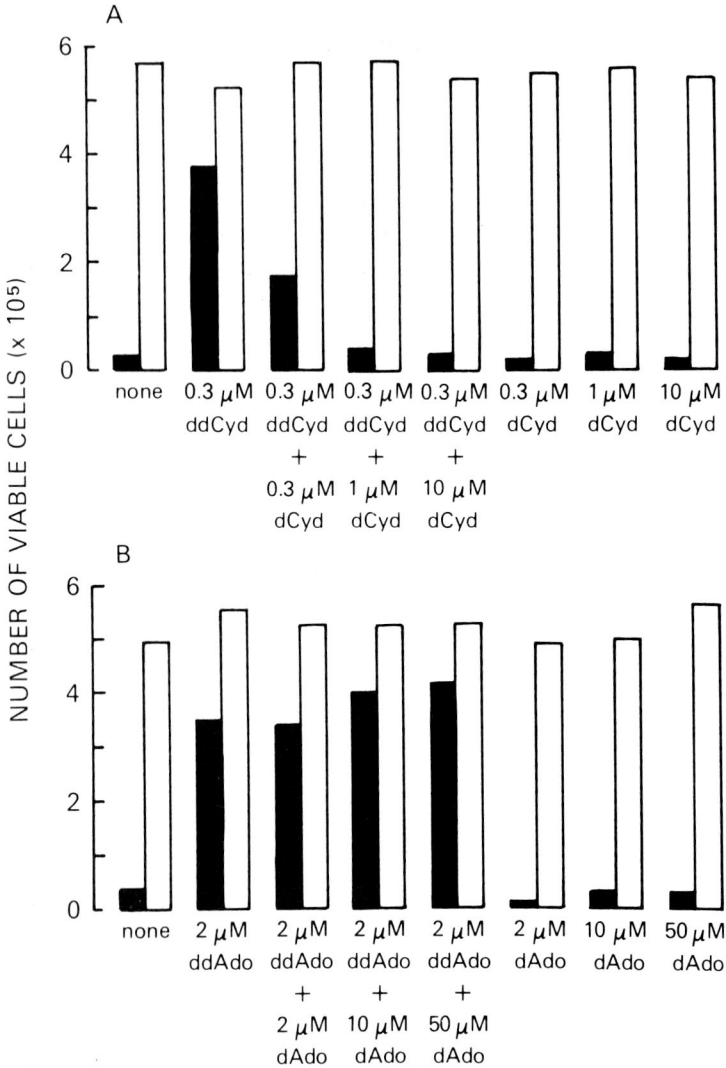

FIGURE 9 Effect of 2′-deoxynucleosides on antiviral activity of 2′,3′-dideoxynucleosides. ATH8 cells (2 × 10⁵) were exposed to HTLV-III$_B$ (2000 virus particles per cell) and cultured in the presence or absence of 2′,3′-dideoxynucleoside and/or 2′-deoxynucleoside. The total viable cells were counted on day 7 of culture. Panel A: Reversal of antiviral effect of 2′,3′-dideoxycytidine (ddCyd) by 2′-deoxycytidine (dCyd). Panel B: No changes in antiviral effect of 2′,3′-dideoxyadenosine (ddAdo) when combined with 2′-deoxyadenosine (dAdo).

"endogenous" nucleosides and the "endogenous" nucleosides might compete with antiviral nucleoside analogues. Moreover, certain levels of nucleic acid precursors are known to circulate in the plasma (although there is a range of values). For example, human plasma levels of 2'-deoxycytidine and thymidine have been reported to be 0.71 μM and 0.75 μM, respectively,[42] while that of 2'-deoxyadenosine has been <0.5 μM.[43] We have quantitated nucleoside and base concentrations in a normal volunteer before and after meal. It was noted that fasting plasma levels of tested nucleosides and bases do not differ substantially from postprandial levels (H. Mitsuya, D. Cooney, and Jayaram, unpublished data). For example, levels of deoxycytidine were 0.8, 0.6, and 0.5 μM in the fasting, 30-min. postprandial, and 120-min. postprandial plasmas, respectively. It is worth stressing that under certain conditions if clinically achievable plasma concentrations of therapeutic agents are below those of normal relevant nucleosides, there might not be a significant effect in vivo.

In Vitro Drug Screening and Clinical Application of Anti-HTLV-III/LAV Agents

Effective anti-HTLV-III/LAV drugs should meet several criteria. A first requirement is sufficient potency for complete inhibition of viral infectivity and replication. In the most ideal case, the antiviral agent may hold the virus in check while the immune system gears up to execute the capacity to eliminate or suppress the virus. In the case of AIDS, however, the patients' humoral and cell-mediated immunity cannot be relied upon to suppress the infectivity/replication of the virus that escaped the drug. If infectivity and replication of HTLV-III/LAV is not sufficiently inhibited, the virus would continue to spread from one cell to another (a process of "internal contagion"), which would result in progressive immunodeficiency. A second requirement is that the drug should have a minimum of toxicity for the host cells and should not suppress the immune reactivity of patients with AIDS. The most important premise of the antiviral treatment of AIDS is that, with the inhibition of the virus's "internal contagion," the uninfected functioning immunocompetent cells grow and restore active immunity in the patient. Under certain circumstances, there will also be a premium on giving drugs to patients as early as possible, before the virus has devastated the immune system. Moreover, the presence of neutralizing antibodies[44,45] might play a role to retard the progression of the disease in the patients with HTLV-III/LAV infection, once a virustatic drug has had a chance to work. Thus, an effective drug should be profoundly active against and highly specific for HTLV-III/LAV, and it should be relatively nontoxic.

Conclusion

In the relatively short time since the discovery of a retrovirus as a causative agent of AIDS and its related diseases, a great deal has been learned about the etiology, immunology, biochemistry, and molecular biology of the retrovirus that causes the disease. Nevertheless, AIDS appears to be difficult to control because of the capacity of HTLV-III/LAV to integrate into the host's genome, to reside in the host in a latent form, and to express heterogeneity in its amino acid and nucleotide sequence. Since AIDS is a widespread disease among risk groups, a vaccine may be appropriate for the control of the disease. The genomic diversity observed is, however, making us less optimistic about an immediate success in development of an effective vaccine. In contrast, in the last two years, more than a dozen drugs have been identified to have anti-HTLV-III/LAV activity,[1,2,37,38,46-52] and chemotherapeutic strategies might have considerable value in attacking this disease. However, these will not be easy undertakings. At least several efficient screening systems for agents active against HTLV-III/LAV have been reported and several drugs identified in these systems have been tested in patients with HTLV-III/LAV infection. One of the highest priorities of the drug discovery effort is to establish a rapid mass-screening system for new antiretroviral agents. We hope that the rapid in vitro screening for agents against HTLV-III/LAV described in this chapter helps focus the search for antiretroviral agents that will be of potential use in the treatment of HTLV-III/LAV diseases.

Acknowledgments

We thank Drs. Ruth Jarrett, Marvin Reitz, Akihiro Yachie, Fulvia Veronese, and M. G. Sarngadharan for their help in these studies, and Drs. Zachary Spigelman, Ronald McCaffrey, Hidetaka Masuda, John Dahlberg, Stuart Aaronson, Robert Yarchoan, Shuzo Matsushita, Jan Balzarini, Erik De Clercq, Takashi Okamoto, Yoshitaka Taguchi, David Cooney, and Dave Johns for helpful suggestions and discussions. We also thank Dr. Robert Gallo for providing HTLV-III/LAV virus and H9 cells; Dr. Piet Herdewijn for providing 3'-azido-2',3'-dideoxyadenosine; Dr. Fritz Eckstein for providing 3'-amino-2',3'-dideoxyadenosine; Drs. Sandra Lehrman and David Barry for providing 3'-azido-3'-deoxythymidine; Dr. Y. Fulmar Shealy for providing carbocyclic nucleoside analogues; and Dr. John Driscoll for helpful advice and critical reading of the manuscript.

Appendix

Generation of Antigen-Specific Helper-Inducer T-Cell Clones

Tetanus-toxoid-specific T-cell clones were generated as follows: 10^6 peripheral blood mononuclear cells (PBM) isolated from heparinized blood of a normal volunteer [who had been immunized with tetanus toxid] were cultured with 2-limit flocculation units per ml of tetanus-toxoid (Commonwealth of Massachusetts Departments of Public Health) in 24-well microculture plates at 37°C in 5% CO_2-containing humidified air in 1 ml of complete media [RPMI 1640 supplemented with 4 mM L-glutamine, 5×10^{-5} M 2-mercaptoethanol, penicillin (50 units/ml), and streptomycin (50 μg/ml)] containing 10% autologous plasma. After 7 days in culture the cells were restimulated with the same concentration of tetanus toxoid plus irradiated (4000 rads) fresh autologous PBM. On day 14 and beyond, the cells were continuously exposed to 15% (vol/vol) interleukin-2 (IL-2, lectin-depleted; Cellular Products) and were stimulated with antigen every 7 days as described above. On day 40 of culture the cells were cloned by limiting dilution. The most rapidly growing clones (T4$^+$ normal T cells) in wells that were plated with 0.5 cells were expanded with 15% IL-2-containing media. These T4$^+$ clones serve as normal target T cells in the screening system. Immortalized T4$^+$ T-cell clones were obtained by cloning a normal tetanus-toxoid-specific T-cell line in the presence of human T-lymphotropic virus type I (HTLV-I)-producing cells as previously described.[11] An HTLV-III/LAV-sensitive T4$^+$ T-cell clone (ATH8) was selected for this study on the basis of its rapid growth (in the presence of IL-2) and readily apparent sensitivity to the cytopathic effect of the virus.

HTLV-III/LAV Cytopathic Effect Inhibition Assay

ATH8 cells are used as target cells without antigen stimulation, while normal cloned T cells (such as clone TM3)[2,53] are stimulated by antigen plus irradiated (4000 rads) fresh autologous PBM in IL-2-containing complete medium 4 to 6 days before assay. 2×10^5 target T cells are pre-exposed to 1 μg/ml polybrene (Sigma) for 30 min, pelleted, exposed to purified HTLV-III/LAV virus (1000 to 5000 virus particles per cell: HTLV-III/LAV was directly concentrated from supernatant of HTLV-III$_B$-producing H9 cells by centrifugation and enumerated by electron microscopy) for 60 min, resuspended in 2 ml IL-2-containing complete media, and cultured in test tube (Falcon 3033) at 37°C in 5% CO_2-containing humidified air. (Each batch of virus needs to be independently standardized for minimum cytopathic effect prior to use). When nucleosides are tested in this system, various concentrations of the compounds are added to the culture following exposure to the virus. When certain compounds that penetrate into target cells slowly or antibodies such as T4 antibodies or possible neutralizing antibodies are tested in this system, target cells are treated with such agents prior to exposure to the virus. Control cells are treated similarly but are not exposed to the virus. In the co-culture experiments, 2×10^5 target cells are pretreated with 1 μg/ml polybrene and are co-cultured with 4×10^5 lethally irradiated (10,000 rad) HTLV-III-producing H9 cells or virus-unexposed H9 cells in the presence or absence of compounds. Cells are continuously exposed to IL-2 and putative drug. At various time points, the viable target cells are counted in a hemocytometer under the microscope by the trypan blue dye exclusion method.

References

1. Mitsuya H, Weinhold KJ, Furman PA, St. Clair MH, Lehrman SN, Gallo RC, Bolognesi D, Barry DW, Broder S. 3'-Azido-3'-deoxythymidine (BW A509U): an antiviral agent that inhibits the infectivity and cytopathic effect of human T-lymphotropic virus type III/lymphadenopathy-associated virus in vitro. Proc Natl Acad Sci USA 1985; 82:7096–7100.

2. Mitsuya H, Broder S. Inhibition of the in vitro infectivity and cytopathic effect of human T-lymphotropic virus type III/lymphadenopathy-associated virus (HTLV-III/LAV) by 2',3'-dideoxynucleosides. Proc Natl Acad Sci USA 1986; 93:1911–1915.

3. Wong-Staal F, Gallo RC. Human T-lymphotropic retroviruses. Nature 1985; 317:395–403.

4. Barré-Sinoussi F, Chermann JC, Rey F, Nugeyre MT, Chamaret S, Gruest J, Dauguet C, Axler-Blin C, Vézinet-Brun F, Rouxioux C, Rozenbaum W, Montagnier L. Isolation of a T cell lymphotropic virus from a patient at risk for acquired immunodeficiency syndrome (AIDS). Science 1983; 220:868–871.

5. Popovic M, Sarngadharan MG, Read E, Gallo RC. Detection, isolation, and continuous production of cytopathic retrovirus (HTLV-III) from patients with AIDS and pre-AIDS. Science 1984; 224:497–500.

6. Gallo RC, Salahuddin SZ, Popovic M, Sherer GM, Kaplan M, Haynes BF, Palker TJ, Redfield R, Oleske J, Safai B, White G, Foster P, Markham PD. Frequent detection and isolation of cytopathic retroviruses (HTLV-III) from patients with AIDS and at risk for AIDS. Science 1984; 224:500–503.

7. Hahn BH, Gonda MA, Shaw GM, Popovic M, Hoxie JA, Gallo RC, Wong-Staal F. Genomic diversity of the acquired immune deficiency syndrome virus HTLV-III: different viruses exhibit greatest divergence in their envelope genes. Proc Natl Acad Sci USA 1985; 82:4813–4817.

8. Veronese FdM, Sarngadharan MG, Rahman R, Markham PD, Popovic M, Bodmer AJ, Gallo RC. Monoclonal antibodies specific for p24, the major core protein of human T-cell leukemia virus type III. Proc Natl Acad Sci USA 1985; 82:5199–5202.

9. Gottlieb MS, Schroff R, Schanker HM, Weisman JD, Fan PT, Wolf FA, Saxon A. *Pneumocystis carinii* pneumonia and mucosal candidiasis in previously healthy homosexual men. Evidence of a new acquired cellular immunodeficiency. N Engl J Med 1981; 305:1425–1431.

10. Broder S, Gallo RC. A pathogenic retrovirus (HTLV-III) linked to AIDS. N Engl J Med 1984; 311:1292–1297.

11. Mitsuya H, Guo HG, Cossman J, Megson M, Reitz MS Jr, Broder S. Functional

properties of antigen-specific T cells infected by human T-cell leukemia-lymphoma virus (HTLV-I). Science 1984; 225:1484–1486.

12. Harada S, Koyanagi Y, Yamamoto N. Infection of HTLV-III/LAV in HTLV-I-carrying cells MT-2 and MT-4 and application in a plaque assay. Science 1985; 229:563–566.

13. Waqar, MA, Evans MJ, Manly KF, Hughs RG, Huberman JA. Effects of 2′,3′-dideoxynucleosides on mammalian cells and viruses. J Cell Physiol 1984; 121:402–408.

14. Robins MJ, Robins RK. The synthesis of 2′,3′-dideoxyadenosine from 2′-deoxyadenosine. J Am Chem Soc 1964; 86:3585–3586.

15. Horwitz JP, Chua J, Noel M. Nucleosides. V. The monomesylates of 1-(2′-deoxy-b-D-lyxofuranosyl)thymidine. J Org Chem 1964; 29:2076–2078.

16. McGovern AM, Jansen M, Cohen SS. Polymer synthesis in killed bacteria: Lethality of 2′,3′-dideoxyadenosine. J Bact 1966; 92:565–574.

17. Horwitz JP, Chua J, Noel M, Donatti JT. Nucleosides. XI. 2′,3′-dideoxycytidine. J Org Chem 1967; 32:817–818.

18. Toji L, Cohen SS. The enzymatic termination of polydeoxynucleotides by 2′,3′-dideoxyadenosine triphosphate. Proc Natl Acad Sci USA 1969; 63:871–877.

19. Glinski RP, Khan MS, Kalamas RL, Sporn MB. Nucleotide synthesis. IV. Phosphorylated 3′-amino-3′-deoxythymidine and 5′-amino-5′-deoxythymidine and derivatives. J Org Chem 1973; 38:4299–4305.

20. Ostertag W, Roesler G, Krieg CJ, Kind J, Cole T, Crozier T, Gaedicke G, Steinheider G, Kluge J, Dube S. Induction of endogenous virus and of thymidine kinase by bromodeoxyuridine in cell cultures transformed by Friend virus. Proc Natl Acad Sci USA 1974; 71:4980–4985.

21. Lin T-S, Prusoff WH. Synthesis and biological activity of several amino acid analogues of thymidine. J Med Chem 1978; 21:109–112.

22. Hahn BH, Shaw GH, Arya SK, Popovic M, Gallo RC, Wong-Staal F. Molecular cloning and characterization of the virus associated with AIDS (HTLV-III). Nature 1984; 312:166–169.

23. Shaw GM, Harper ME, Hahn BH, Epstein LG, Gajdusek DC, Price RW, Navia BA, Petito CK, O'Hara CJ, Groopman JE, Cho E-S, Oleske JM, Wong-Staal F, Gallo RC. HTLV-III infection in brains of children and adults with AIDS encephalopathy. Science 1985; 227:177–182.

24. Cooney DA, Dalal M, Mitsuya H, McMahon JB, Nadkarni M, Balzarini J, Broder S, Johns DG. Initial studies on the cellular pharmacology of 2′,3′-dideoxycytidine, an inhibitor of HTLV-III infectivity. Biochem 1986 (in press).

25. Waqar MA, Evans MJ, Huberman JA. Effect of 2′,3′-dideoxythymidine-5′-triphosphate on Hela cell in vitro DNA synthesis: evidence that DNA polymerase alpha is the only polymerase required for cellular DNA replication. Nucleic Acids Res 1978; 5:1933–1946.

26. Miller MR, Chinault DN. Evidence that DNA polymerase alpha and beta participate differentially in DNA repair synthesis induced by different agents. J Biol Chem 1982; 257:46–49.

27. Krokan H, Schaffer P, DePamphilis ML. Involvement of eukaryotic acid polymerase

alpha and gamma in the replication of cellular and viral deoxyribonucleic acid. Biochemistry 1979; 18:4431–4443.

28. Smoller D, Molineux I, Baltimore D. Direction of polymerization by the avian myeloblastosis virus deoxyribonucleic acid polymerase. J Biol Chem 1971; 246: 7697–7700.

29. Faras AJ, Taylor JM, Levinson WE, Goodman HM, Bishop JM. RNA-directed DNA polymerase of Rous sarcoma virus: initiation of synthesis with 70 S viral RNA as template. J Mol Biol 1973; 79:163–183.

30. Chiu I-M, Yaniv A, Dahlberg JE, Gazit A, Skunitz SF, Tronick SR, Aaronson SA. Nucleotide sequence evidence for relationship of AIDS retrovirus to lentiviruses. Nature 1985; 317:366–368.

31. Dahlberg J, Chiu I-M, Yaniv A, Gazit A, Tronick SR, Aaronson SA. Molecular cloning of equine infectious anemia virus and detection of genetic relatedness to lentivirus and HTLV-III/LAV. Sci Proc 10th Pan Am Veterinary Congress 1986 (in press).

32. Atkinson MR, Deutscher MP, Kornberg A, Russel AF, Moffatt JG. Enzymatic synthesis of deoxyribonucleic acid. XXXIV. Termination of chain growth by 2',3'-dideoxyribonucleotide. Biochemistry 1969; 8:4897–4904.

33. Sanger F, Nickson S, Coulson AR. DNA sequencing with chain-terminating inhibitors. Proc Natl Acad Sci USA 1977; 74:5463/5467.

34. Yarchoan R, Klecker RW, Weinhold KJ, Markham PD, Lyerly HK, Durack DT, Gelmann E, Lehrman SN, Blum RM, Baryy DW, Shearer GM, Fischl MA, Mitsuya H, Gallo RC, Collins JM, Bolognesi DP, Myers CE, Broder S. Administrataion of 3'-azido-3'-deoxythymidine, an inhibitor of HTLV-III/LAV replication, to patients with AIDS or AIDS-related complex. Lancet 1986; i:575–580.

35. Shealy YF, O'Dell CA, Shannon WM, Arnett G. Carbocyclic analogues of 5-substituted uracil nucleosides: Synthesis and antiviral activity. J Med Chem 1983; 26:156–161.

36. Shealy YF, Clayton JD, Arnett GH, Shannon WM. Synthesis and antiviral evaluation of carbocyclic analogues of ribofuranosides of 2-amino-6-substituted-purines and of 2-amino-6-substituted-8-azapurines. J Med Chem 1984; 27:670–674.

37. Mitsuya H, Popovic M, Yarchoan R, Matsushita S, Gallo RC, Broder S. Suramin protection of T cells in vitro against infectivity and cytopathic effect of HTLV-III. Science 1984; 226:172–174.

38. Mitsuya H, Matsushita S, Harper ME, Broder S. Pharmacological inhibition of infectivity of HTLV-III in vitro. Cancer Res 1985; 45(Suppl):4583s–4587s.

39. Broder S, Yarchoan R, Collins JM, Lane HC, Markham PD, Mitsuya H, Hoth DF, Gelmann E, Groopman JE, Resnick L, Gallo RC, Myers CE, Fauci AS. Effects of suramin on HTLV-III/LAV infection presenting as Kaposi's sarcoma or AIDS-related complex: clinical pharmacology and suppression of virus replication in vivo. Lancet 1985; ii:627–630.

40. Chu MY, Fischer GA. A proposed mechanism of action of 1-β-D-arabinofuranosyl-cytosine as an inhibitor of the growth of leukemic cells. Biochem Pharm 1962; 11:423–430.

41. Evans JS, Mengel GD. The reversal of cytosine arabinoside activity in vivo by deoxycytidine. Biochem Pharm 1964; 13:984–994.

42. Dudman NPB, Deveski WB, Tattersall MHN. Radioimmunoassays of plasma thymidine, uridine, deoxyuridine, and cytidine/deoxycytidine. Anal Biochem 1980; 115:428–437.
43. Major PP, Agarwal RP, Kufe DW. Clinical pharmacology of deoxycoformycin. Blood 1981; 58:91–96.
44. Weiss RA, Clapham PR, Cheingsong-Popov R, Dalgleish AC, Carne CA, Weller IVD, Tedder RS. Neutralization of human T-lymphotropic virus type III by sera of AIDS and AIDS-risk patients. Nature 1985; 316:69–72.
45. Robert-Guroff M, Brown M, Gallo RC. HTLV-III-neutralizing antibodies in patients with AIDS and AIDS-related complex. Nature 1985; 316:72–74.
46. McCormick JB, Getchell JP, Mitchell SW, Hicks DR. Ribavirin suppresses replication of lymphadenopathy-associated virus in culture of human adult lymphocytes. Lancet 1984; ii:1367–1369.
47. Groopman GE, Gottlieb MS, Goodman J, et al. Recombinant alpha-2 interferon therapy for Kaposi's sarcoma associated with the acquired immunodeficiency syndrome. Ann Int Med 1984; 100:671–676.
48. Rosenbaum W, Dormont D, Spire B, Vilmer E, Gentilini M, Griscelli C, Montagnier L, Barré-Sinoussi F, Chermann JC. Antimoniotungstate (HPA 23) treatment of three patients with AIDS and one with prodrome. Lancet 1985; i:450–451.
49. Sandstrom EG, Kaplan JC, Byington RE, Hirsch MS. Inhibition of human T-cell lymphotropic virus type III in vitro by phosphonoformate. Lancet 1985; i:1480–1482.
50. Sarin PS, Taguchi Y, Sun D, Thornton A, Gallo RC, Oberg B. Inhibition of HTLV-III/LAV replication by forscarnet. Biocehm Pharm 1985; 34:4075–4079.
51. Ho DD, Harshorn KL, Rota TR, Andrews CK, Kaplan JC, Shooley RT, Hirsch MS. Recombinant human interferon alpha suppressed HTLV-III replication in vitro. Lancet 1985; i:602–604.
52. Sarin PS, Gallo RC, Scheer DI, Crews F, Lippa AS. Effects of a novel compound (AL 721) on HTLV-III infectivity in vitro. N Engl J Med 1985; 313:1289–1290.
53. Jarrett RF, Mitsuya H, Mann DL, Cossman J, Broder S, Reitz MS. Configuration and expression of the T cell receptor β chain gene in human T-lymphotropic virus I-infected cells. J Exp Med 1986; 163:383–399.

Strategies for the Pharmacological Intervention Against HTLV-III/LAV

Robert Yarchoan
Samuel Broder
Clinical Oncology Program
National Cancer Institute
National Institutes of Health
Bethesda, Maryland

Acquired immunodeficiency syndrome (AIDS) was first recognized in 1981 as an unexplained, life-threatening immunodeficiency disorder appearing in certain individuals with risk factors.[1-3] At the same time, a high incidence of Kaposi's sarcoma (KS) was observed in individuals with similar risk factors,[4] and it became apparent that this was part of the same syndrome. Since 1981, the incidence of AIDS has increased in an exponential fashion, and over 20,000 recognized cases have been identified in the United States. In the absence of an identified etiological agent, early attempts at the treatment of AIDS were directed at the clinical manifestations, in particular, therapy for the opportunistic infections,[5] with attempts at immunological reconstitution,[6] and cytotoxic chemotherapy for KS.[4,7] While some of these approaches resulted in transient improvement in certain patients, accompanied by an improved quality of life, none appeared to halt the underlying disease process.

Three years after the recognition of AIDS as a clinical disorder, Gallo and his co-workers at the National Cancer Institute provided formal proof that this disease was caused by a newly discovered exogenous human retrovirus called human T-cell lymphotropic virus type III (HTLV-III)[8,9] or lymphadenopathy-associated virus (LAV).[10] The discovery of this virus has permitted the testing for antibodies to HTLV-III (an indication of prior exposure and probable infection with HTLV-III), and screening of the blood supply in this manner has almost eliminated blood transfusion as a means of spreading this disease. It is now thought that at least one million persons in the United States are infected with HTLV-III and have the potential to develop AIDS. The identification of an etiological agent has also formed the basis for possible development of a vaccine (for persons not yet exposed to the virus) and for consideration of specific antiviral therapy for those who are already infected. In this chapter, we will discuss the rationale for the use of antiviral agents in patients with HTLV-III infection, outline a strategy that has been used to develop drugs with potential clinical application, and report on the status of several drugs that are presently under investigation.

Potential Strategies for the Antiviral Therapy of HTLV-III Infection

To develop therapeutic strategies for the treatment of HTLV-III-induced disease, one must first consider the life cycle of the etiological agent. HTLV-III belongs to the family of RNA viruses known as retroviruses, which replicate through a DNA intermediate (i.e., at one step of their cycle of replication, genetic information flows from RNA to DNA, a reverse or "retro" direction). The first step in infection of a cell by HTLV-III is the binding to the target cell receptor (Table 1). In the case of helper-inducer cells, this receptor is thought to be near or on the CD4 antigen,[11-14] but other receptors may possibly be used by HTLV-III in infecting other cell types. This binding step may be inhibitable by antibodies either to the virus or to the receptor (Table 1). It is known that there is a great deal of variation in the envelope from one viral isolate to another. Alteration in the envelope binding site, however, is most likely constrained by the need to bind to CD4 (which is relatively constant), and antibody directed at this site would probably bind to (and neutralize) most strains of HTLV-III. Thus, monoclonal antibodies to HTLV-III may have a therapeutic role in patients with HTLV-III disease. A potential difficulty of this approach, however, is that lymphocytes are mobile and can make direct cell–cell contacts; binding may thus elude inhibition by antibodies. It has been shown that disease can occur in the presence of neutralizing antibodies to HTLV-III, although whether this occurs because the titers of such neutralizing antibodies are low is a topic for future research.[15,16] After binding, HTLV-III

TABLE 1 Stages in the Life Cycle of HTLV-III That May Be Susceptible to Therapeutic Intervention

Stage	Potential intervention
Binding to target cell	Antibodies to virus or cell receptor; or oligopeptide blockers
Entry into target cell	Drugs (e.g., amantadine for influenza virus) Antibodies to virus or cell receptor
Transcription of RNA to DNA by reverse transcriptase	Reverse transcriptase inhibitors (includes many drugs being studied)
Integration of DNA into host genome	Drugs which inhibit polymerase-mediated integration?
Transcription of DNA to RNA	Inhibitors specific for retrovirus not yet available
Translation of RNA	"Anti-sense" constructs Inhibitors of the *tat*-III protein
Viral component production and assembly	Glycosylation and protease inhibitors?
Budding of virus	Interferons

enters the target cell by a poorly defined mechanism, perhaps by a fusion process. It is possible that drugs may be identified that block this entry step; in the case of influenza virus, for example, it has been shown that amantadine can inhibit viral entry.[17]

After HTLV-III enters a suitable cell, the viral DNA polymerase (i.e., the reverse transcriptase [RT]) makes a minus-strand DNA copy of the viral RNA and, in addition, the same enzyme can catalyze the production of a positive-strand DNA copolymer.[18,19] RT is the enzyme that characterizes the family of retroviruses, but is generally not expressed in normal eukaryotic cells. Because of its essential and unique role in retroviral replication, RT is a potential target for antiviral therapy and, as will be noted, a number of drugs that inhibit RT have been shown to block infection of cells with HTLV-III.

The DNA copy of HTLV-III is circularized soon after its formation, and can either remain in an unintegrated form or become integrated into the host cell genome. At some later time, perhaps after activation of the infected cell, the DNA is transcribed to RNA using host RNA polymerases, and this RNA is then translated to form viral proteins, again using the machinery of the host cell.[19] It has recently been shown that HTLV-III is one of several retroviruses in which a retroviral product (called the *tat*-III protein) markedly enhances the production of viral proteins; unlike other viruses in which *trans*-activation has been observed, the *tat*-III protein is thought to increase translation of the viral

RNA, rather than affecting transcription per se.[20-22] The *tat*-III protein is thought to provide the virus with a positive feedback loop in infected cells by which a viral product can, in turn, increase production of itself and other viral proteins. The *tat*-III product is a small (86 amino acids long) protein with a cluster of positively charged amino acids, suggesting that it interacts directly with viral RNA;[22] it is possible that drugs or other agents may be found which inhibit this process.

One possible approach that may inhibit the translation of viral products would be the use of an "anti-sense" oligodeoxyribonucleotide. In principle, this can be a short sequence of DNA (or DNA that is chemically modified to enable better cell penetration and resistance to enzymatic degradation) that is complementary to a viral segment of the HTLV-III messenger RNA;[23-27] by binding to this segment, such oligodeoxyribonucleotides could potentially block expression of the viral genome through hybridization arrest or possibly by interfering with the binding of a regulatory protein such as *tat*-III. This could be delivered to the cell either directly as an oligodeoxyribonucleotide or alternatively as an "anti-sense" virus (i.e., one that contains a genetically engineered inverted sequence of the HTLV-III genome so that a complementary strand of viral mRNA is produced which "neutralizes" the expression of the original virus).

The final stages in the replicative cycle of HTLV-III involve the secondary processing of viral proteins by cleavage and glycosylation, assembly of the virus, and budding from the cell surface. Interferons have been shown to interfere with the budding of other retroviruses, and may act to interfere with this stage of HTLV-III replication. Other strategies for interfering with cleavage and glycosylation are currently being investigated.

The Disease Process of HTLV-III Infection:
Implications for Antiviral Therapy

Even if one were able to successfully block a particular step in the replication of HTLV-III, clinical improvement would not necessarily result. For example, in the case of another retroviral disease in humans, HTLV-I-induced lymphoma, it is unlikely that antiviral therapy alone would be successful once malignant transformation had occurred. What then, are the features of the pathogenesis of AIDS that may potentially render it treatable by antiviral therapy?

The most important premise on which the antiviral treatment of AIDS is based is that continued viral replication is important in the pathogenesis of the disease. The hallmark feature of HTLV-III infection is a progressive depletion of helper-inducer (OKT4$^+$ or Leu 3$^+$) T cells, eventually resulting in profound cellular immunodeficiency.[1-3,28,29] It is thought that, at least in part, this depletion is the result of a gradual spread of HTLV-III from one cell to another by a process of "internal contagion" and the subsequent death of these cells from the cytopathic effect of HTLV-III.[9,30] It is unclear, however, whether a direct cytopathic effect of the virus HTLV-III can completely explain the immunodeficiency. With available technology (specifically Southern blot hybridization and in situ hybridization), it appears that only a minority of OKT4[+] T cells contain *and* express HTLV-III at any one time.[19,31] (It is worth stressing that HTLV-III can also infect macrophages and B cells under some conditions.) In addition, the existing OKT4[+] cells in these patients do not appear to function normally.[32] Finally, there is recent evidence that a lymphokine produced by the infected cells or a viral product may directly interfere with T-cell function.[33,34] Thus, the direct destruction of helper-inducer T cells and, in addition, secondary factors (and even a true autoimmune phenomenon) may contribute to the immunodeficiency in AIDS once HTLV-III infection has become established in an individual.

Another point to consider is that while most helper-inducer T cells die soon after their infection with HTLV-III,[9,30] a subset of normal T cells may remain infected with HTLV-III in a latent form and produce virus when stimulated at a later time.[35-37] As mentioned, other cells, particularly Epstein-Barr-infected B cells[38] and macrophages (M. Popovic, personal communication) may harbor HTLV-III, and such cells might be somewhat more resistant to the cytopathic effect of the virus than helper-inducer T cells. Thus, while the continuous spread of HTLV-III from cell to cell is probably important in the development of AIDS, long-lived infected cells may provide a reservoir of virus, even in the face of potent antiviral therapy.

Improvement in immune function from antiviral therapy can only occur if the immune system has a regenerative potential in these patients. This will depend in part on the existence of uninfected stem cells, a point which has not been demonstrated, and on residual thymic function. Also, if long-lived virally infected cells are a source of toxic lymphokines in these patients, or if virally-driven autoimmune phenomena contribute to the disease process, immunological improvement may not necessarily occur. The age of the patient at the time of disease development may be one factor determining the level of regenerative capacity that one can expect. Considerations such as these provide a rationale for exploring bone marrow transplantation (and other kinds of cellular replacement therapy) in combination with antiviral chemotherapy.[6] Drs. A. Fauci and H. C. Lane at the National Institute of Allergy and Infectious Diseases are currently pursuing this line of research.

It has recently been observed that patients with HTLV-III infection develop dementia or other central nervous system (CNS) symptoms, and that these are at least partly the result of infection of cells in the CNS with HTLV-III.[39-41]

The brain may be infected early in the disease, in some cases even before immunodeficiency can be diagnosed. Indeed, Southern blot technology has shown that there is more viral DNA in the brain than in any other tissue.[39] Preliminary data suggest that it is the microglial elements in the brain that most readily express the virus (M. Popovic, personal communication).

From a therapeutic perspective, one can conceptualize the brain as an important target for HTLV-III infection in its own right, and a sanctuary for viral escape from therapy. It is not clear if the infected cells in the CNS are quickly destroyed by HTLV-III or are long-lived reservoir cells; in either case, drugs that do not penetrate into the CNS will probably be of only limited usefulness if used alone. Also, it is unclear as to what extent the CNS pathology in this disease may be reversible; even if largely irreversible, however, antiviral therapy may prevent progression of CNS disease.

The ability of HTLV-III to integrate into the host genome and exist in a latent form suggests that antiviral therapy in patients with HTLV-III disease will have to be administered for a long time, perhaps for the lifetime of the patient (at least on an intermittent basis). In addition, the existence of cells that can produce virus over a long period of time without dying[35-38] indicates that agents that block early steps of viral replication (reverse transcription or earlier) may affect a different subset of cells than those agents that act at later stages. For this reason, it is likely that the combination of an early-acting and a late-acting agent may be more effective than either used alone.

Drug Development in HTLV-III-Induced Diseases

With this background, one can begin to appreciate the features that are theoretically desirable in an antiviral agent for use in AIDS and other HTLV-III-induced diseases. As shown in Table 2, effective inhibition of viral replication (either before or after transcription to DNA) and lack of toxicity are the most critical properties. Because it is anticipated that an antiviral agent would have to be given for a prolonged period of time, perhaps the life of the patient, it is essential that the drug be tolerated even over a prolonged period of time. Other desirable features include penetration into the CNS, suitability for oral administration, and a half-life that is sufficiently long to permit sustained plasma levels with a convenient schedule of administration (Table 2).

Although it is less than 3 years since the identification of HTLV-III/LAV as the causative agent in AIDS,[8,9] there are a number of drugs that have been shown to block the replication of HTLV-III in vitro, and several of these have already entered clinical trial (Table 3). This rapid progress has, in part, been attainable because of previous work on identifying drugs that inhibit the reverse transcriptases of other retroviruses. Reverse transcriptase was dis-

TABLE 2 Desirable Properties in an Antiviral Agent for Use in HTLV-III Diseases

1. Effective inhibition of HTLV-III replication at levels that are attainable in vivo
2. Minimal toxicity, particularly after long-term usage
3. Penetration into the CNS
4. Suitability for oral administration
5. Relatively long half-life in the body (at least > 30 minutes)
6. Low cost

covered by Temin and Baltimore in 1972,[42,43] and as retroviruses have been known to cause tumors in certain animals and reverse transcriptase activity was found in certain tumors,[44] it was thought that inhibitors of reverse transcriptase might play a role in antitumor therapy. With this impetus, effort has been directed at identifying substances that inhibit the RT of avian and murine retroviruses.[45-48] In the case of retrovirally-induced tumors, however, it is not clear that continued viral replication or RT activity has a role once malignant transformation has occurred. With the advent of AIDS, however, in which continued viral replication appears to be required for disease progression, there has been a renewed interest in such drugs.

The in vitro screening for drugs with activity against HTLV-III is the subject of another chapter of this book (see the chapter by Mitsuya and Broder) and will not be discussed in detail here. Briefly, the National Cancer Institute has utilized a variety of approaches in the screening of drugs for potential usefulness in HTLV-III disease. One is the determination of whether a drug blocks the cytopathic effect of HTLV-III; an HTLV-I-infected T-cell line (ATH8) developed by Dr. Mitsuya, which is quite sensitive to the cytopathic effect of HTLV-III, has been used for this purpose.[49,50] This enables the simultaneous determination of inhibition of viral infection and a lack of toxicity. Other in vitro screening has involved examining: (1) inhibition of viral protein expression, viral RNA synthesis, and pro-viral DNA formation in susceptible lines exposed to HTLV-III; (2) testing of several isolates of HTLV-III to determine if there are differences in the effect among the isolates; (3) testing for toxicity of the drugs on a variety of lymphocyte functions, including proliferation and antibody production; and (4) testing for changes in production of RT or viral proteins in chronically infected lines, which are then exposed to the drugs being tested. This last test is potentially useful for screening drugs that may act at the later stages of viral replication.

Except for those drugs that have been used previously in humans (e.g., suramin), testing for toxicity in animals must, of course, be undertaken before

TABLE 3 Certain Drugs Being Studied for Possible Use in HTLV-III–Induced Diseases

Drug	Proposed mode of action	In vitro inhibition	In vivo effects	Comments
Suramin	RT inhibition?	25–50 μM	Virustatic; probably no clinical improvement	No penetration into CSF; renal and adrenal toxicity
HPA-23	RT inhibition?	Observed	Virustatic; probably no clinical improvement	Thrombocytopenia; short half-life
AZT	Chain termination	1–10 μM	Virustatic; short-term immunological and clinical improvement	Excellent CSF penetration; induces pyrimidine starvation at high doses leading to megaloblastic anemia and increased mean corpuscular volume of erythrocytes
Dideoxycytidine	Chain termination	0.5–5 μM	Not tested	
Ribavirin	? interference with 5′-mRNA capping	100 μg/ml (partial)	Being tested	Useful in patients with Lassa fever and other viral diseases
Phosphonoformate	RT inhibition	132–680 μM	Being tested	Serum levels of up to 450 μM attainable in humans; acute renal failure can occur
Rifabutine	RT inhibition?	10–100 μg/ml (partial)	Being tested	Activity against M. avium
AL-721	Alters viral binding to cells	100 μg/ml (partial)	Being tested	Lipid compound; likely to have very low toxicity
Alpha-interferon	Unknown Inhibits budding?	4–1024 U/ml (partial)	Some activity against KS	Unclear if activity against KS is due to antiviral activity

any drug that appears to have in vitro action is used in humans. It may, under some circumstances, also be useful to test a drug in animal retroviral infections (e.g., feline immunodeficiency disease or murine retroviral infections) before they are used in humans.[51-53] Many of the drugs that inhibit the RT of one retrovirus will be effective in others, and infection with certain animal retroviruses (e.g., feline leukemia virus) is easier to monitor than is monitoring of HTLV-III infection in humans (see the following section). It should be noted, however, that we do not have enough experience at this point to know how predictive these animal models will be for the use of drugs in HTLV-III disease.

Evaluation of Antiviral Drugs in Patients with HTLV-III Disease

In certain viral illnesses, there is a direct relationship between the replication of the virus and the clinical manifestation of the illness; in the case of animals inoculated with vaccinia virus, for example, the number and size of the pox lesions have a direct relationship to the inoculum used. In the case of AIDS, however, most of the salient clinical manifestations (e.g., opportunistic infections, Kaposi's sarcoma, or lymphoma development) are not directly caused by HTLV-III replication, but instead are mediated indirectly. Because of this, one must undertake the evaluation of antiviral drugs in this disease with an understanding of the disease process and an awareness of the limitations of the tools at hand.

The parameters that one can follow in patients with HTLV-III disease can be divided into three broad categories: clinical, immunological, and virological. In terms of the clinical parameters, one can and should observe the patients for their longevity and for the development of opportunistic infections. In addition, for those patients with Kaposi's sarcoma, one can follow the progression of the lesions. At present, however, it is unclear what role HTLV-III plays in the pathogenesis of KS, and it is theoretically possible that progression of KS could occur in spite of effective antiviral therapy. KS has been observed to develop in certain patients on immunosuppressive therapy, and resolution of the KS has then occurred several weeks or months after the immunosuppression was discontinued.[54] Thus, KS may be affected by changes in the immune system in these patients. In addition, one must remember that the KS lesions may be directly affected by the antitumor activity of a putative antiviral drug.

Many patients with HTLV-III infection have poor appetite, weight loss, low-grade fevers, night sweats, and general feelings of malaise. The fevers and malaise are seen in acute HTLV-III infection[55] and may be caused directly by the viral replication. These parameters, thus, may improve following antiviral therapy; they are quite nonspecific, however, and may be influenced by the strong placebo effect in patients with life-threatening disorders who are receiving experimental treatment. Finally, CNS symptomatology, including dementia, is frequently seen in HTLV-III disease, and may be affected by antiviral therapy.

In terms of immunological parameters, there are a number of tests of cellular immunity that are abnormal in patients with HTLV-III infection and that are suitable for monitoring. Perhaps the most useful to follow is the absolute number of helper-inducer (OKT4$^+$ or Leu 3$^+$) T-lymphocytes.[28-30] It should be kept in mind, however, that many factors can affect the number of helper-inducer T cells, that drug toxicity may directly decrease the number of these cells, and that increases can be observed only in those patients whose immune system still has reconstitutive potential. Assays of T-cell function, including antigen- or mitogen-induced proliferation,[32] cytotoxic responses to virally infected autologous cells,[56] and delayed-type cutaneous hypersensitivity reactions[1-3,6] are markedly abnormal in patients with AIDS, and can provide a measure of the status of the remaining T cells. If repeated skin-testing is performed, it must be remembered that repeated testing with certain antigens (including *Candida*, streptokinase-streptodornase, and tetanus) can induce an increase in the size of positive reactions,[57,58] although it is unusual for positive tests to develop in previously anergic persons as a result of repeated skin testing[57] or to develop with PPD.[58] This problem can be minimized if skin testing is done at infrequent intervals (more than 7 weeks apart)[57] or if the multitest system is used.[59]

Assessment of changes in the viral load would appear to be the most direct means of evaluating whether a putative antiviral agent had an in vivo virustatic effect. In most patients with AIDS, however, only a minority of peripheral blood cells (1/1000 or less) express HTLV-III at any given point in time,[31] and there is, at present, no sensitive and quantitative assay available to assess the viral load in these patients. The most frequently employed method at present is culture of the peripheral blood cells in interleukin-2 (IL-2)-enriched medium after stimulation by a mitogen such as phytohemagglutinin (PHA).[8,9,60] Allogeneic mononuclear cells from a normal donor or a cell line that is easily infected by HTLV-III (such as H9 or Jurkat) can, after a couple of days, be added to ensure that adequate numbers of cells which can support viral replication are present.[60] The production of HTLV-III can be monitored by measuring precipitable RT in the supernatant, by measuring a virally-encoded protein (such as p24 *gag* protein) in the supernatant, or examining the cells periodically for viral proteins using immunofluorescence.[8,9,60] While this method is reasonably sensitive, it is only semiquantitative and cannot differentiate between cells actively producing virus and those that only produce virus upon stimulation in vitro. In addition, it can be affected by the number and viability of the circulating helper-inducer T-lymphocytes; this may be the reason that patients with late AIDS yield a lower percentage of positive cultures than do patients with ARC.[9]

Other methods that can detect HTLV-III include Southern blot technology,[31] in situ hybridization,[31,39] and immunofluorescence of circulating cells for HTLV-III-encoded proteins.[9,60] Although occasional cells in the peripheral blood can be shown to be producing HTLV-III by in situ hybridization,[31] the number is generally too low to reliably permit detection of changes that may occur as a result of antiviral therapy. Neither Southern blot technology nor immunofluorescence are sensitive enough to directly detect HTLV-III in the peripheral blood cells of most patients, and while HTLV-III can sometimes be detected in brain or lymph node preparations by these techniques, the virus is unevenly distributed[31,39] and neither of these sites are suitable for serial sampling. Another approach being tested is the use of immunological assays (ELISA or radioimmune assays) to detect circulating viral proteins (usually p24). However, patients frequently have high titers of antibodies to these proteins, which can interfere with these assays. Thus, at present, there is no ideal method available for virological assessment of HTLV-III load in patients receiving antiviral drugs. Until such an assay is developed, virological monitoring must be undertaken only with a critical awareness of the limitations of the presently available techniques.

Drugs Being Investigated for Possible Use in the Treatment of AIDS

With this background, then, we can discuss certain antiviral agents that are presently under investigation for use in the treatment of HTLV-III disease (Table 3). In the 2 years since HTLV-III/LAV was shown to be the etiological agent of AIDS, almost a dozen drugs have been shown to at least partially block the infectivity of HTLV-III in vitro, and several of these are presently being evaluated in clinical trials. It should be noted that many of these agents are believed to act by inhibition of reverse transcriptase.

Suramin

The first drug that was reported to block the infectivity of HTLV-III in vitro was suramin.[61] This drug was first synthesized by the chemists at Bayer in 1920, and was shown to be an effective agent for use in trypanosomiasis; it is presently used for treatment of East African trypanosomiasis and onchocerciasis.[62,63] It is a large (MW 1429) urea of the aminoaphthalene-sulfonic type, which can bind to and inhibit the function of a variety of proteins.[62] In 1979, de Clercq[48] showed that suramin inhibited the RT of a number of murine and avian retroviruses. Because of the clinical experience with this drug, this was one of the first drugs we chose for screening at the National Cancer Institute, primarily because the agent could be used in clinical trials without delay if found to have in vitro activity.

In vitro testing revealed that suramin (in fetal calf serum-containing cultures) could block the expression of MW 24,000 viral *gag* proteins in H9 cells exposed to HTLV-III, and at 25 to 50 μg/ml, suramin blocked the cytopathic effect of HTLV-III on a helper-inducer T-cell clone.[61] At concentrations of 100 μg/ml or higher, it inhibited lymphocyte proliferation.[61] Additional testing showed that suramin could also inhibit the infection of cells with HTLV-I,[64] and that when administered to mice inoculated with Rauscher murine leukemia virus, it could partially inhibit virus-induced splenomegaly.[53] While suramin was originally chosen for testing because of its reported inhibition of RT, it is not clear that this is the mechanism for its effect on HTLV-III; while it inhibits the RT of HTLV-III (Refs. 65, 66, and L. Arthur, personal communication), it also inhibits mammalian DNA polymerase alpha at similar concentrations.[65,66] In addition, the estimated intracellular free suramin levels are lower than those at which HTLV-III RT is inhibited (R. Yarchoan, R. Klecker, J. C. Myers, S. Broder, and J. Collins, unpublished observations). It is possible that suramin enters the cell in a vacuole with HTLV-III, and that the local concentration is relatively high. Alternatively, suramin may act by a completely different mechanism.

Based on these in vitro results, we initiated a joint National Cancer Institute/National Institute of Allergy and Infectious Diseases/Walter Reed Medical Center trial of suramin in 10 patients with AIDS or ARC.[67] A regimen similar to that used to treat onchocerciasis was chosen; patients received a 0.2 gm test dose, followed by 6 weekly 1 gm doses, each dose being given intravenously over 20 minutes. Analysis of suramin concentrations in plasma samples showed that the half-life of suramin was 44 to 54 days, and that plasma levels of 100 μg/ml or greater were maintained for several weeks on this regimen.[67,68] (It is likely that the free suramin level is the determinant of drug effect, and because of its extensive binding to proteins [approximately 99.7% in plasma],[68] drug levels in fetal calf serum-enriched media cannot be directly compared with drug levels in vivo.) A number of the patients experienced toxic reactions including fevers up to 40°C, macular rashes, burning sensations of the skin, proteinuria, pyuria, and elevations in transaminase levels.[67] Many of these occurred early in the course of therapy and became less severe, even with additional administration of the drug; all were reversible after the drug was discontinued. One patient developed adrenal failure after being given a second 9 gm course of suramin,[69] and this may be the dose-limiting toxicity with this drug in larger trials now being conducted at several centers.

HTLV-III was detected in primary cultures from four of the patients at entry into this study, and in each case, virus was either undetectable or substantially diminished at times when the plasma suramin level was over 100 μg/ml; after administration of the drug, the virus was again detectable in each case.[67] One patient given a second course of suramin again had decreased virus as detected by primary culture (R. R. Redfield, P. D. Markham, R. Yarchoan, and S. Broder, unpublished observations). In spite of this apparent virustatic effect, however, there was no evidence of clinical improvement or immunological reconstitution in the patients who received suramin. In particular, there was no general increase in the number of helper-inducer T cells, no reconstitution of delayed-type cutaneous hypersensitivity, and no clearing of KS lesions.[67] Other clinical trials with suramin in patients with HTLV-III infection have been initiated in the United States and abroad. Saimot and co-workers[70] in the Hospital St. Claude Bernard in Paris, and Levine and co-workers in the University of Southern California (Dr. A. Levine, personal communication) have both seen a virustatic effect in the patients as assessed by culture of peripheral lymphocytes. Several patients with ARC in Rwanda[71] and several of Dr. Levine's patients had weight gain after being given suramin, and one patient (of Dr. Levine) with AIDS and lymphoma had a complete remission after being given suramin (Dr. A. Levine, personal communication); otherwise, no clinical responses were noted. The reason for the lack of immunological or clinical benefits in most of these patients is unclear, although it is likely that only a partial virustatic effect is attained and that, in addition, the lymphotoxicity of suramin acts to inhibit immunological reconstitution. A similar failure of in vitro activity to translate into clinical efficacy has been observed with other antiviral drugs; 5-iodo-2'-deoxyuridine (IUDR), for example, is virustatic for *Herpesviruses,* but has not been shown to improve the outcome of patients with herpes simplex encephalitis.[17] The preliminary results with suramin thus suggest that it does not have a role as a single agent in the treatment of HTLV-III disease. In addition, suramin does not penetrate into the CNS;[62,63] as we now know (but did not when suramin was first considered for use in AIDS), central nervous system involvement is an important component in HTLV-III-induced diseases, and this further limits its potential usefulness. It is possible, however, that suramin may still have some role when combined with other antiviral agents or with immunoreconstitutive therapy.[6,67]

HPA-23

Ammonium 21-tungsto-9-antimoniate (HPA-23) is a large (MW 6800) compound that has been shown to be an inhibitor of murine oncornaviruses.[72] It is believed to act as a competitive inhibitor of RT[73] and has been shown to have an in vivo effect on Friend virus-induced leukemia in mice.[72]

HPA-23 has a half-life of approximately 20 minutes in man. In initial clinical studies reported by Rozenbaum et al.,[74] four patients who had HTLV-III detectable by culture at entry each received a 3 hour daily infusion of HPA-23 for 15 consecutive days. In each case, virus could not be isolated at the end of the 15 days on drug. Virus was detected in follow-up cultures initiated 30 days after HPA-23 administration, suggesting that the drug had a transient virustatic effect.[74] The primary toxicity observed was thrombocytopenia; three of the patients also developed transient transaminase elevations.[74] As in the case with suramin, there was no evidence of immunological improvement in the patients. Phase I/II trials with HPA-23 are presently underway in France and the United States.

3'-Azido-3'-deoxythymidine (AZT) and Other Chain Terminators

We have been quite intrigued by the observations that some compounds that are chain terminators for DNA synthesis can act as potent inhibitors of retroviral replication.[49,50] One such drug is AZT (also called "compound S" and "BW A509 U"). AZT is a thymidine analog in which the 3'-hydroxy (-OH) group is replaced by an azido (-N_3) group (Fig. 1).[75] Mitsuya et al.[49] in the Clinical Oncology Program have recently shown that this drug inhibits the in vitro infectivity and cytopathic effect of HTLV-III at 1 to 3 μM; lymphocyte proliferation in vitro was not inhibited at these concentrations and, in fact, was not affected at concentrations below 15 μM. The antiviral effect of AZT is a function of target cell susceptibility and viral dose.

AZT is converted by cellular enzymes to a triphosphate form, which is utilized by RT. Because of the 3' modification, subsequent 5' → 3' phosphodiester linkages cannot be added, and AZT can act as a chain terminator for DNA synthesis.[49,76,77] Cellular DNA polymerase alpha is approximately 100-fold less susceptible to inhibition by AZT-triphosphate as compared with HTLV-III RT (P. A. Furman, personal communication),[76,77] and this difference is one basis (but not necessarily the only basis) for the antiviral activity of AZT against HTLV-III. Animal studies in rats and dogs have revealed little toxicity at doses of 80 mg/kg per day or greater (K. Ayers, personal communication). Based on the results of these in vitro and animal data, a Phase I trial of AZT in patients with AIDS and ARC was recently initiated at the National Cancer Institute and Duke University Medical Center in collaboration wtih Wellcome Research Laboratories.[78]

Initially, the patients received AZT intravenously. It was subsequently shown that the drug was well absorbed when given orally (60% bioavailability) and AZT, therefore, appears to be suitable for oral administration. Pharmacokinetic studies showed that peak levels of 1.5 to 2 μM were attained after an in-

THYMIDINE

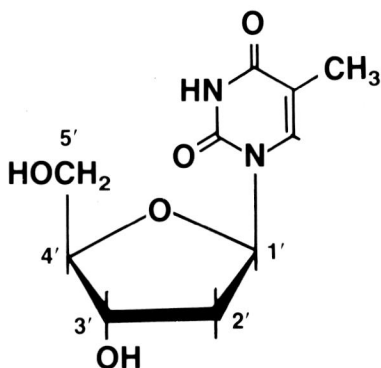

3′-AZIDO-3′- DEOXYTHYMIDINE

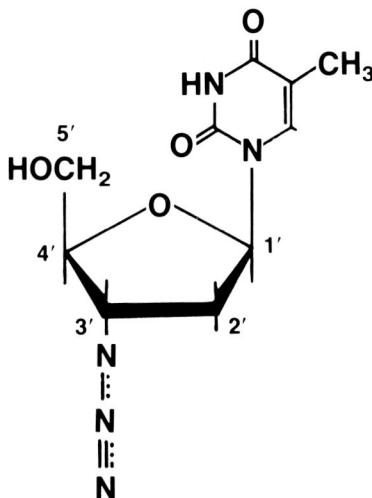

FIGURE 1 Structure of thymidine (left) and 3′-deoxy-3′azidothymidine (right). The drug is a 2′,3′-dideoxythymidine with an azido substituent at the 3′-carbon of the sugar.

fusion of 1 mg/kg or oral administration of 2 mg/kg, and that the drug has a half-life of approximately 1 hour. Increased doses of the drug yielded proportionally increased peak levels; for example, 5 mg/kg given intravenously yielded a peak level of 6 to 10 μM. In addition, sampling of the cerebral spinal fluid (CSF) showed penetration of AZT; CSF levels have ranged from 15 to 70% of simultaneously measured plasma levels (R. W. Klecker, J. M. Collins, R. Yarchoan, S. Broder, and C. E. Myers, unpublished observations).[78]

Nineteen patients have so far been studied on this Phase I trial. This was an escalating dose trial, and patients received 3, 7.5, 15, or 30 mg/kg per day intravenously for 2 weeks, followed by twice that dose given orally for 4 weeks. For the first two dose schedules, the drug was administered three times per day. For the last two dose schedules, it was divided into six doses spaced 4 hours apart. This scheduling modification was made because of the relatively short half-life of AZT. The drug was, in general, well tolerated; during short-term administration, side effects were: (1) greater than 10% hematocrit drops in three patients; (2) headaches in approximately half the patients, (3) tremors and confusion in one patient who was simultaneously receiving trimethoprim-sulfamethoxazole, and (4) decrease in the total white blood count in two of the four patients on the highest dose.

While the primary purpose of this study was to determine if AZT could be tolerated in patients with HTLV-III infection, the results also indicated that immunological and/or clinical responses were observed in some of the patients during the 6 weeks of therapy. In particular, 15 of the 19 patients had increases in the absolute number of circulating helper-inducer T-lymphoctyes, six of the 16 patients who were anergic at entry developed positive skin tests while on AZT, and one patient who was serially studied had the restoration of a cytotoxic response to influenza virus-infected autologous cells. The immunological improvement was most consistently observed in patients receiving 7.5 or 15 mg/kg per day intravenously (followed by twice that dose given orally); at the highest dose tested (30 mg/kg per day) only two of the four patients had increases in their helper-inducer T-cells, and two of the patients had decreases in their total white blood cells, suggesting that drug-induced toxicity may have been occurring at that dose.

In addition to the partial immunological reconstitution observed in these patients, clinical improvement was seen in some. Two patients who had chronic nailplate fungal infections at entry had clearing of these infections without specific antifungal therapy (Fig. 2). In addition, one patient who had debilitating aphthous stomatitis before therapy had healing of the lesions, 13 of the 19 patients had weight gains of 2 kg or greater (not explainable by fluid retention and associated with an increase in appetite), and six patients noted that their fevers stopped or had an improved sense of well-being. One patient had lower extremity weakness and dysesthesia, accompanied by electromyelographic abnormalities that were atttributed to HTLV-III infection. After receiving AZT, his symptoms resolved, and a repeat electromyelogram was normal. Finally, one patient with an expressive aphasia and one patient with severe impairment of cognitive functions appeared to improve on AZT therapy.

During the 6 weeks of AZT, however, no decrease in the progression of KS was observed in the patients, and one patient died from aggressive visceral KS since entry into the trial. In addition, three of the patients developed nonlife-threatening infections (localized herpes zoster, sinusitis, and pneumonia) during the 6-week period of the initial protocol, which responded to appropriate therapy.

In spite of the clinical and immunological improvements on the middle two doses of AZT, HTLV-III could be isolted from several of the patients on the lower doses using the technique of PHA-stimulated lymphocyte culture.[78] However, at the highest does (30 mg/kg per day IV followed by 60 mg/kg per day orally), virus was not detected in the patients on therapy, suggesting that a virustatic effect was attained at that dose.

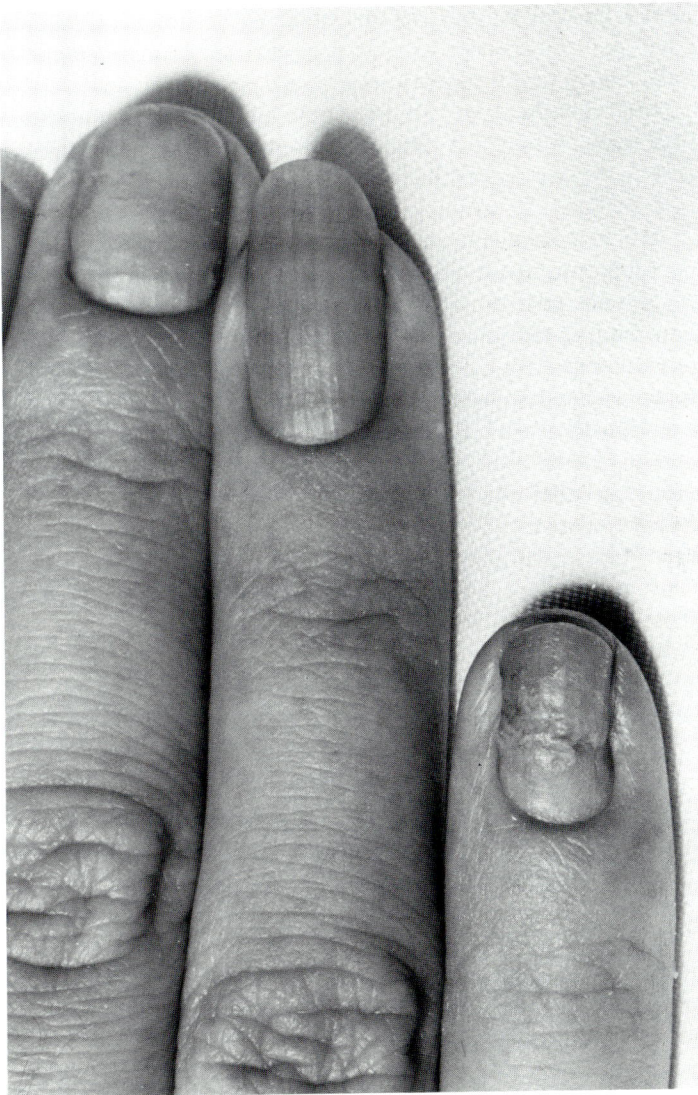

FIGURE 2 Clearing of a chronic nailbed infection in a patient with AIDS 3 months after beginning therapy with AZT. The nail of the fifth finger (on the right) shows evidence of clearing of a fungal nailbed infection (onychomycosis). The older part of the nail is deformed due to the fungal infection, while the newer nail growth is normal. The time of the change to normal nail growth corresponds to the time this patient began taking AZT. The patient did not receive any systemic antifungal therapy.

The earliest patients entered into this trial were taken off AZT for 1 month and then restarted on the drug; later patients were continued on the drug after the initial 6 weeks and, in many cases, an escalating dose regimen was used. At the National Cancer Institute, we are presently following 11 patients on extended AZT therapy. While this study is presently ongoing, preliminary results suggest that the number of helper-inducer T cells reaches a plateau after 6 weeks of therapy and then, in some patients, declines. Six of the patients being followed have KS, and of these, one has had a complete remission of his KS (confirmed by biopsy), and three patients have had some clearing of their lesions. Interestingly, the patient with a complete remission initially had worsening of his lesions while on AZT, but had clearing starting in the 8th week of therapy. Two of the AIDS patients who had had PCP prior to entry developed a second episode of PCP (one responded to pentamidine and the other to trimethoprim-sulfamethoxazole) several months after their initial entry into the study; one of these patients also developed localized herpes zoster 4 months after entry.

Thus, extended treatment with AZT was associated with a complete response of KS in at least one patient, and partial clearing in three others. However, the number of helper-inducer lymphocyte cells plateaued after an initial rise, and often fell in the patients whose daily dose was escalated. At the same time, patients developed megaloblastic changes in the bone marrow (not explainable by vitamin deficiencies) and decreased numbers of total white blood cells, and these changes (including the late depression of lymphocytes) most likely represent a cumulative drug toxicity. Recent in vitro studies indicate that cells exposed to high concentrations of AZT have decreased levels of thymidine triphosphate, and AZT-induced pyrimidine starvation may be one factor in causing this late toxicity (J. Balzarini, D. A. Cooney, D. G. Johns, and S. Broder, unpublished observations). Thus, strategies aimed at redicing this depletion of normal pyrimidine pools may permit long-term therapy with AZT without unacceptable toxicity. It may also be possible to monitor the increase in the red blood cell mean corpuscular volume (MCV) as an indication of impending drug toxicity. We are currently exploring regimens that take these factors into consideration.

These initial results with AZT suggest that it can, at least for a 6-week period, induce immunological improvement in patients with HTLV-III disease and in some, also yield potential clinical benefits. A randomized double-blind placebo-controlled study of orally administered AZT is presently being organized by Burroughs Wellcome Co. in several medical centers throughout the United States to further evaluate this drug, and specifically to determine whether it can be tolerated for 6 months, whether it can yield immunological benefits over this time period, and whether it can reduce the morbidity and mortality of patients with AIDS

As noted, AZT is one member of a family of nucleoside analogs that can act as chain terminators. It has recently been shown that several other analogs with 3' modifications are equal or more potent inhibitors of HTLV-III replication on a molar basis than is AZT.[50] (Also see the chapter by Mitsuya and Broder). At least one of these, namely 2',3'-dideoxycytidine, is presently being tested in animals as a first step towards being tested in patients. Several dideoxynucleosides have been found to have activity against a spectrum of animal and human retroviruses (S. Aaronson, J. Dahlberg, S. Matsushita, H. Mitsuya, and S. Broder, unpublished observations), and we believe these agents might have important potential in human and veterinary medicine. It might be worth mentioning that these drugs are activated (phosphorylated) by host cell kinases. Thus, unlike the situation with acyclovir and herpes virus, retroviruses cannot adopt a strategy of mutation in a kinase to develop drug resistance to dideoxynucleosides.

Other Drugs with In Vitro Activity Against HTLV-III

In addition to the drugs just noted, several other substances have been shown to have in vitro activity against HTLV-III. Some of these are now undergoing initial testing in patients with HTLV-III disease, and others are being considered for clinical trials.

Ribavirin: Ribavirin is a guanosine analog that has activity against several RNA viruses in vitro, and which has recently been shown to partially inhibit RT production by T cells exposed to HTLV-III.[79] The mechanism of action of ribavirin against HTLV-III is unknown; one proposed mechanism for its action against other viruses is interference with the capping of virus-specific RNA by inhibition of messenger RNA guanylyl transferase activity.[80] Ribavirin has been used clinically for the therapy of respiratory syncytial virus infection,[81] Lassa fever,[82] and influenza A.[83] It can be administered orally, with the main toxicities being anemia and liver enzyme elevations. One potential drawback of its use in patients with HTLV-III infection is that only partial inhibition of HTLV-III replication was attained in vitro, even at the highest doses tested (100 μg/ml).[80] If it acts at a different step other than by interfering with RT, however, it may be potentially useful when combined with other drugs, even if not completely effective when used alone. Clinical trials with ribavirin in HTLV-III disease are presently underway in the United States.

Phosphonoformate: Another agent that has previously been administered to humans and has recently been shown to inhibit HTLV-III replication in vitro is trisodium phosphonoformate, also called foscarnet.[84,85] This drug had previously been shown to be an inhibitor of the reverse transcriptase of a number of animal retroviruses.[86] Recent studies[84] have demonstrated that at a concentration of 132 μM, it partially inhibits RT production by H9 cells exposed to HTLV-III, and at 680 μM, it completely inhibits RT production. Foscarnet is also an inhibitor of the DNA polymerase of certain human herpes viruses,[87] and has already been administered to patients with CMV infection.[84] Clinical trials in patients with AIDS are presently underway with foscarnet in the United States and Europe. Acute renal failure is one potential side effect of this agent.

Rifabutine: In the mid-1970s, it was shown by Ting and co-workers[45] that certain rifamycin analogs were inhibitors of RT. More recently, it has been shown that one such derivative, rifabutine (ansamycin LM 427), can inhibit HTLV-III replication.[88] This drug has activity against *Mycobacterium avium*,[89] and interestingly has been administered to AIDS patients for experimental therapy of this organism. Efforts are now underway to determine if it has activity against HTLV-III in the patients with AIDS

Drugs Other than Nucleoside Analogs or Reverse Transcriptase Inhibitors: Most of the drugs just mentioned are nucleoside analogs or drugs that were selected as potential RT inhibitors. Mention should be made, as well, of two agents that have activity against HTLV-III, but do not fall into either of those two groups. One is the lipid substance AL-721, which has been shown to have in vitro activity against HTLV-III.[90] A second is alpha-interferon (IFN). Even before it was known that a retrovirus was the etiological agent of AIDS, clinical trials with alpha-IFN were initiated in patients with KS. These trials were undertaken because of the antitumor action of alpha-IFN, and because it was thought that its antiviral effect may be beneficial in this disease; the results indicated that while there was no improvement in immunological function, a percentage of patients with KS, particularly those with early disease limited to the skin, went into complete remission.[91-93] In the initial description of HTLV-III, it was noted that virus production by infected cell lines was increased by the addition of antibody to alpha-IFN to the culture media[9] and, more recently, it has been shown that exogenous alpha-IFN can inhibit HTLV-III production in vitro.[94] It is presently unknown if alpha-IFN is virustatic when administered to patients.

Conclusion

In the brief period since HTLV-III/LAV was identified as the etiological agent of AIDS, a number of drugs have already been shown to have activity against the virus and at least one (AZT) has been shown to induce immunological improvement when administered over a short period of time. While these preliminary results are encouraging, the high number of persons infected with HTLV-III and the high mortality rate once the infection progresses to frank AIDS add a sense of urgency to research on drug development in this field. The general field of antiviral drug development is in its infancy, and HTLV-III has several characteristics that make it potentially difficult to control; namely, its ability to integrate into the host genome and lie dormant, its tendency to mutate, and its ability to infect at least one organ (the brain) with limited regenerative potential.

Initial clinical trials will most likely be targeted at determining whether single agents have a clinical effect in patients. Because of the ability of HTLV-III to lie dormant and mutate, however, it is possible that combination drug therapy may ultimately be more effective in these patients than the use of one drug alone. Using two or more drugs together may allow simultaneous interference with two steps of viral replication, may lessen the chance of viral resistance developing by mutation, and may permit additive antiviral activity without additive toxicity of the drugs. Such therapy has been shown to be essential in the treatment of certain cancers and of *Mycobacterium* infections, and this may be a logical next step in clinical AIDS therapeutic research.

Combination antiviral therapy, however, can only be based on the finding of single agents that are effective against the virus. As can be seen, a good start has been made in this area. It likely that as we learn more about HTLV-III, its molecular biology, and the effect of drugs on its replication, we can more rationally develop drugs or even design recombinant DNA constructs that will be of use in the treatment of HTLV-III disease.

References

1. Gottlieb MS, Schroff R, Schanker HM, et al. *Pneumocystis carinii* pneumonia and mucosal candidiasis in previously healthy homosexual men: evidence of a new acquired immunodeficiency. N Engl J Med 1981; 305:1425–1430.
2. Masur H, Michelis MA, Greene JB, et al. An outbreak of community acquired *Pneumocystis carinii* pneumonia: initial manifestations of cellular dysfunction. N Engl J Med 1981; 305:1431–1438.
3. Siegal FP, Lopez C, Hammer GS, et al. Severe acquired immunodeficiency in male homosexuals, manifested by chronic perianal ulcerative herpes simplex lesions. N Engl J Med 1981; 305:1439–1444.
4. Hymes KB, Cheung T, Greene JB, et al. Kaposi's sarcoma in homosexual men—a report of eight cases. Lancet 1981; ii:598–600.
5. Masur H. New concepts in the therapy of infections in the acquired immunodeficiency syndrome. In: Fauci AS, moderator. The acquired immunodeficiency syndrome: an update. Ann Intern Med 1985; 102:802–804.
6. Lane HC, Masur H, Longo DL, et al. Partial immune reconstitution in a patient with the acquired immunodeficiency syndrome. N Engl J Med 1984; 311:1099–1103.
7. Lewis B, Abrams J, Ziegler J, et al. Single agent or combination chemotherapy of Kaposi's sarcoma (KS) in acquired immunodeficiency syndrome (AIDS). Proc Am Soc Clin Oncol 1983; 2:59.

8. Popovic M, Sarngadharan MG, Reed E, Gallo RC. Detection, isolation, and continuous production of cytopathic retroviruses (HTLV-III) from patients with AIDS
   and pre-AIDS. Science 1984; 224:497–500.
9. Gallo RC, Salahuddin SZ, Popovic M, et al. Frequent detection and isolation of
   cytopathic retroviruses (HTLV-III) from patients with AIDS and at risk for AIDS.
   Science 1984; 224:500–503.
10. Barré-Sinoussi F, Chermann JC, Rey F, et al. Isolation of a T cell lymphocytic virus
    from a patient at risk for acquired immunodeficiency syndrome (AIDS). Science
    1983; 220:868–871.
11. Dalgleish AG, Beverly PCL, Clapham PR, et al. The CD4 (T4) antien is an essential
    component of the receptor for the AIDS retrovirus. Nature 1984; 312:763–767.
12. Klatzmann D, Champagne E, Chamerat S, et al. T-lymphocyte T4 molecule behaves
    as the receptor for human retrovirus LAV. Nature 1984; 312:767–768.
13. Popovic M, Gallo RC, Mann DL. OKT-4 antigen bearing molecule is a receptor for
    the human retrovirus HTLV-III. Clin Res 1984; 33:560A.
14. McDougal JS, Kennedy MS, Slight JM, et al. Binding of HTLV-III/LAV to T4+ T
    cells by a complex of the 110K viral protein and the T4 molecule. Science 1986;
    231:382–385.
15. Weiss RA, Clapham PR, Cheingsong-Popov R, et al. Neutralization of human T-
    lymphotropic virus type III by sera of AIDS and AIDS-risk patients. Nature 1985;
    316:69–72.
16. Robert-Guroff M, Brown M, Gallo RC. HTLV-III-neutralizing antibodies in patients
    with AIDS and AIDS-related complex. Nature 1985; 316:72–74.
17. Dolin R. Antiviral chemotherapy and chemoprophylaxis. Science 1985; 227:1296–
    1303.
18. Broder S, Gallo RC. A pathogenic retrovirus (HTLV-III) linked to AIDS. N Engl J
    Med 1984; 311:1292–1297.
19. Wong-Staal F, Gallo RC. Human T-lymphotropic retroviruses. Nature 1985; 317:
    395–403.
20. Sodroski JG, Rosen CA, Wong-Staal F, et al. Trans-acting transcriptional regulation
    of human T-cell leukemia virus type III long terminal repeat. Science 1985;
    227:171–173.
21. Rosen CA, Sodroski JG, Haseltine WA. The location of the cis-acting regulatory
    sequences in the human T cell lymphotropic virus type III (HTLV-III/LAV) long
    terminal repeat. Cell 1985; 41:813–823.
22. Rosen CA, Sodroski JG, Goh WC, et al. Post-transcriptional regulation accounts for
    the trans-activation of the human T-lymphotropic virus type III. Nature 1986;
    319:555–559.
23. Stephenson ML, Zamecnik PC. Inhibition of Rous sarcoma viral RNA translation by
    a specific oligodeoxyribonucleotide. Proc Natl Acad Sci USA 1978; 75:285–288.
24. Izant JG, Weintraub H. Inhibition of thymidine kinase gene expression by anti-
    serase RNA: a molecular approach to genetic analysis. Cell 1984; 36:1007–1015.
25. Pestka S, Daugherty BL, Jung V, et al. Anti-mRNA: specific inhibition of translation
    of single mRNA molecules. Proc Natl Acad Scie USA 1984; 81:7526/7528.
26. Murikami A, Blake KR, Miller PS. Characterization of sequence-specific oligo-

deoxyribonucleoside methylphosphonates and their interaction with rabbit globin mRNA. Biochemistry 1985; 24:4041–4046.

27. Wickstrom E, Simonet WS, Medlock K, Ruiz-Robles I. Complementary oligonucleotide probe of vesicular stomatitis virus matrix protein mRNA translation. Biophys 1986; 49:15–17.

28. Fahey JL, Prince H, Weaver H, et al. Quantitative changes in T helper or T suppressor/cytotoxic lymphocyte subsets that distinguish acquired immunodeficiency syndrome from other immune subset disorders. Am J Med 1984; 76:95–100.

29. Nicholson JKA, McDougal JS, Spira TJ, et al. Immunoregulatory subsets of the T helper and T suppressor cell populations in homosexual men with chronic unexplained lymphadenopathy. J Clin Invest 1984; 73:191–201.

30. Klatzmann D, Barré-Sinoussi F, Nugeyre MT, et al. Selective tropism of lymphadenopathy associated virus (LAV) for helper-inducer T lymphocytes. Science 1984; 225:59–63.

31. Shaw G, Hahn BH, Arya SK, et al. Molecular characterization of human T cell leukemia (lymphotropic) virus type III in the acquired immunodeficiency syndrome. Science 1984; 226:1165–1171.

32. Lane HC, Depper JM, Greene WC, et al. Qualitative analysis of immune function in patients with the acquired immunodeficiency syndrome. N Engl J Med 1985; 313:79–84.

33. Laurence J, Gottlieb AB, Kunkel HG. Soluble suppressor factors in patients with acquired immunodeficiency syndrome and its prodrome: elaboration in vitro by T lymphocyte-adherent cell interactions. J Clin Invest 1983; 72:2072–2081.

34. Pahwa S, Pahwa R, Saxinger C, Gallo RC, Good RA. Influence of the human T-lymphotropic virus/lymphadenopathy-associated virus on functions of human lymphocytes: evidence for immunosuppressive effects and polyclonal B-cell activation by banded preparations. Proc Natl Acad Sci USA 1985; 82:8198–8202.

35. Hoxie JA, Haggarty BS, Rackowski JL, et al. Persistent noncytopathic infection of normal human T lymphocytes with AIDS-associated retrovirus. Science 1985; 229:1400–1402.

36. Folks T, Powell DM, Lightfoote MM, et al. Induction of HTLV-III/LAV from a non-virus producing T-cell line: implications for latency. Science 1986; 231:600–602.

37. Zagury D, Bernard J, Leonard R, et al. Long-term cultures of HTLV-III-infected T cells: a model of cytopathology of T-cell depletion in AIDS. Science 1986; 231:850–953.

38. Montagnier L, Gruest J, Chamaret S, et al. Adaptation of lymphadenopathy associated virus (LAV) to replicate in EBV-transformed B lymphoblastoid lines. Science 1984; 225:63–66.

39. Shaw GM, Harper ME, Hahn BH, et al. HTLV-III infection in brains of children and adults with AIDS encephalopathy. Science 1985; 227:177–182.

40. Ho DD, Rota TR, Schooley RT, et al. Isolation of HTLV-III from cerebrospinal fluid and neural tissues of patients with neurologic syndromes related to the acquired immunodeficiency syndrome. N Engl J Med 1985; 313:1493–1497.

41. Resnick L, DiMarzo-Veronese F, Schüpbach J, et al. Intra-blood-brain barrier synthesis of HTLV-III-specific IgG in patients with neurologic symptoms associated with AIDS or AIDS-related complex. N Engl J Med 1985; 313:1498–1504.

42. Baltimore D. RNA-dependent DNA polymerase in virions of RNA tumour viruses. Nature 1970; 226:1209–1211.
43. Temin MH, Mizutani S. RNA-directed DNA polymerase in virions in Rous sarcoma virus. Nature 1970; 226:1211–1213.
44. Gallo RC, Yang SS, Ting RC. RNA-dependent DNA polymerase of human acute leukemic cells. Nature 1970; 228:927–929.
45. Ting RC, Yang SS, Gallo RC. Reverse transcriptase, RNA tumor virus transformation and derivatives of rifamycin SV. Nature New Biol 1972; 236:163–166.
46. Chandra P, Demirhan I, Ebener U, et al. Modulation of retrovirus DNA polymerase activity by polynucleotides and their analogs. In: Becker Y, ed. Antiviral drugs and interferon: the molecular basis for their activity. Boston: Martinus Nijhoff Publishing, 1984:173–189.
47. Chandra P, Demirhan I, de Clercq E. A study of antitemplate inhibition of mammalian, bacterial, and viral DNA polymerases by 2- and 2'-substituted derivatives of polyadenylic acid. Cancer Let 1981; 12:181–193.
48. de Clercq E. Suramin: a potent inhibitor of the reverse transcriptase of RNA tumor viruses. Cancer Let 1979; 8:9–22.
49. Mitsuya H, Weinhold KJ, Furman PA, et al. 3'-azido-3'-deoxythymidine (BW A509U): an antiviral agent that inhibits the infectivity and cytopathic effect of human T-lymphotropic virus type III/lymphadenopathy-associated virus in vitro. Proc Natl Acad Sci USA 1985; 82:7096–7100.
50. Mitsuya H, Broder S. Inhibition of the in vitro infectivity and cytopathic effect of HTLV-III/LAV by 2',3'-dideoxynucleosides. Proc Natl Acad Sci USA 1986; 83: 1911–1915.
51. Grant CK, de Noronha F, Tusch C, et al. Protection of cats against progressive fibrosarcomas and persistent leukemia virus infection by vaccination with feline leukemia cells. J Natl Cancer Inst 1980; 65:1285–1292.
52. Essex M, Klein G, Snyder AP, Harrold JB. Correlation between humoral antibody and regression of tumours induced by feline sarcoma virus. Nature 1971; 233:195–196.
53. Ruprecht RM, Rossoni LD, Haseltine WA, Broder S. Suppression of retroviral propagation and disease by suramin in murine systems. Proc Natl Acad Sci USA 1985; 82:7733–7737.
54. Harwood AR, Osoba D, Hofstader SL, et al. Kaposi's sarcoma in recipients of renal transplants. Am J Med 1979; 67:759–765.
55. Cooper DA, Gold J, Maclean P, et al. Acute AIDS retrovirus infection. Definition of a clinical illness associated with seroconversion. Lancet 1985; i:537–540.
56. Shearer GM, Salahuddin SZ, Markham PD, et al. Prospective study of cytotoxic T lymphocyte responses to influenza and antibodies to human T lymphotropic virus-III in homosexual men. J Clin Invest 1985; 76:1699–1704.
57. Hogan TF, Border EC, Freeberg BL, et al. Enhancement in recall antigen responses by frequent, repetitive skin testing with candida, mumps, and streptokinase-streptodornase in 38 normal adults. Cancer Immunol Immunother 1980; 10:27–31.
58. Keystone EC, Demerieux P, Gladman D, et al. Enhanced delayed hypersensitivity skin test reactivity with serial testing in healthy volunteers. Clin Exp Immunol 1980; 40:202–205.
59. Lesourd B, Winters WD. Specific immune responses to skin test antigens following

repeated multiple antigen skin tests in normal individuals. Clin Exp Immunol 1982; 50:635–643.

60. Markham PD, Salahuddin SZ, Popovic M, et al. Advances in the isolation of HTLV-III from patients with AIDS and AIDS-related complex and from donors at risk. Cancer Res 1985; 45(Suppl):4588s–4591s.

61. Mitsuya H, Popovic M, Yarchoan R, et al. Suramin protection of T cells in vitro against infectivity and cytopathic effect of HTLV-III. Science 1984; 266:172–174.

62. Hawking F. Suramin: with special reference to onchocerciasis. Adv Pharm Chemother 1978; 15:289–322.

63. Hawking F. Chemotherapy of filariasis. Antibiot Chemother 1981; 30:135–162.

64. Yarchoan R, Mitsuya H, Matsushita S, Broder S. Implications of the discovery of HTLV-III for the treatment of AIDS. Cancer Res 1985; 45(Suppl):4684s–4688s.

65. Chandra P, Vogel A, Gerber T. Inhibitors of retroviral DNA polymerase: their implication in the treatment of AIDS. Cancer Res 1985; 45(Suppl):4677s–4684s.

66. Basu A, Modak MJ. Observations on the suramin-mediated inhibition of cellular and viral DNA polymerases. Biochem Biophys Res Comm 1985; 128:1395–1402.

67. Broder S, Yarchoan R, Collins JM, et al. Effects of suramin on HTLV-III/LAV infection presenting as Kaposi's sarcoma or AIDS-related complex: clinical pharmacology and suppression of virus replication in vivo. Lancet 1985; ii:627–630.

68. Collins JM, Klecker RW, Yarchoan R, et al. Clinical pharmacokinetics of suramin in patients with HTLV-III/LAV infection. J Clin Pharmacol 1986; 26:22–26.

69. Stein CA, Saville W, Yarchoan R, et al. Hypoadrenalism after suramin treatment. Ann Intern Med 1986; 104:286–287.

70. Saimot AG, Matheron S, le Port C, et al. An open trial of suramin in AIDS patients: suppression of HTLV-III/LAV replication and clinical outcome. In: E.C. Workshop, EORTC. Brussels: Raven Press (in press).

71. Rouvroy D, Bogaerts J, Habyarimana JB, et al. Short term results with suramin for AIDS-related conditions. Lancet 1985; i:878–879.

72. Jasmin C, Chermann JC, Raybaud M, et al. In vivo inhibition of murine leukemia and sarcoma viruses by heteropolyanion 5-tungsto-2-antimoniate. J Natl Cancer Inst 1974; 53:469–474.

73. Chermann JC, Sinoussi F, Jasmin C. Inhibition of RNA-dependent DNA polymerase of murine oncornaviruses by 5-tungsto-2-antimoniate. Biochem Biophys Res Comm 1975; 65:1229–1236.

74. Rozenbaum W, Dormont D, Spire B, et al. Antimoniotungstate (HPA 23) treatment of three patients with AIDS and one with prodrome. Lancet 1985; i:450–451.

75. Lin TS, Prusoff WH. Synthesis and biological activity of several amino acid analogues of thymidine. J Med Chem 1978; 21:109–112.

76. St. Clair MH, Weinhold K, Richards CA, et al. Characterization of HTLV-3 reverse transcriptase and inhibition by the triphosphate of BW A509U. Program and abstracts of the twenty-fifth interscience conference on antimicrobial agents and chemotherapy. Minneapolis: American Society for Microbiology, 1985:172.

77. Furman PA, St. Clair M, Weinhold K, et al. Selective inhibition of HTLV-3 by BW A509U. In: Program and abstracts of the twenty-fifth interscience conference on antimicrobial agents and chemotherapy. Minneapolis: American Society for Microbiology, 1985:172.

78. Yarchoan R, Klecker RW, Weinhold KJ, et al. Administration of 3'-azido-3'-

deoxythymidine, an inhibitor of HTLV-III replication, to patients with AIDS or AIDS-related complex. Lancet 1986; i:575–580.

79. McCormick JB, Getchell JP, Mitchell SW, Hicks DR. Ribavirin suppresses replication of lymphadenopathy-associated virus in cultures of human adult T lymphocytes. Lancet 1984; ii:1367–1369.

80. Goswami BB, Borek E, Sharma OK, et al. The broad spectrum antiviral agent ribavirin inhibits capping of mRNA. Biochem Biophys Res Commun 1979; 89:830–836.

81. Hall CB, McBride JT, Walsh EE, et al. Aerosolized ribavirin treatments of infants with respiratory syncytial virus infection: a randomized double-blind study. N Engl J Med 1983; 308:1443–1447.

82. McCormick JB, King IJ, Webb PA, et al. Lassa fever: effective therapy with ribavirin. N Engl J Med 1986; 314:20–26.

83. Knight V, McClung HW, Wilson SZ, et al. Ribavirin small-particle aerosol treatment of influenza. Lancet 1981; 2:945–949.

84. Sandstrom EG, Kaplan JC, Byington RE, Hirsch MS. Inhibition of human T-cell lymphotropic virus type III in vitro by phosphonoformate. Lancet 1985; i:1480–1482.

85. Sarin PS, Taguchi Y, Sun D, et al. Inhibition of HTLV-III/LAV replication by foscarnet. Biochem Pharm 1985; 34:4075–4079.

86. Sundquist B, Öberg B. Phosphonoformate inhibits reverse transcriptase. J Gen Virol 1979; 45:273–281.

87. Helgstrand E, Eriksson B, Johansson NG, et al. Trisodium phosphonoformate, a new antiviral compound. Science 1978; 201:819–821.

88. Anand R, Moore J, Feorino P, et al. Rifabutine inhibits HTLV-III. Lancet 1986; ii:97–98.

89. Woodley CL, Kilburn JO. In vitro susceptibility of *Mycobacterium avium* complex and *mycobacterium tuberculosis* strains to a spiro-piperidyl rifamycin. Am Rev Resp Dis 1982; 126:586–587.

90. Sarin PS, Gallo RC, Scheer DI, et al. Effects of a novel compound (AL 721) on HTLV-III infectivity *in vitro*. N Engl J Med 1985; 313:1289–1290.

91. Krown SE, Real FX, Cunningham-Rundles S, et al. Preliminary observations on the effect of recombinant leukocyte A interferon in homosexual men with Kaposi's sarcoma. N Engl J Med 1983; 308:1071–1076.

92. Groopman JE, Gottlieb MS, Goodman J, et al. Recombinant alpha-2 interferon therapy for Kaposi's sarcoma associated with the acquired immunodeficiency syndrome. Ann Intern Med 1984; 100:671–676.

93. Gelmann EP, Preble OT, Steis R, et al. Human lymphoblastoid interferon treatment of Kaposi's sarcoma in AIDS: clinical response and prognosis parameters. Am J Med 1985; 78:737–741.

94. Ho DD, Hartshorn KL, Rota TR, et al. Recombinant human interferon alpha (A) suppresses HTLV-III replication in vitro. Lancet 1985; i:602–604.

Index

Acute HTLV-III infection, 139
Adults, AIDS incidence in, 77–79
Adult T-cell leukemia/lymphoma
    (ATLL), epidemiology of, 10–
    11
African Kaposi's sarcoma, 220–221
AIDS (a new kind of epidemic immu-
    nodeficiency), see Epidemic im-
    munodeficiency
AIDS cases
  by half-year of diagnosis (1981–
    1985), 100
  by sex and age at diagnosis, 101
AIDS-related complex (ARC), 13, 136–
    138

[AIDS-related complex (ARC)]
    psychiatric and psychosocial effects
      of AIDS on patients with, 128
AIDS-related malignant B-cell lym-
      phomas, 233–244
    analysis for Epstein-Barr virus, 240
    analysis for HTLV-III/LAV, 238–240
    clinical manifestations, 236–237
    course of disease, 240–241
    epidemiological history, 235
    immunological studies, 237–238
    past medical history, 234–235
    pathological characteristics of the
      disease, 235–236
    potential pathogenesis, 241–242

[AIDS-related malignant B-cell lymphomas]
  response to treatment, 240–241
  survival, 240–241
AL-721, 342, 354
Alpha-interferon (IFN), 342, 354
Animal models of HTLV-III/LAV infection and AIDS, 63–73
  experimental infection of HTLV-III/LAV in chimpanzees, 69–70
  feline leukemia viruses, 64
  simian T-lymphotropic viruses, 64–69
  STLV-I, 65–66
  STLV-III, 66–69
Antigen-specific helper-inducer T-cell clones, generation of, 328–329
Anti-HTLV-III activity, in vitro assessment of, 303–333
  activities of other 2′,3′-dideoxynucleoside analogues, 319–320
  antiretroviral activities of 2′,3′-dideoxynucleosides, 308–311
  development of screening system for antiretroviral agents, 304–305
  generation of HTLV-III/LAV cytopathic effect-sensitive T-cell clone, 305–308
  inhibition of HTLV-III/LAV DNA synthesis and RNA expression T cells exposed to virus, 313
  in vitro antiviral effect of combinations of putative drugs, 320–325
  in vitro drug screening and clinical application of anti-HTLV-III/LAV agents, 327
  mechanisms of antiretroviral activity of 2′,3′-dideoxynucleosides, 316–317
  reversal of 2′,3′-dideoxynucleoside protection, 325–327
Antiviral therapy, 33
  desirable properties in agents for use in, 341

[Antiviral therapy]
  disease process of infection, 338–340
  strategies for, 336–338
AZT (3′-azido-3′-deoxythymidine), 342, 348–353

Bacteria, 148, 155
B-cell lymphomas, 139–141
  malignant, AIDS-related, 233–244
    analysis for Barr-Epstein virus, 240
    analysis for HTLV-III/LAV, 238–240
    clinical manifestations, 236–237
    course of disease, 240–241
    epidemiological history, 235
    immunological studies, 237–238
    past medical history, 234–235
    pathological characteristics of the disease, 235–236
    potential pathogenesis, 241–242
    response to treatment, 240–241
    survival, 240–241
Biopsy-proven lymphoid interstitial pneumonia associated with pediatric AIDS, 254
Blood transplantation-associated AIDS, 109–110
Brain abscess, 266

Campylobacter fetus, 198
Candida albicans, 195–196
Carcinomas, 160, 294
Cardiomyopathies associated with pediatric AIDS, 257
CDC definition of AIDS, 113
Central nervous system (CNS) infections, 191–195
Central nervous system lymphoma, 139
Cerebral mass lesions, 170–171
Children, AIDS incidence in, see Pediatric AIDS

Classical Kaposi's sarcoma, 221–223
Cotrimoxazole, 188
Cryptosporidium, 196–198
Cutaneous infections, 198–199
  See also Mucocutaneous infections
Cytopathicity, HTLV-III and, 45–46

Dermatological (non-Kaposi's sarcoma)
    manifestations, 285–302
  drug eruptions, 286, 294–296
  granuloma annulare-like eruptions,
    286, 299
  malignancies, 286, 293–294
    carcinomas, 294
    lymphomas, 293–294
  mucocutaneous infections, 286,
    287–293
    fungi, 286, 291–293
    viruses, 286, 287–291
  oral hairy leukoplakia, 286, 296–
    298, 299
  primary HTLV-III/LAV infection,
    286, 296
  seborrheic dermatitis, 286, 296
Diarrhea, 196
Dideoxycytidine, 342
2′,3′-Dideoxynucleosides
  anti-HTLV-III/LAV activities of,
    308–311, 319–320
  antiretroviral activity mechanisms
    of, 316–317
  reversal of protection against HTLV-
    III/LAV by, 325–327
Disseminated infections, 199–200
DNA
  HTLV-III/LAV and, 313
  recombinant, development of immu-
    nodiagnostic reagents for AIDS
    and, 46
  retroviruses and, 3, 4
Drug eruptions, 286, 294–296
Drugs
  putative, in vitro antiviral effect by,
    320–325

[Drugs]
  See also Pharmocological interven-
    tion against HTLV-III/LAV;
    names of drugs

Encephalitis, 266
Encephalopathies, HTLV-III/LAV-re-
    lated, 270–275
Encephalopathy syndromes associated
    with pediatric AIDS, 257
env genes, 54, 57
  AIDS virus and, 32–33
  role played in HTLV-III-induced
    pathogenesis by, 59–60
  role played in virus life cycle by, 59
Epidemic immunodeficiency (AIDS as
    new kind), 75–90
  in adults, 77–79
  background, 76
  in children, 79–80
  incidence rates and premature mor-
    tality, 80–81
  modes of transmission, 82–84
  other manifestations of infection
    with AIDS virus, 81–82
  outlook for the future, 85–86
  prevention efforts, 84–85
  search for a cause, 76
  surveillance, 76–77
Epidemiology of human retroviruses,
    91–121
  history and nomenclature, 91–93
  HTLV-I, 95–98
  HTLV-II, 98
  HTLV-III and AIDS, 98–111
    epidemiology of clinically related
      conditions, 98–99
    natural history, 105–106
    pathogenesis, 104–105
    risk groups, 102–104
    seroepidemiology, 106–111
    surveillance and registry data, 99–
      102
  prospecting the future, 111–113
  serology, 93–95

Epstein-Barr virus (EBV), 199, 200
 malignant B-cell lymphomas and,
 240
Extra-CNS non-Hodgkin's lymphoma,
 139

Feline leukemia viruses (FeLV), 64
Fungi, 148, 155–157
 dermatological manifestations of,
 286, 291–293
Future prospects for treatment, 85–86,
 111–113
 pediatric AIDS and, 258–260

gag genes, 54–57
 role played in HTLV-III-induced
 pathogenesis by, 59–60
 role played in virus life cycle by, 59
Gastrointestinal infections, 195–198
Granuloma annulare-like eruptions,
 286, 299

Health care workers, psychiatric and
 psychosocial effect of AIDS on,
 131–132
Hematological lesions associated with
 AIDS, 144–147
Hemophiliacs, seroepidemiology of
 AIDS in, 108–109
Hepatitis syndrome associated with pe-
 diatric AIDS, 257
Herpesvirus CMV, 196
Herpesvirus HSV, 196
Heterosexual transmission,
 seroepidemiology of AIDS by,
 110–111
High-risk groups, psychiatric and psy-
 chosocial effects of AIDS on,
 128–130
Histoplasma capsulatum, 200
Hodgkin's disease, 159–160
 HTLV-III infection and, 140–141

Homosexual men, seroepidemiology of
 AIDS in, 107–108
HPA-23 (ammonium 21-tungsto-9-
 antimoniate), 342, 347–348
HTLV-I, 12–13
 characteristics of the disease associated with, 9–10
 epidemiology of, 95–98
 genetic structure of, 40–41
 HTLV-III and, 18
 mechanism of T-cell transformation
 of, 11–12
 origin and spread of, 10–11
 transcriptional regulation of cellular
 genes by, 42–45
HTLV-II, 12–13
 epidemiology of, 98
 genetic structure of, 40–41
 HTLV-III and, 18
 transcriptional regulation of cellular
 genes by, 42–45
HTLV-III/LAV, 18
 AIDS and, 13–15, 98–111
 epidemiology of clinically related
 conditions, 98–99
 natural history, 105–106
 pathogenesis, 104–105
 projecting the future, 111–113
 risk groups, 102–104
 seroepidemiology, 106–111
 surveillance and registry data, 99–
 102
 -associated diseases, 15–16
 cytopathic effect on T4 cells of, 16–
 17
 cytopathicity and, 45–46
 development of screening system for
 agents active against, 305
 genetic polymorphism of, 46–48
 genetic structure of, 40–41
 heterogeneity of, 16–17
 infection spectrum of, 135–142
 acute HTLV-III infection, 139
 AIDS-related complex (ARC),
 136–138

[HTLV-III/LAV]
  associated neoplasms, 139–141
  in chimpanzees of, 69–70
  malignant B-cell lymphomas and,
    238–240
  nervous system diseases, 138–
    139
  molecular biology of, 53–62
    gag, pol, and *env* genes, 54–57
    other puzzles and prospects, 60–
      61
    sor, tat, and 3'*orf* genes, 58–60
    unusual features of the virus life
      cycle and disease, 57–58
  pharmacological intervention
    against, 335–360
  prevention and treatment of infec-
    tion, 17–18
  therapeutic intervention during
    stages in life cycle of, 337
HTLV-III/LAV cytopathic effect inhibition assay, 329–330
HTLV-III/LAV cytopathic effect-sensitive T-cell clone (ATH8), 305–
  308
HTLV-III/LAV-related neurological disease, 263–283
  acute neurological disease related to
    primary infection, 268–270
  diagnosis and treatment, 279–281
  encephalopathy, 270–275
  myelopathy, 275–276
  neurotropism, 265–266
  peripheral neuropathy, 276–279
Human retrovirus epidemiology, 91–
  121
  history and nomenclature, 91–93
  HTLV-I, 95–98
  HTLV-II, 98
  HTLV-III and AIDS, 98–111
    epidemiology of clinically related
      conditions, 98–99
    natural history, 105–106
    pathogenesis, 104–105
    risk groups, 102–104

[Human retrovirus epidemiology]
    seroepidemiology, 106–111
    surveillance and registry data, 99–
      102
  prospecting the future, 111–113
  serology, 93–95
Human T-lymphotropic retroviruses,
  1–21
  background, 2
  characteristics of leukemic cells and
    of the disease associated with
    HTLV-I, 9–10
  cytopathic effect of HTLV-III on T4
    cells, 16–17
  general biology, 3–6
  general features, 6–7
  heterogeneity of HTLV-III, 16–17
  HTLV-III and the origin of AIDS,
    13–15
  HTLV-III-associated diseases, 15–16
  mechanism of HTLV-I T-cell trans-
    formation, 11–12
  origin and spread of HTLV-I and
    epidemiology of ATLL, 10–11
  prevention and treatment of HTLV-
    III infection, 17–18
  remarks on HTLV-I and HTLV-II,
    12–13
  remarks on HTLV-III, 18

Immunodeficiency,
  diseases considered at least moder-
    ately indicative of, 113–114
  See also Epidemic immunodeficiency
Immunodiagnostic reagents for AIDS,
  recombinant DNA technology
  and, 46
Immunosuppressive drug therapy, Kaposi's sarcoma associated with,
  223–224
Incidence of AIDS in the U.S. (1981–
  1985), 77
Incidence rates of AIDS, premature
  mortality and, 80–81

Infection spectrum of HTLV-III, 135–142
acute HTLV-III infection, 139
AIDS-related complex (ARC), 136–138
associated neoplasms, 139–141
nervous system diseases, 138–139
Infection syndrome associated with pediatric AIDS, 256
Infectious complications of AIDS, 185–203
central nervous system infections, 191–195
cutaneous infections, 198–199
disseminated infections, 199–200
gastrointestinal infections, 195–198
opportunistic infections, 185–187
pulmonary infections, 187–191
Interstitial pneumonitis syndrome associated with pediatric AIDS, 254
In vitro assessment of antiretroviral activity, 303–333
activities of other 2',3'-dideoxynucleoside analogues, 319–320
antiretroviral activities of 2',3'-dideoxynucleosides, 308–311
development of screening system for antiretroviral agents, 304–305
generation of HTLV-III/LAV cytopathic effect-sensitive T-cell clone, 305–308
inhibition of HTLV-III/LAV DNA synthesis and RNA expression T cells exposed to virus, 313
in vitro antiviral effect of combinations of putative drugs, 320–325
in vitro drug screening and clinical applications of anti-HTLV-III/LAV agents, 327
mechanisms of antiretroviral activity of 2',3'-dideoxynucleosides, 316–317
reversal of 2',3'-dideoxynucleoside protection, 325–327

Kaposi's sarcoma (KS), 15, 78, 98, 139, 141, 157–159, 205–232
in the AIDS pandemic, 219–232
African Kaposi's sarcoma, 220–221
in the AIDS patient, 224–229
associated with immunosuppressive therapy, 223–224
classical Kaposi's sarcoma, 221–223
prospects, 229
classical and epidemic forms, 205–218
associated diseases, 212–214
clinical manifestations and course of the disease, 208–211
epidemiology, 207–208
histogenesis, 214–215
histopathology, 211–212
history, 206–207
pediatric AIDS and, 249

Lentiviruses, 2
AIDS virus as, 28–30
prospects of handling diseases caused by, 32
Lesions, lymphoid and hematological, associated with AIDS, 144–147
Leukemic cells, diseases associated with HTLV-I and, 9–10
Leukemogenesis
mechanisms of, 43
two-step, by HTLV-I, 44
Lymphadenopathy/AIDS virus, 23–37
AIDS virus as lentivirus, 28–30
antiviral therapy, 33
env variation, 32–33
link between virus and disease, 23–24
prospects of handling lentivirus diseases, 32
relevance of visna groups to AIDS, 31–32
vaccination, 33
viral genome, 24–28

Lymphadenopathy-associated virus
(LAV), 13
associated with pediatric AIDS, 257
See also HTLV-III/LAV; HTLV-III/LAV-related neurological
disease
Lymphoid lesions associated with
AIDS, 144–147
Lymphomas, 293–294
extra-CNS non-Hodgkin's, 139
See also B-cell lymphomas

Malignancies, 157–161
dermatological manifestations of,
286, 293–294
Hodgkin's disease, 158–160
Kaposi's sarcoma, 157–159
other malignancies, 160–161
small cell carcinomas, 160
Malignant B-cell lymphomas, AIDS-related, see B-cell lymphomas,
malignant, AIDS-related
MAI (group II mycobacterium), 199
Meningitis, 266
Metabolic disorders, 267
Microglial nodules (MN), 161–164
Modes of transmission, 82–84
Molecular biology
of HTLV-III, 53–62
gag, pol, and env genes, 54–57
other puzzles and prospects, 60–
61
sor, tat, and 3'orf genes, 58–60
unusual features of the virus life
cycle and disease, 57–58
of the HTLV family, 39–52
development of immunodiagnostic
reagents for AIDS by recombinant DNA technology, 46
genetic polymorphism of HTLV-
III and prospects for a vaccine,
46–48
genetic structure of HTLV-I, HTLV-
II, and HTLV-III, 40–41
HTLV-III and cytopathicity, 45–46

[Molecular biology]
putting together the genes for transactivation, 41–42
summary and perspectives, 48–49
transcriptional regulation of cellular
genes by HTLV-I and HTLV-II,
42–45
Mucocutaneous infections, 286, 287–
293
Mycobacterium tuberculosis, 200
Myelopathic complications, 266–267
HTLV-III/LAV-related, 275–276
Myositis, 267

Natural history, 105–106
Neoplasms associated with HTLV-III
infection, 139–141
Nervous system disease-associated
HTLV-III, 138–139
Neurological diseases
HTLV-III and, 16
See also HTLV-III/LAV-related
neurological diseases
Neuropathology of AIDS, 161–173
cerebral mass lesions, 170–171
microglial nodules, 161–164
pediatric cases, 172–173
peripheral nerve involvement, 171–
172
specific secondary infections, 166–
170
subacute encephalitis, 164–166
Neurotropism, HTLV-III/LAV-related,
265–266
Nonsexual/nonblood transmission of
AIDS, 111
Nucleosides
in vitro anti-HTLV-III/LAV activity
of, 318
See also 2',3'-Dideoxynucleosides

Opportunistic infections in AIDS patients, 147–157
bacteria, 148, 157

[Opportunistic infections in AIDS pa-
tients]
fungi, 148, 155–157
protozoa, 147–153
viruses, 148, 153–155
Oral hairy leukoplakia, 286, 296–298,
299
3′orf genes, 58–59
Organic mental syndromes, 125

Pathology of AIDS, 143–184
lymphoid and hematological lesions
associated with AIDS, 144–147
malignancies and AIDS, 157–161
Hodgkin's disease, 159–160
Kaposi's sarcoma, 157–159
other malignancies, 160–161
small cell carcinomas, 160
neuropathology of AIDS, 161–173
cerebral mass lesions, 170–171
microglial nodules, 161–164
pediatric cases, 172–173
peripheral nerve involvement,
171–172
specific secondary infections,
166–170
subacute encephalitis, 164–166
opportunistic infections in AIDS patients, 147–157
bacteria, 148, 157
fungi, 148, 155–157
protozoa, 147–153
viruses, 148, 153–155
Patients, psychiatric and psychosocial
effects of AIDS on, 124–128
Pediatric AIDS, 79–80, 245–262
clinical features in syndromes associated with, 256–257
clinical presentation and diagnosis,
246–251
epidemiology and natural history,
251–255
future prospects for prevention,
treatment, and immu-
noprophylaxis, 258–260

[Pediatric AIDS]
neurological manifestations in, 172–
173
pulmonary syndromes associated
with, 254
virology, 255–257
Pentamidine isoethionate, 188
Peripheral nervous system (PNS) disease, 171–172
HTLV-III/LAV-related, 276–279
Pharmacological intervention against
HTLV-III/LAV, 335–360
disease process of HTLV-III infection, 338–340
drug development in HTLV-III-induced diseases, 340–343
drugs being investigated for AIDS
treatment, 342, 345–354
evaluation of antiviral drugs in patients with HTLV-III disease,
343–345
potential strategies for antiviral
therapy, 336–338
Phosphonoformate, 342, 353–354
Pneumocystis carinii pneumonia (PCP),
75–76, 78, 98, 149–150, 187–
190
pol genes, 54–57
Positive individuals (HTLV-III antibody), psychiatric and psychosocial effects of AIDS on, 128–129
Premature mortality, incidence rates of
AIDS and, 80–81
Prevention efforts, 84–85
Primary HTLV-III infection, 286, 296
Protozoa, 147–153
Psychiatric and psychosocial aspects of
AIDS, 123–134
for health care workers, 131–132
for high-risk groups, 128–130
AIDS-related complex (ARC), 128
HTLV-III antibody (positive individuals), 128–129
worried well, 129–130
for patients, 124–128
for the public, 130

Pulmonary infections, 187–191
Pulmonary syndromes associated with
    pediatric AIDS, 254
Putative drugs, in vitro antiviral effect
    of, 320–325

Retinitis, 195
Retroviruses, 2
    general features of, 6–7
    genetic structure and proposed clas-
      sification of, 5
    life cycle of, 4
    See also Human retrovirus epi-
      demiology; Human T-lympho-
      tropic retroviruses
Ribavirin, 342, 353
Rifabutine, 342, 354
Risk groups, 102–104
    psychiatric and psychosocial effects
      of AIDS on, 128–130
RNA
    HTLV-III/LAV and, 313
    retroviruses and, 3, 4

Salmonella typhimurium, 198
Seborrheic dermatitis, 286, 296
Secondary infections, 166–170
Seroepidemiology, 106–111
Simian T-lymphotropic viruses
    (STLV), 64–69
Small cell carcinomas, 160
sor genes, 58–59
STLV-I, 65–66

STLV-III, 66–69
Subacute encephalitis, 164–166
Suramin, 342, 345–347

tat genes, 58–59
    role played in HTLV-III-induced
      pathogenesis by, 59–60
    role played in virus life cycle by, 59
Toxoplasmosis, 78, 192
Transfusion-associated AIDS, 109–111
Transmission modes, 82–84
Trimethoprim-sulfamethoxasole, 188

United States (U.S.), incidence of
    AIDS in (1981–1985), 77

Vaccination, 33
    genetic polymorphism of HTLV-III
      and, 46–48
Vascular complications, 267
Viruses, 148, 153–155
    dermatological manifestations of,
      286, 287–291
Visna group, relevance to AIDS of, 31–
    32

Wasting syndrome associated with pe-
    diatric AIDS, 256
Worried well groups, psychiatric and
    psychosocial effect of AIDS on,
    129–130